NUTRITION UPDATE

NUTRITION UPDATE

Volume 1

Edited by

JEAN WEININGER, Ph.D.

GEORGE M. BRIGGS, Ph.D.

Department of Nutritional Sciences
University of California, Berkeley

A Wiley-Interscience Publication
JOHN WILEY & SONS
New York • Chichester • Brisbane • Toronto • Singapore

Library of Congress Cataloging in Publication Data:

Main entry under title:

Nutrition update.

"A Wiley-Interscience publication."
Includes bibliographical references and index.
1. Nutrition disorders. 2. Nutrition. 3. Nutrition
policy—United States. I. Weininger, Jean. II. Briggs,
George M. (George McSpadden), 1919-   . [DNIM:
1. Nutrition. QU 145 N976]
RC620.N85   1983   613.2   82-20085
ISBN 0-471-09607-5

Printed in the United States of America

10 9 8 7 6 5 4 3 2 1

Series Preface

It is our intention that the *Nutrition Update* series will greatly assist people with diverse backgrounds and interests to keep informed about the latest breakthroughs, developments, and controversies in the fast moving field of human nutrition.

Nutrition Update is written primarily for the nutrition practitioner rather than for the nutrition scientist. The series will be of special use to nutrition educators, dietitians, college teachers of nutrition and related fields, public health nutritionists, and nutrition students at all levels. In addition, the subjects are chosen to be of interest to all types of health professionals and practitioners (including nurses, physicians, dentists, and public health workers), home economists, food scientists and technologists, and nutritionists working in academic institutions, industry, governmental agencies, agricultural extension, and other areas.

For the most part, *Nutrition Update* is written with a minimum of scientific jargon; its language is readily understood. Therefore, we feel it will be valuable for large numbers of lay people who have an interest in their own nutrition and health and who want to keep up with new discoveries. Nutrition educators can recommend this series to those lay people who are looking for readable sources of reliable nutrition information.

This series is an outgrowth of an annual summary of current nutrition information that we started in 1974 as "Nutrition Update" articles for the *Journal of Nutrition Education*. That series continued until 1979. From the feedback we learned of the real need for an annual update of current nutrition developments in one volume, written so that it can be understood by and be useful to scientists and nonscientists. It is our regular practice to cover almost all of the world's nutrition literature in the original journals—updating, building up extensive files, and looking for topics and authors for *Nutrition Update*.

We have asked well-qualified scientists and professionals to bring us up to date in their field of expertise, to explore new ideas and controversies, to give their interpretation of the facts, and to provide practical dietary advice wherever possible. Many of our contributors are internationally known; some are younger

v

people with new approaches in their field. All of them have excellent credentials and the respect of their colleagues. Each chapter is written specifically for *Nutrition Update*. These are not papers given at a symposium and then put together in a book.

In addition to serving as a reference book, each volume can serve as a textbook in courses on current issues and as supplementary reading material for undergraduate and graduate students in nutrition courses, and for students of medicine, nursing, and related health areas.

As the science of nutrition evolves, we intend to bring to the readers of this series researchers and thinkers who are on the leading edge of nutrition and who will address difficult questions: Where do we stand in nutrition today? What really matters in nutrition today? How can the results of nutrition research be translated into action in a way that contributes to the health, well-being, and quality of life of people all over the world?

Taken as a whole, we hope that these volumes will be a valuable record of the history of nutrition and, even more important, will help to point out how much we do *not* know and what remains to be discovered.

JEAN WEININGER
GEORGE M. BRIGGS

April 1983

Preface

There are literally scores of topics, and experts to discuss them, that we could have chosen to include in this first volume of the *Nutrition Update* series. The field of nutrition is so rich and varied that numerous subjects would qualify as "hot topics." However, we had to settle on a manageable number and select those that we felt were particularly important, interesting, and of practical significance.

We asked each contributor to write in a way that was comfortable for her or him. There are different styles and approaches, and different levels of writing, even though there are common features of organization. We consider this variety to be a *plus*—a positive feature of this book—and we hope the readers will enjoy the diversity.

We have grouped the chapters in this volume into four sections:

1. Chapters in "Issues in Nutrition" cover some of the fastest moving and most controversial areas, such as caffeine, that have captured the public attention and that require close watching for updated information. As we go to press, the Food and Drug Administration's rulemaking process on the GRAS status of caffeine is expected to conclude at any time. The chapters on alcohol and fructose are of particular use to physicians and those in a clinical setting, although they have broad public health implications as well. The discussions on food additives and behavior, sodium and hypertension, and hazards in the food supply underscore how natural and added substances in our food can directly affect our physical and mental health.

2. In "Update on Nutrients," leading authorities discuss the mushrooming research on zinc and selenium, two trace elements whose role in human nutrition is being clarified, and dietary fiber, which is not in the strictest sense a "nutrient" but which nevertheless appears to be essential for optimal health.

3. At different stages of life there are different areas of nutritional concern. Chapters in "Nutrition in the Life Cycle" focus on current knowledge about nutrition and developmental disabilities, dietary risks during pregnancy, infant nutrition, and the nutritional factors contributing to bone loss as we grow older.

4. Three historical and thought-provoking essays are presented in "Nutrition Policy and Food Advertising." The two chapters on nutrition policy tie together the many reports, guidelines, and dietary recommendations that have come out in the past few years and give the authors' perspectives on how research can be utilized in policymaking. *Diet, Nutrition, and Cancer,* a report published by the National Academy of Sciences after these chapters were submitted, will be discussed in Volume 2 of this series. The final chapter examines the enormous impact of food advertising on our nutrition.

Among those topics we expect to include in the next volume are: food choices for cancer prevention; weight-reducing diets; cultural aspects of eating and weight; "ultra" trace elements; trace elements in hair; cholesterol and health; vegetarian diets; adolescent nutrition; inborn errors of metabolism; determinants of breast feeding; maternal nutrition, fertility, and reproductive performance; nutrition and contraception; nutrition and diabetes; the astronauts' diet; nutrition and the elderly; wild foods; nutrition education—advances in accessibility and effectiveness; literature resources in nutritional sciences; and nutrition and the media.

Your suggestions for future topics, and your constructive evaluation of any of the chapters, will be sincerely appreciated. Please feel free to write to either of the editors.

JEAN WEININGER
GEORGE M. BRIGGS

Department of Nutritional Sciences
University of California
Berkeley, California 94720

April 1983

Acknowledgments

The editors are deeply grateful to numerous people who have contributed directly and indirectly to this book. In particular, we would like to thank Stan and Judith Kudzin and many others at John Wiley & Sons, for providing their expertise and encouragement in all phases of production; Henry Mooney, for converting the manuscript into camera-ready copy, and Jane-Ellen Long, for proofreading it; Dominic Federico, Al Silbowitz, Virginia LeRoux, Catherine and Ron Browning, and Michael Zimmerman, for their direct personal support; and especially all the contributors, for their hard work and great patience during the development of this first volume of the *Nutrition Update* series.

Contents

NUTRITION UPDATE

Issues in Nutrition

1

Caffeine and Health

CURRENT STATUS

STUART L. NIGHTINGALE, M.D.
Associate Commissioner for Health Affairs

W. GARY FLAMM, Ph.D.
Deputy Associate Commissioner for Health Affairs (Science)

Food and Drug Administration
Rockville, Maryland

Address correspondence to Stuart L. Nightingale, M.D., Associate Commissioner for Health Affairs, Food and Drug Administration, Rockville, Maryland 20857.

ABSTRACT

Caffeine, in one dietary form or another, has been consumed by humans throughout the world for centuries. In the United States, the single greatest source of caffeine is coffee. For one segment of the population, young children, soft drinks constitute the major dietary sources of caffeine. Caffeine is both a natural and an added ingredient in soft drinks. The safety of caffeine has been challenged by a committee established by the Federation of American Societies for Experimental Biology which, under contract with the Food and Drug Administration, has reviewed the scientific literature on caffeine. Recent studies that show that caffeine can induce birth defects in rats also bring the safety of caffeine into question. Human studies neither support nor refute the findings in animals, and concern remains that caffeine may increase the risk of birth defects for humans. Because of this concern the Food and Drug Administration has proposed to remove caffeine from the list of substances generally recognized as safe and to regulate the added uses of caffeine to food and beverages on an interim basis, providing that additional studies are undertaken that relate to the question of caffeine's safety. In the meantime, the Food and Drug Administration has recommended prudence on the part of pregnant women in the use of caffeine products, stressing that these further studies may take 2—4 years to complete.

BACKGROUND

Throughout the centuries humans have searched for stimulants in their food and beverages. The coffee bean was discovered in Arabia; the tea leaf in China; the kola nut in West Africa; the cocoa bean in Mexico; the ilex plant, which provides mate, in Brazil; and the cassina or

---

The views and assessments expressed by the authors are based solely on the data and information identified and do not represent the final decisions of the Food and Drug Administration, nor do they reflect a consideration of any comments received by the FDA in the course of its administrative proceedings relating to the proposed interim listing of caffeine as a food additive.

4

Christmas berry tree in North America. All contain caffeine, which accounts for their stimulant properties and, at least to some extent, their consumer acceptance. The popular coffee beverage spread from Arabia to Ethiopia, Turkey, then to Near Eastern and other North African regions, and finally to Europe and North and South America. When initially introduced, coffee was considered potentially dangerous to health, but, despite early medical warnings and efforts to suppress it, coffee became a welcomed and socially acceptable drink. However, the controversy over the health aspects of coffee continues (1).

Today, for many persons, the consumption of caffeine in one form or another begins at an early age and continues for much of their lifetimes. Most people are aware that a cup of coffee or tea contains caffeine. Perhaps not as many persons realize that this drug is also in many soft drinks, and even fewer may realize they are ingesting caffeine when they drink a cup of cocoa, eat a chocolate bar, or take pills for a headache or cold.

Caffeine is very much a part of the human diet today. It is a natural ingredient in coffee, tea, cocoa, and some soft drinks. The Food and Drug Administration (FDA) requires it as an ingredient in cola and pepper-type beverages and permits it in other soft drinks such as orange soda; it is used in cold, headache, allergy, stay-awake, and other over-the-counter drugs, and in some prescription drugs as well; and it is used in some baked goods, frozen dairy products, soft candies, gelatins, and puddings.

Despite caffeine's well-known stimulant properties, its use as an added ingredient in soft drinks and other foods has been regarded as generally recognized as safe (GRAS). Indeed, the FDA's regulations formally list added caffeine as a GRAS ingredient in cola-type soft drinks. The GRAS status of caffeine has exempted it over the years from the food additive sections of the federal Food, Drug, and Cosmetic Act that require a food additive be proven safe to FDA by a sponsor prior to its being granted approval for marketing.

As part of its program to review the safety of all substances listed in its regulations as GRAS, the FDA has reviewed the safety of caffeine and has identified several questions about its safety that need to be addressed (2). In addition, there are questions that should be asked about the purpose for which caffeine is added to food, especially soft drinks. The above concerns were summarized in a proposal to modify the official regulatory status of caffeine pending further studies (2).

CURRENT DIETARY SOURCES AND USES OF CAFFEINE

Caffeine is an alkaloid structurally identified as 1,3,7-trimethylxanthine. It is one of several xanthine derivatives that occur naturally in coffee beans, tea leaves, kola nuts, and cocoa beans. Theophylline (1,3-dimethylxanthine) and theobromine (3,7-dimethylxanthine) are also found in significant amounts in these plant products. Caffeine is present at up to 1.5% in the leaves of tea (*Camellia sinensis*). Caffeine is a natural component of chocolate (*Theobroma cacao*) and the kola nut (*Cola acuminata* and related species).

The vast majority of the caffeine present in the American diet is imported. The major sources and amounts brought into the United States in 1972 are listed in Table 1 (3). Coffee was by far the most important source. After considering losses during preparation and serving, coffee accounted for about 25–30 million of the 35 million pounds of caffeine consumed; that is, it represented about 75–80% of total caffeine consumption. Tea was next in importance, contributing about 3.8 million pounds of caffeine. Cola beverages ranked third, with caffeine coming approximately one-half from the kola nut and one-half from added caffeine. Tea and cocoa, although only minor sources of caffeine, together contributed about 6.0 million pounds of theophylline and 7.7 million pounds of theobromine (3), respectively.

Table 1. Caffeine Imported into the United States in 1972

Product[a]	Billion Pounds of Product	Caffeine Content (%)	Million Pounds of Caffeine
Coffee	2.5	1.30	35
Tea	150	4.0	6
Kola nut	200	1.0	2
Caffeine	2	100	2
Cocoa	625	0.3	0.187

[a]dry basis.

The predominant use of caffeine as an added ingredient in food is in soda-water beverages (soft drinks). Most of that use (approximately 80–90%), according to the National Soft Drink Association, is in cola-type soft drinks. Under the current version of the FDA's standard of identity for soda-water beverages, caffeine from kola nut extract and/or other natural caffeine-containing extracts is a mandatory ingredient in cola-type or soda-water beverages, and additional caffeine from any source, natural or synthetic, may be used as an optional ingredient in any soda-water beverage up to a total of 0.02% of the marketed product.

The Federation of American Societies for Experimental Biology (FASEB) in its 1977 report to the FDA presented data (4) concerning the levels of exposure to caffeine experienced by consumers from soft drinks. Using survey data on the frequency of consumption of these beverages among various age groups and the average serving size and assuming a caffeine level of 0.01% in the soft drink, FASEB reported the mean consumption of caffeine to be 0.17 mg/kg of body weight per day in the 0–11-month age group; 0.49 mg/kg/day in the 1–5-year age group; 0.31 mg/kg/day in the 6–11-year age group; 0.21 mg/kg/day in the 12–17-year age group; and 0.18 mg/kg/day in the 18 and older age group. For those in the upper 90–100 percentile for soft drink consumption, exposure levels are significantly higher: 1.8 mg/kg/day in the 1–5-year group; 1.1 mg/kg/day in the 6–11-year age group; 0.71 mg/kg/day in the 12–17-year age group; and 0.66 mg/kg/day in the 18 and older age group. It is worthy of note that the highest exposure to caffeine from soft drinks on a mg/kg/day basis is among young children, especially those in the 1–5-year age group.

FASEB also presented data comparing the levels of caffeine exposure from soft drinks with levels of caffeine exposure from all food sources. Persons in the 18 and older category who consume an average amount of soft drinks get the smallest proportion of their total dietary exposure to caffeine from soft drinks: 0.18 mg/kg/day of their total 2.4 mg/kg/day exposure (or 7.5%) is from soft drinks. On the other extreme, children in the age category of 1–5 years who are in the 90–100 percentile of consumption of soft drinks get 1.8 mg/kg/day of their total 3.0 mg/kg/day exposure (or 60%) from soft drinks. Limited data exist concerning exposure to caffeine by pregnant women. Data collected by the Market Research Corporation of America indicated that the mean consumption of caffeine among pregnant women from coffee alone is approximately 2.9 mg/kg/day.

The exact amount of caffeine in various products varies and depends on such factors as how they are prepared and the brands used. Dietary caffeine is consumed almost entirely in beverages (Table 2) (5). Relatively insignificant amounts enter the diet through other foods, such as coffee-flavored ice cream, chocolate bars, and other chocolate-flavored foods.

Table 2.   Caffeine Content of Beverages

Beverage	Quantity (ounces)	Amount (mg caffeine)
Coffee	8	75–155
Decaffeinated coffee	8	3–5
Instant coffee	8	66
Tea	8	50
Cocoa	8	5
Cola beverage	12	48

PHARMACOLOGY OF CAFFEINE

Caffeine is a pharmacologically active substance that is used in a number of prescription and over-the-counter drugs. The major pharmacologic effect of caffeine is on the central nervous system, but it can also stimulate the heart and increase cardiac output. Caffeine with sodium benzoate used to solubilize the caffeine is given by physicians subcutaneously or intramuscularly in dosages of 0.5–1.0 grams as a central nervous system stimulant. In addition to its use in prescription drugs, caffeine is the active ingredient in many over-the-counter drugs used to maintain wakefulness (Table 3) (5). The dosage level in these over-the-counter (OTC) stimulants is usually 100–200 mg per tablet. Caffeine is also used in a variety of OTC analgesic, diuretic, cold, and diet-aid preparations at single dose levels ranging from approximately 15–200 mg (Table 3).

Table 3.   Over-the-Counter Sources of Caffeine

OTC Product	Milligrams/Tablet
Cold tablets	15
Allergy relief	30
Headache relief	32
Stay-awake tablets	100–200

TOXICITY OF CAFFEINE

Intoxication and Overdose

Animals given a lethal dose of caffeine develop convulsions and die from respiratory failure. In humans, the fatal oral dose of caffeine is estimated to be about 10 grams (6). Untoward central nervous system and circulatory system reactions following ingestion of 1 gram or more of caffeine do occur. These include insomnia, restlessness, excitement progressing to mild delirium, tremulousness, and increased heart and respiratory rate (6).

Other forms of caffeine toxicity occur at lower doses and are more subtle and difficult to detect and measure. These are listed below.

Birth Defects

Due to recently developed evidence concerning the ability of caffeine to cause birth defects in rats, the FDA's primary concern about caffeine has shifted from caffeine's potential behavioral effects (see below) to its potential teratogenicity—its ability to induce birth defects. Although much uncertainty still exists about whether caffeine actually increases the risk of birth defects in humans, the data now available from animal studies are significant enough to be of serious concern and to justify additional research directed toward resolving, as quickly as possible, the uncertainties about caffeine's potential teratogenicity in humans.

In 1979 the FDA reviewed all information available in the literature on the ability of caffeine to produce birth defects in experimental animals (7). It was reported in the FDA's review that the administration of caffeine by various routes to pregnant mice indicated that caffeine may be capable of producing toxic effects among the unborn offspring (fetotoxicity) and, possibly, the production of birth defects as well. In fact, these studies revealed a variety of effects which might have been due to caffeine administration; that is, cleft palate, digital defects, muscular disorders, facial deformities, anophthalmia (absence of eyes), and exencephaly (the brain lying outside of the skull) (8–10). The picture in rats was somewhat similar to that reported in mice, namely, delayed or incomplete bone ossification in the offspring, and, with higher doses, missing digits (9), cleft palates (11), and other unspecified abnormalities (12). No evidence of caffeine-induced birth defects was seen among hamsters that were treated with relatively low doses of caffeine, whereas ectrodactyly (partial or complete absence of digit or digits) was reported in the rabbit.

Despite the strong suggestion that caffeine is capable of producing birth defects among mice, rats, and rabbits when administered at relatively high doses, all of the studies suffered from certain deficiencies such as lack of proper control animals, lack of concurrent control animals, small numbers of animals, and insufficient information on procedures. Nevertheless, when considered in totality, the studies did indicate that at sufficiently high levels of exposure, well above human exposure, caffeine can cause birth defects. The studies were not adequate to determine with any degree of confidence a no-effect level for the teratogenic effect of caffeine in animals. No-effect levels are important in animal studies because they are used in determining the safe human dose of the substance being tested.

Due to these uncertainties, in 1979 the FDA undertook two new studies of teratogenic effects of caffeine in rats, hoping to resolve the question of whether caffeine has the ability to produce birth defects and to determine the dosage level at which these defects occur. In the first study, caffeine was administered by gavage, that is, the forced feeding of measured amounts of the substance (dissolved in an aqueous solution) through a stomach tube. This study has been fully analyzed and reviewed and has revealed that high doses of caffeine result in the death and resorption of embryos, significant decreases in fetal weights, and reduction in crown-rump distances. Ectrodactyly was also observed at the higher dosage levels, as were an assortment of other skeletal anomalies: reduced pubis size, reduced dorsal arch, missing hind digits. Delayed or incomplete ossification of the sternebrae (segments of the sternum, or breast bone) was observed at high, middle, and low doses. In the second study, which is still being analyzed, caffeine was administered in drinking water consumed *ad libitum*.

The first study raised serious concerns about caffeine. It was the first large study of its kind on caffeine that showed irreversible birth defects (missing digits) at levels as low as 80 mg/kg of body weight and other adverse effects (incomplete ossification of sternebrae) at levels as low as 6 mg/kg. It is possible that these effects occur at somewhat lower levels as well, but additional studies would be needed to determine that. In any case, it is apparent that the effects seen at birth were caused by exposures to caffeine which were within a factor of 10 or less times the caffeine levels humans might be expected to consume.

In the determination of the significance of the FDA gavage study for humans, the major question becomes whether animal studies of teratogenic effects can accurately predict the occurrence of human birth defects. Interpretation of the relevance of teratology studies to humans is affected by many considerations that combine to make the interpretation of such studies complex, difficult, and uncertain (13). These considerations, which are the same whenever one attempts to extrapolate teratogenic response observed in one species to another species, include the following:

1. Physiologic and biochemical differences that affect the absorption, metabolism, and excretion of the substance.
2. Variability in placental barriers.
3. Differences in susceptibility to chemical interactions at the cell, tissue, organ, and organ system levels.
4. Variability in background incidence of birth defects.
5. Variability in the sequence of gestational development.

These factors must be taken into account, to the extent that the available data permit, when one attempts to assess the relevance to humans of any specific study of teratogenic effects conducted in a particular species with a particular chemical.

It is known that similar doses of caffeine on a mg/kg basis given to humans, as opposed to experimental animals, expose the maternal organism and the developing fetus to widely different levels of caffeine and to different kinds and amounts of caffeine metabolites. It is not known to what extent these differences in metabolism and pharmacokinetics between the rat and humans relate to the observed birth defects in the rat. These differences do raise serious questions, however, about the ability of the animal studies to predict the response of humans to caffeine.

At this time, there are insufficient data to determine whether caffeine per se and/or one of its metabolites is the causative agent for the teratogenic effects observed in experimental animals. In the absence of an answer to that question and in the absence of more complete information on the comparative metabolism and pharmacokinetic handling of caffeine in humans and animals, especially the rat, we cannot determine with confidence what, if any, potential risk exists for humans.

There have been six human epidemiologic studies that deal at least partially with the teratogenic effects of caffeine (14–18). All of these studies, to some degree, were directly or indirectly concerned with exposure to caffeine and an increased risk of complications of pregnancy. Unfortunately, most, if not all, of these studies have methodologic problems associated with them that make it difficult to draw any reasonably valid inferences from the results. In general, these studies are flawed by a failure to control important variables that could have altered study results. These variables include measurements made for exposure (amount and length of time of caffeine consumption), intake of alcohol, smoking habits, age at pregnancy, and level of prenatal care. As a consequence, the available human studies, whether taken as a group or singly, do not conclusively determine the relationship between caffeine consumption and teratogenic effects.

Carcinogenicity

Two studies conducted to evaluate whether or not caffeine causes cancer found no increase in carcinogenicity in rats given rations containing instant coffee (19, 20). The animals were tested for 2 years, and their rations contained up to about 0.18% caffeine. In a lifetime study, mice given fresh brewed coffee instead of drinking water did not show any increased incidence of cancer (21).

In a recent study (22), no increase in neoplastic (cancerous) or preneoplastic (precancerous) lesions was observed in a group of 20 male rats given 0.5% caffeine in the diet for up to 75 weeks. Because the animals in this experiment were killed after only 75 weeks, the time for tumor formation may not have been long enough for the expression of cancer. The quality and sensitivity of the study is further undermined by the fact that only one sex was studied and that the number of animals used was not sufficient, by contemporary standards, for adequate testing for carcinogenicity.

Human epidemiologic studies have not demonstrated a causal relationship between caffeine consumption and cancer (22–25). Kihlman (26) believes that most of the available evidence suggests that caffeine may have anticarcinogenic effects rather than being a carcinogen. However, a higher incidence of bladder cancer has been detected among coffee drinkers as compared to matched controls (27), and a correlation has been perceived between coffee consumption and national mortality rates from carcinoma of the kidney (28). More recently, MacMahon et al. (29) reported an association between coffee consumption and an increase in cancer of the pancreas. Even if this observation proves to be reproducible, it is unlikely that the effect is attributable to the caffeine in coffee since the consumption of tea was not associated with an increase in pancreatic cancer.

The data on both animals and humans concerning the potential carcinogenicity of caffeine are inadequate and incomplete. There are no lifetime feeding studies on caffeine in animals that meet currently accepted toxicologic testing criteria for the testing of carcinogenesis. Moreover, there are no fully acceptable and replicated epidemiologic data linking human exposure to caffeine with a significant increase in the incidence of cancer.

Behavioral Effects

The neuropharmacologic properties of caffeine have been under investigation for several decades. Numerous behavioral, neurochemical, and neurophysiologic studies have been conducted to characterize the neuropharmacologic effects of caffeine in humans and in animals (6, 30, 31). Most of the studies were designed to consider caffeine as a drug and have dealt with the acute or short-term effects of caffeine in the mature, adult organism. There is only limited information about the neurobehavioral effects of chronic or long-term exposure or about the effects on the young, immature organism.

In studies with adult animals, caffeine has been shown to exert varying effects on the neurochemical and neurophysiologic systems and to influence such behaviors as learning and memory, motor performance, sensory function, and emotional reactivity at acute dose levels as low as 0.5–2.5 mg/kg (32–34). Recently, evidence of physiologic withdrawal has been reported in rats following several weeks of parenteral exposure to caffeine (35).

Little experimental attention has been given to the consequences of prolonged dietary exposure to caffeine on the functional capacity of the nervous system. In a single study recently reported by Estler et al. (36), caffeine was given in the drinking water to mice for 6 weeks at a daily dose of 150 mg/kg. In contrast to the effects of a single dose, prolonged exposure to the caffeine resulted in detrimental effects, including diminished capacity to perform exhaustive work (swimming) under stressful conditions, impaired thermoregulation, as well as reduced weight gain. Spontaneous activity was unaffected, and motor coordination was even facilitated. Similar detrimental effects on work capacity were reported earlier (37) following prolonged exposure of mice to coffee.

In explaining its conclusion that caffeine in cola-type beverages should no longer be generally recognized as safe, FASEB emphasized the potential behavioral effects of caffeine in children (4). FASEB suggested that the concerns about the behavioral effects of caffeine are less for adults ". . . than for children where there can be chronic consumption of caffeine in cola-type beverages during the period of brain growth and development. It is during this period of plasticity that the developing central nervous system is most sensitive to the effects of all aspects of the environment. The estimated levels of caffeine intake at these ages are near those levels that are known to cause central nervous system effects in adults."

Although FASEB acknowledged that the available data were not adequate to answer the question of whether chronic exposure to caffeine in cola-type beverages poses a potential hazard to children and others, FASEB stated that it ". . . views with concern the continued addition of caffeine to cola-type beverages, representing as it does a unique addition to food of a pharmacologically active central nervous system stimulant." FASEB said: ". . . there is a possibility that behavioral effects in children from infancy through adolescence exist, even though these potential effects are neither adequately documented nor are their consequences clear."

The FDA shares FASEB's concern about the addition to food of a pharmacologically active agent and FASEB's uncertainty about the potential behavioral effects of caffeine, especially in young children. The FDA also is proposing to adopt FASEB's basic conclusion that questions about the safety of caffeine make it no longer appropriate to continue the listing of added caffeine as a GRAS substance.

Many of the observed neurobehavioral effects, with the notable exception of effects on intellectual ability, have also been shown to occur to some extent in humans following acute or short-term dosing. The usual active oral dose in man is approximately 200–240 mg caffeine (3–4 mg/kg). Its effects range from those considered therapeutically desirable, such as improved motor performance, decreased fatigue, enhanced sensory acuity, mild cerebral stimulation, and increased alertness, to those considered nominal or inconsequential, such as irritability, nervousness, or prolonged time required to fall asleep.

LEGAL AND REGULATORY STATUS

In order to clarify the legal status of many substances that were being used in food in 1958 when the Food Additives Amendment was added to the federal Food, Drug, and Cosmetic Act, the FDA established lists of substances that the agency considered to be GRAS. The FDA's decisions to place substances on the original GRAS lists were based on the data available at the time and on the then current state of knowledge in the field of toxicology.

During the ensuing years, however, as more data became available on the properties of particular substances and as the science of toxicology developed, it became apparent that, in order to ensure the safety of the food supply, the agency's earlier safety determinations should be reviewed and modified where appropriate. To this end, the FDA initiated the GRAS review program in 1970.

To carry out the GRAS review, the FDA conducted surveys of food manufacturers and searched the scientific literature to collect current data on the levels of consumption and the toxicity of substances that were listed as GRAS. Under a contract with the FDA, the Federation of American Societies for Experimental Biology (FASEB), acting through its Select Committee on GRAS Substances (SCOGS), compiled and evaluated the data and made recommendations to the agency concerning the appropriate action with respect to each substance under review. To date SCOGS has reviewed hundreds of substances.

If the FDA, after thorough review of the FASEB report on a particular substance, concludes that the substance is GRAS, it proposes to delete the substance from the original GRAS list and to add it to the Code of Federal Regulations, where the substance's GRAS status will be affirmed and the conditions of use for which the substance is considered GRAS will be specified. If FDA concludes that a substance can no longer be considered GRAS, the agency's usual course of action is to propose to delete the substance from the GRAS list and to declare that the substance is a food additive that cannot be used in food unless approved as a food additive under the conditions specified in section 409 of the Food, Drug, and Cosmetic Act.

There is, however, an intermediate step the agency can take, under appropriate circumstances, when it decides that a substance can no longer be considered GRAS. Under part 180 of the Code of Federal Regulations, the FDA can permit the use of such a substance on an interim basis, notwithstanding the safety question(s) that preclude affirming GRAS status, if the agency finds that "... there is a reasonable certainty that the substance is not harmful and that no harm to the public health will result from the continued use of the substance for a limited period of time while the question raised is being resolved by further study." Substances allowed to be marketed on this basis are referred to as "interim food additives." As stated at the beginning of this chapter, the FDA has recently proposed to remove caffeine from the GRAS list and to place caffeine that is added to food in the interim listing status. Final action by the FDA must await the receipt of public comments on this proposal, this being the standard agency practice for revising current regulations and adopting new regulations.

At this time, the FDA has not initiated any action concerning caffeine as a constituent of food or as an ingredient in OTC or prescription drug products.

NEED FOR ADDITIONAL STUDIES

The continued use of caffeine as a food additive under the proposed interim food additive regulation would depend on the execution of those studies necessary to resolve questions concerning the safety of caffeine and its purpose as an added food ingredient. The FDA's proposal specified that these studies should include:

1. Pharmacokinetic studies, both acute and chronic, in human volunteers and in appropriate animal species, including the rat, to determine the comparative patterns of absorption, biotransformation, and excretion of caffeine in humans and animals.
2. Studies necessary to determine whether the teratogenic effects of caffeine seen in rats are caused by caffeine per se or by one of its metabolites, and whether any metabolites of caffeine that are unique to humans are teratogenic in appropriate animal models.
3. Multigeneration reproductive and neurobehavioral studies in appropriate animal species to resolve questions about the effects of prolonged exposure to caffeine on the mammalian reproductive and nervous system.
4. Definitive chronic feeding studies in two appropriate animal species that will be adequate to resolve questions that have been raised about the potential carcinogenicity of caffeine.
5. Chronic feeding studies to determine whether or not caffeine can cause chronic, pathologic effects other than cancer.
6. Appropriate epidemiologic studies on caffeine performed in accordance with the epidemiology guidelines of the Interagency Regulatory Liaison Group.
7. Appropriate studies demonstrating the need for added caffeine in soda-water and other foods.

ADVICE ON CAFFEINE

In September 1980, the FDA warned the public of caffeine's possible dangers to unborn children. Pregnant women were urged to be prudent in the use of caffeine products. The agency stressed that further studies, which may take 2–4 years, will provide more information about the implications of caffeine's effects on humans and advised that "while further evidence is being gathered on the possible relationship between caffeine and birth defects, a prudent and protective mother-to-be will want to put caffeine on her list of unnecessary substances which she should avoid."

Statements by the FDA also noted that caffeine is a stimulant which has a definite pharmacologic effect, and advised that, as a general rule, pregnant women should avoid all substances that have drug-like effects at levels consumed in food.

REFERENCES

1. P. E. Stepheson, Physiologic and psychotropic effects of caffeine on man. *J. Am. Diet. Assoc.* **71**, 240 (1977).
2. Department of Health and Human Services, Food and Drug Administration. Soda water; standard of identity and caffeine; deletion of GRAS status; proposed declaration the no prior sanction exists; and use on an interim basis pending additional study; proposed regulations. *Fed. Regist.* **45**, 69816 (1980).
3. D. M. Graham, Caffeine—its identity, dietary sources, intake and biological effects. *Nutr. Rev.* **336**, 97 (1978).
4. Select Committee on GRAS Substances. Evaluation of the health aspects of caffeine as a food ingredient. *Federation of American Societies for Experimental Biology Rep.; 1977.* (Available from National Technical Information Service, Order no. PB 283-441/AS) (1977).
5. U.S. Department of Health and Human Services, Food and Drug Administration, Office of Public Affairs, HHS Pub. no. (FDA) 81-1081, 1981.
6. J. M. Ritchie, Central nervous system stimulants: the xanthines. In L. S. Goodman and A. Gilman, eds., *The Pharmacological Basis of Therapeutics*, 5th ed., Macmillan, New York, 1975, p. 368.
7. T. F. X. Collins, Review of reproduction and teratology studies of caffeine. *FDA By-Lines* **9**, 352 (1979).
8. H. Nishimura and K. Nakai, Congenital malformations in offspring of mice treated with caffeine, *Proc. Soc. Exp. Biol. Med.*, **104**, 140 (1960).
9. M. Bertrand, J. Girod, and M. F. Rigaud, Ectrodactylie provoquée par la caféine chez les rongeurs: Rôle des facteurs spécifiques et génétiques, *C.R. Soc. Biol.* **164**, 1488 (1970).
10. Groupe d'Etude des Risques Tératogènes, Tératogénèse expérimentale: étude de la caféine chez la souris, *Thérapie* **24**, 575—580 (1969).
11. F. Leuscher and W. Schwerdtfeger, On the influence of caffeine and other methylxanthines on the reproduction of Wistar rats. In *Coffeine und andere Methylxantine,* F. D. Schanttaur Verlag, Stuttgart, 1969, pp. 209—215.

12. F. Leuschner and G. Czok, Reversibility of prenatal injuries induced by caffeine in rats, *Colloq. Int. Chim. Cafes [C.R.]* 5, 388 (1973).
13. J. G. Wilsonn and F. G. Fraser, eds., *Handbook of Teratology, Vol. 1. General Principles and Etiology,* Plenum Press, New York, 1974.
14. M. M. Nelson and J. O. Forfar, Associations between drugs administered during pregnancy and congenital abnormalities of the fetus. *Br. Med. J.* 1, 523 (1971).
15. B. J. van den Berg, Epidemiologic observations of prematurity: effects of tobacco, coffee, and alcohol. In D. M. Reed and F. J. Stanley, eds., *The Epidemiology of Prematurity*, Urban & Schwarzenberg, Baltimore, 1977, pp. 157–176.
16. O. P. Heinonen, D. Slone, and S. Shapiro, Caffeine and other Xanthine derivatives. In *Birth Defects and Drugs in Pregnancy,* Publishing Sciences Group, Littleton, Mass., 1977.
17. A. P. Streissguth, H. M. Barr, D. C. Martin, and C. S. Herman, Effects of maternal alcohol, nicotine, and caffeine use during pregnancy on infant mental and motor development at eight months. *Alcoholism: Clin. Exp. Res.* 4, 152–164 (1980).
18. I. Borlee, M. F. Lechat, A. Bouckaert, and C. Mission, Coffee: risk factor during pregnancy. *Louvain Med.* 97, 279–284 (1978).
19. H. P Wurzner, E. Lindstrom, L. Vuataz, and A. Luginbuhl, Two-year feeding study of instant coffees in rats. II. Incidence and types of neoplasms. *Food Cosmet. Toxicol.* 15, 289 (1977).
20. B. R. Zeitlin, Coffee and bladder cancer. *Lancet* 1, 1066 (1972).
21. A. R. Bauer, Jr., R. K. Rank, R. Kerr, R. L. Stratley, and J. D. Mason, The effects of prolonged coffee intake on genetically identical mice. *Life Sci.* 21, 63 (1977).
22. M. A. Weinberger, L. Friedman, T. M. Farber, F. M. Moreland, E. L. Peters, C. E. Gilmore, and M. A. Khan, Testicular atrophy and impaired spermatogenesis in rats fed high levels of the methylxanthines caffeine, theobromine, or theophylline. *J. Environ. Pathol. Toxicol.* 15, 289 (1977). The lower urinary tract. *Lancet* 1, 1335 (1971).
23. J. F. Fraumeni, J. Scotto, and L. J. Dunham, Coffee-drinking and bladder cancer. *Lancet* 2, 1204 (1971).
24. B. Armstrong, A. Garrod, and R. Doll, A retrospective study of renal cancer with special reference to coffee and animal protein consumption. *Br. J. Cancer* 33, 127 (1976).
25. P. Stocks, Cancer mortality in relation to national consumption of cigarettes, solid fuel, tea and coffee. *Br. J. Cancer* 24, 215 (1970).

26. B. A Kihlman, *Caffeine and Chromosomes*, Elsevier Scientific Publications, Amsterdam, 1977.

27. R. Schmauz and P. Cole, Epidemiology of cancer of the renal pelvis and ureter. *J. Nat. Cancer Inst.* **52**, 1431 (1974).

28. D. H. Shennan, Renal carcinoma and coffee consumption in 16 countries. *Br. J. Cancer* **28**, 473 (1973).

29. B. MacMahon, S. Yen, D. Trichopoulos, K. Warren, and G. Nardi, Coffee and cancer of the pancreas. *N. Engl. J. Med.* **304**, 630 (1981).

30. B. Weiss and V. G. Laties, Enhancement of human performance by caffeine and the amphetamines. *Pharmacol. Rev.* **14**, 1–36 (1962).

31. D. Efron, ed., *Psychopharmacology: A Review of Progress, 1957-1967*, U.S. Government Printing Office, Washington, D.C., 1967.

32. H. Rahman, Influence of caffeine on memory and behavior in golden hamsters. *Pflugers Archiv* **276**, 384 (1963).

33. W. M. Kallman and W. Isaac, The effects of age and illumination on the dose—response curves for three stimulants. *Psychopharmacology* **40**, 313 (1975).

34. K. R. Kirsh, M. G. Pinzone, and J. H. Forde, Spontaneous locomotor activity changes evoked by caffeine in mice. *Fed. Proc.* **33**, 466 (1974).

35. M. V. Vitello and S. C. Woods, Evidence for withdrawal from caffeine by rats. *Pharmacol. Biochem. Behav.* **6**, 553 (1977).

36. C. Estler, H. Ammon, and C. Herzog, Swimming capacity of mice after prolonged treatment with psychostimulants. *Psychopharmacology* **58**, 161 (1978).

37. K. Neumann, Tierversuche zur Frage Korperlichen Leistungsvermogens nach Aufnahme von Koffein. *Med. Klin. (Munich)* **60**, 13354 (1965).

ADDITIONAL RECENT REFERENCES

P. B. Dews, Caffeine. In W. J. Darby, H. P. Broquist, and R. E. Olson, eds., *Annual Review of Nutrition*, Vol. 2, Annual Reviews Inc., Palo Alto, 1982.

L. Rosenberg, A. A. Mitchell, S. Shapiro, and D. Slone, Selected birth defects in relation to caffeine-containing beverages. *J. Am. Med. Assoc.* **247**, 1429 (1982).

2

The Behavioral Toxicity of Food Additives

BERNARD WEISS, Ph.D.
University of Rochester School of Medicine and Dentistry
Rochester, New York

Address correspondence to Bernard Weiss, Ph.D., Professor of Toxicology, Division of Toxicology, Department of Radiation Biology and Biophysics, and Environmental Health Sciences Center, University of Rochester School of Medicine and Dentistry, Rochester, New York 14642.

ABSTRACT

Debates about the safety of food additives have taken on a new dimension with claims (the Feingold hypothesis) that certain additives may evoke behavioral disturbances, especially in children. In evaluating such claims, one must recognize that food additive safety evaluation typically excludes behavior as a criterion of toxicity. Even before Feingold's assertions, moreover, the medical literature had recorded many instances of adverse somatic reactions to substances such as synthetic food dyes and flavors. Scientific studies of the Feingold hypothesis indicate that adverse behavioral reactions may also be evoked by additives, especially in younger children. Such studies emphasize the need to include behavioral testing in food additive safety evaluations. They also suggest that the nutrition and medical communities take steps to eliminate cosmetic, nonfunctional additives from the food supply.

Our food supply travels a winding route from producer to consumer. The product we eat or cook may bear only the most remote relation to what the farmer ships to the middleman or processor. Such transformations, moreover, are not a novel feature of modern technology. For thousands of years, foodstuffs have been altered from their natural state to preserve them, to ripen them, to improve their texture or appearance, or to modify their flavor. Only the scale is different now. The breadth of contemporary chemical technology is perhaps nowhere exemplified so stunningly as in food processing. How many of our grandmothers would have foreseen a synthetic chicken soup?

This explosion in technology is arousing resistance—often bitter, sometimes strident—among consumer advocates and some health professionals. The media immerse us in a bewildering mélange of claims and counterclaims. The food industry proffers reassurance and proclaims its devotion to the public welfare. And government officials, sometimes trapped by legislation and ancient regulations, twist into an uneasy armistice with both sides. The debate, however, has grown in

22

scope and intensity with the injection of a new theme: do these processes and additives impair behavioral functions?

TYPES OF ADDITIVES

About 3000 agents are approved for use as food additives (1). They are distinguished from substances that may be added inadvertently, such as pesticides and other environmental contaminants. Regulations define an additive as a substance deliberately added to foodstuffs during production, processing, storage, or packaging. Sugar and salt are among the most common additives and are often used to replace flavors lost through processing. They also are added generously to combinations such as sauces and puddings. Table 1 shows that about 2000 of the currently approved additives are flavors, of which 1500 are artificial; that is, they are the results of commercial syntheses and do not exist in nature. Many consist of mixtures; artificial pineapple flavor, for example, contains 17 different components.

Table 1.   Classification of Intentional Additives

Additive	Number
Preservatives	33
Antioxidants	28
Sequestrants	45
Surface active agents	111
Stabilizers, thickeners	39
Bleaching and maturing agents	24
Buffers, acids, alkalies	60
Food colors	34
Nonnutritive and special dietary sweeteners	4
Nutritive supplement	117
Flavorings, synthetic	1610
Flavorings, natural	502
Miscellaneous: yeast foods, texturizers, firming agents, binders, anticaking agents, enzymes	157
Total Number of Additives	2764

The other additives fall into four broad divisions. Preservatives are the most traditional additives, but newer chemical agents have largely supplanted the more traditional treatments such as smoking, drying, fermenting, souring, seasoning, and cooling. Antioxidants such as butylated hydroxytoluene (BHT) and butylated hydroxyanisole (BHA) are added to many fat-containing products, such as oil, lard, potato chips, and crackers, to prevent rancidity. Mold inhibitors, such as calcium propionate, are added to baked goods, sulfur dioxide to wine and dried fruit, and nitrates and nitrites to sausage and bacon to prevent contamination by microbial toxins, especially botulinus toxin. Texturing agents include the emulsifiers, stabilizers, and thickeners. They are used extensively in baked goods, ice cream, frozen desserts, toppings, margarine, and soft drinks. Some additives serve as buffers and neutralizing agents, others as bleaching and maturing agents for flour, and others as crisping agents. Although only a few synthetic colors are approved for use in food, they are widely distributed and preferred in most cases to coloring agents from natural sources because of their stability during processing and their strong coloring potency.

Despite regulations issued by the Food and Drug Administration, labeling can be misleading and sometimes totally uninformative. For instance, BHT-impregnated wrappers for prepared cereals and certain "natural" ice creams need not be acknowledged on the label. Certain products, such as mayonnaise, operate under what is called a Standard of Identity, so that certain additives need not be listed on the label. Bakers who use BHT-treated shortening may overlook that ingredient on their own labels.

SAFETY TESTING

An extensive body of legislation and regulation guides the use of food additives. The original Food and Drug Act of 1906 was revised and supplemented many times and finally replaced by the Food, Drug and Cosmetic Act of 1938. The Food Additives Amendment of 1958 called for prior approval by the Food and Drug Administration of new, commercially added food ingredients. With the passage of the 1958 act, however, many substances were retained, under a special clause, on the GRAS list (Generally Regarded As Safe) without undergoing further toxicity testing. It was assumed that since they already had been marketed and used without signs of overt toxicity, they did not offer a substantial health risk. If, at a later time, the Food and Drug Administration did find evidence of such a risk, they could be removed. A recent review of the GRAS concept by a panel of toxicologists noted its discrepancies with current knowledge and practice (2).

Conventional toxicity testing is directed mainly at pathology. Since evaluation of carcinogenicity is a critical phase of food additive testing, a significant part of toxicity assessment is a long-term feeding study in rodents. The main purpose of such an investigation is to mimic human exposure, which may last a lifetime. Such studies typically last 18 months in mice and 2 years in rats. Observations on growth and longevity and evidence of tissue damage constitute the main bases for safety evaluation. More contemporary assessments of toxicity also include reproduction, embryotoxicity, and teratogenicity, complemented by a bacterial assay method such as the Ames Test for evaluating mutagenicity. Although such quick assay procedures may play an important role in the early screening of additives, their predictive power has not yet been established.

BEHAVIOR AS A CRITERION OF TOXICITY

The dominance of pathology in safety evaluation is receding as other criteria emerge into increasing prominence. We recognize now that functional defects can be just as significant for the individual. Long-term, low-level exposures to environmental contaminants such as heavy metals may produce injurious behavioral effects without clinically detectable damage. The current debate about air quality standards and lead focuses on lead's behavioral and neurologic toxicity. Children with moderately elevated body burdens of lead, but who display no other evidence of toxicity, may perform less well on psychologic tests, such as those assessing intelligence; reveal conduct disturbances, such as distractibility, in the classroom; and may even show covert neurologic abnormalities, such as depressed nerve conduction velocity. The recognition that behavioral impairment may be a subtle consequence of toxic exposure has introduced a new set of perspectives into toxicology, which, in some cases, has been embodied in legislation or regulation. The Toxic Substances Control Act of 1976, which mandates the premarket evaluation of all new chemicals introduced into commerce, specifies behavior as one of the criteria by which risk to health is to be estimated.

Such a recognition arose only recently within the context of food additive hazard evaluation. The inertia stemmed from protocols for safety testing established long before behavioral toxicology penetrated toxicologic thinking. With the standardization of protocols, testing approaches inevitably petrified. It was not until the publicity generated by the Feingold hypothesis that we became aware of the current limitations to food additive safety testing. Feingold is the pediatric allergist who alleged that many of the children diagnosed as hyperactive or suffering from minimal brain dysfunction actually were the victims of an elevated sensitivity to certain constituents in the diet (3). He singled out synthetic food colors and flavors and certain natural constituents, notably salicylates, as the chief offenders. Colors and flavors were specified, not because they were the only offenders, but because they offered no gain in nutritional quality and were the easiest to avoid. Salicylates were singled out because of a role that had been ascribed to them by allergists.

PREDECESSORS TO FEINGOLD

A surprising range of behavioral complaints is blamed on adverse reactions to food. Table 2 lists some that I have extracted from the allergy literature. Most are subjective and nonspecific and are based on anecdotes and clinical impressions rather than on experimental trials. If nothing else, however, these entries reveal how quick we are to attribute such symptoms to diet. Their amorphous quality naturally tempts psychologic explanations but hardly precludes constitutional origins. The discipline of behavioral toxicology, in fact, arose in part because such complaints often had been observed during the early stages of many toxic episodes. They serve as early warning signals.

Table 2. Neurobehavioral Reactions Attributed to Food Allergy

Migraine	Transient blindness
Hyperkinesis	Recurrent neuritis
Sluggishness	Blurred vision
Photophobia	Meniere's disease
Depression	Hyperesthesia
Irrational behavior	Neuralgia
Feeling of unreality	Insomnia
Inability to concentrate	Fatigue
Dizziness	Nervousness
Paranoid ideas	Nervous tics

The approach to toxicity exemplified by "early warning systems" is especially apt for foodstuffs. Unlike occupational exposures, which can be confined and monitored, there are immense variations in food selection and consumption. Occupational exposure levels mandated by regulatory agencies, moreover, not only take into account marked variations in individual susceptibility, but also introduce safety factors based upon the earliest manifestations of toxicity. These are most likely, if they involve the central nervous system, to be vague and nonspecific, just like the entries on the list.

Even as early as 1948, allergists were discussing adverse reactions to food dyes and devising elimination diets excluding such agents. Some of the earlier history is reviewed in Feingold's text (4). Tartrazine (FD & C Yellow no. 5) often was reported as an offending dye. Clinicians made the connection with salicylates because they had noted that patients with aspirin hypersensitivity also seemed to respond adversely to food dyes. Juhlin et al. (5) reported that seven of eight aspirin-sensitive patients, who reacted with asthma or urticaria (hives) to aspirin ingestion, gave similar responses to a rather small amount of tartrazine. Some of the patients also reacted to benzoic acid derivatives, substances often employed as preservatives and which resemble salicylates structurally. Later, Michaelsson et al. (6) described seven patients who suffered the symptoms of allergic vascular purpura (purplish or brownish red discolorations caused by hemorrhage into the tissues) after the ingestion of certain food dyes, including tartrazine, and benzoic acid derivatives. Noid et al. (7), at the Mayo Clinic, noted that many patients with urticaria benefit from a salicylate-free diet. Such a diet excludes prepared foods containing tartrazine or containing salicylate or salicylate-type compounds. Certain fruits and vegetables are also excluded. As I noted before, however, salicylates are used somewhat metaphorically in the allergy literature; substances unrelated structurally to salicylates, such as the drug indomethacin, can precipitate an equivalent spectrum of symptoms in sensitive subjects, and salicylates have not been demonstrated unequivocally in the excluded foods. A recent experimental test was undertaken by Neuman et al. (8) in 97 patients with allergic disorders who were challenged with a 50-mg dose of tartrazine, a realistic challenge given the quantities in soft drinks and other foods. About one-third of their population experienced adverse reactions, including general weakness, heat waves, palpitations, blurred vision, and more conventional hypersensitivity reactions.

The mechanisms of such responses are not known. They probably are not immunologic in character; that is, they do not seem to be the result of antigen—antibody reactions. Instead, they resemble an intolerance reaction whose nature is more like the response to a drug.

The testing of food additives for such reactions is still a crude technology. The Food and Drug Administration's select committee to investigate the status of food additive safety (2) acknowledges this defect in testing standards. Given this history, Feingold's hypothesis should have been perceived, in retrospect, as less outrageous than it was by the biomedical community.

CURRENT EVIDENCE ON THE FEINGOLD HYPOTHESIS

Feingold's assertions stirred enormous interest in parents whose children had navigated endless diagnostic and treatment procedures without success. It was surely to be expected that parents who had abandoned hope after disappointing experiences with standard practices should have turned with enthusiasm to a program as clear and appealing as Feingold's. Many successes were reported, mainly in the form of testimonials and clinical reports. Feingold, of course, was criticized for not having submitted his hypothesis to a rigorous experimental test, namely, controlled trials in which both the patient and the evaluators are unaware of the timing and nature of the patient's particular treatment. Such an experimental design aims to eliminate the bias kindled by the enthusiastic adoption of a new therapy. Enough controlled studies have now been conducted, however, to allow at least a provisional evaluation of the Feingold hypothesis.

Two investigations examined the Feingold Elimination Diet as a total therapy. Conners et al. (9) studied 15 boys who had been diagnosed as hyperactive. The parents were given diet lists from which they were required to select food items. One list contained foods with additives; the other excluded such items as well as salicylate-containing fruits and vegetables. Basing his data on a widely used rating scale of his own design, Conners reported improvement on the diet according to parent and teacher scores on the hyperactivity assessment scale. This was mainly the contribution of four or five subjects. Each phase of the diet (experimental and control) lasted several weeks, with some subjects following one sequence and the others the opposing sequence. Most of the positive responders were in the sequence control-experimental.

A more extensive test was undertaken at the University of Wisconsin by Harley et al. (10). These investigators provided all of the food for the participating families. In the first phase, 36 school-age hyperactive boys spent several weeks on the control diet and several weeks on the elimination diet. Half followed the sequence experimental-control, half the reverse sequence. Thirteen boys improved on the Feingold diet according to mothers' ratings on the Conners Scale. Most of these were in the sequence control-experimental, a finding that led Harley et al. to reject the Feingold hypothesis. I view that rejection as premature, unwarranted, and based on a faulty analysis of the data. A second experiment tested preschool boys under the age of 6. All 10 of these subjects, irrespective of sequence, improved on the diet, by 10% or more, according to mothers' ratings on the Conners Scale. Such a finding cannot simply be attributed to chance or to dietary sequence. The Wisconsin investigators rejected the implications of these findings as well, partly because of the younger ages of the subjects. They failed to grasp the toxicologic implications of the enhanced sensitivity of the younger subjects.

Since total dietary control by the experimenter is expensive and difficult, other investigators have challenged children already maintained on the diet with one or a blend of food dyes. Food color challenges are simplified because so few are approved for use in food (the current dyes are restricted to eight). Selecting an appropriate blend from 1500 synthetic flavors would stagger even the food industry.

I will review only a few of the pertinent studies here because I have reviewed the Feingold literature in detail elsewhere (11). One of the most intriguing sets of studies was also performed at Pittsburgh (12). Children already maintained on the Feingold Diet were challenged with a blend of eight food colors, totalling about 27 mg, in the form of two cookies supplied by the Nutrition Foundation. This quantity was estimated to be the mean daily U.S. intake of food colors in 1968. A sequence of three experiments found that some children showed impaired perceptual-motor performance and elevations in hyperactive behavior. These disorders tended to occur within 3 hours of dye ingestion and to be most visible in the youngest subjects. In Toronto, Williams et al. (13) examined the combined effects of stimulant drugs (amphetamine or methylphenidate) and color challenges in 24 children diagnosed as hyperactive. They relied on Conners scale ratings by both parents and teachers as the criterion. Each child underwent a different sequence of four experimental conditions, each lasting 1 week. These conditions were (1) medication with placebo cookies, (2) medication with challenge cookies (27 mg/day), (3) placebo medication with placebo cookies, (4) placebo medication with challenge cookies. Williams et al. concluded that between three and eight of the children were sensitive to color. My analysis of the raw data highlighted a cluster of subjects (about 25%) showing evidence of food dye sensitivity and one marked responder.

Two, more recent, studies also bear on this issue. Neither was directed toward the Feingold hypothesis as a therapeutic intervention. Both were published at the same time in *Science.* Swanson and

Kinsbourne (14) studied 20 hyperactive children who were positive responders to amphetamine and 20 children who showed adverse effects to the drug. Seventeen of the 20 positive drug responders suffered performance declines on a learning task after the ingestion of 100 or 150 mg of a dye blend. An earlier investigation had detected no response, at least by group statistics, to 26 mg of a dye blend. Swanson and Kinsbourne raised the challenge dose after a Food and Drug Administration survey estimated mean daily intake at 75 mg. These data indicate a dose-response function. The study in which I took part (15) was conducted with a group of 22 younger children, none of whom were clinically hyperactive, but with aversive behaviors that the parents believed were attenuated by the Feingold diet. We administered the 35-mg dye blend as a soft drink, rather than as a cookie, to reduce the calories consumed by the children and to conceal the added color more effectively. The challenge drink was given eight times during an 11-week experimental period. On intervening days, the child consumed the identical-appearing control drink. The parent responsible for making the observations filled out a form every day on which she or he recorded a number of different behavioral indices, most of which consisted of counting or rating 10 target behaviors individually selected for each child. The observers also completed the Conners scale, maintained diet diaries, and provided other information. This experiment uncovered two responders, a 3-year-old boy and a 34-month-old girl. The 34-month-old girl, a dramatic responder, showed significant and striking elevations on five of the seven aversive target behaviors (Table 3) and a marked elevation in Conners scale scores on challenge days. Table 4 contains the mother's comments on those days she correctly guessed as challenge days.

Table 3.   Target Behaviors Aggravated by Food Dyes in a 34-Month-Old Girl

---

Short attention span

Acts as if driven by a motor

Runs away

Throws and breaks things

Whines

Table 4.   Extracts of Mother's Comments on Correctly Guessed Color Challenge Days

Day	Comments
23	Morning very good. In afternoon more and more wound up. Activity to activity.
31	Good morning. Acting "hyper" 1 hour after drink. 1-1/2 hours to fall asleep. Carryover to next day.
37	After lunch (drink) was monster. Would not do anything I asked.
38 (Day after challenge)	Woke up like a motor.
54	Fine morning. Monster in afternoon. Twenty minutes after drink, smeared toothpaste. Constant motion.
58	Super morning. About 12:30 (drink at 11:20) turned into monster. Like a motor.

The conclusions from the human studies are consistent, as even Feingold's most severe critics concede (16, 17): (1) some children benefit from the elimination diet; (2) some children respond adversely to food dyes; (3) the most sensitive children seem to be the youngest. Although Feingold's critics argue with his estimates that perhaps 50% of hyperactive children benefit from the elimination diet, scaling their estimates far below his, they do not contradict the basic premise of sensitivity in some proportion of the population. This premise is further supported by work with laboratory animals. Two studies with neonatal rats indicate that behavioral impairment can occur with doses of food dyes equivalent to those consumed by humans (18, 19).

OTHER ADDITIVES

The doubts incited about food additive safety by the Feingold hypothesis are not unique to colors and flavors. Although caffeine is the most widely consumed drug in the world, only recently has it come under scrutiny as a possible source of unrecognized adverse behavioral effects. Caffeine is consumed in the form of coffee, tea, and soft drinks for its central nervous system stimulant properties. Some individuals, as we all know, consume enormous amounts of it, apparently without harm, although the specter of pancreatic cancer recently has been raised. Despite its extended and pervasive use, however, we know relatively little about caffeine's long-term toxicologic effects. As with food additives and many other drugs and chemicals, concerns about its safety have been stirred less by adult patterns of consumption than by the possibility of adverse effects in children. There is only scant evidence of a fetal caffeine syndrome paralleling that produced by alcohol. But the elevated sensitivity to toxic insult of the developing organism, and, especially, the developing brain, is provoking questions about the consequences of caffeine ingestion during pregnancy and early childhood. Some young children consume large quantities of soft drinks containing caffeine. And the fetus and nursing infant may be exposed through maternal consumption. Is there a durable aftermath? The Food and Drug Administration, responding to these concerns, has proposed that caffeine no longer be required in cola and pepper drinks. Decades ago, these rules were imposed as a precaution against the substitution in cola drinks of substances other than those derived from coca (which contains caffeine). They no longer are required, especially because they have led producers of other soft drinks, as part of marketing strategy, to include caffeine.

Monosodium glutamate (MSG) has stimulated almost as much debate within the biomedical community as has the Feingold hypothesis. MSG is added to processed foods and in cooking as a flavor enhancer. It may be used without label declaration in mayonnaise and salad dressing. Current world production is close to 300,000 tons. Glutamic acid, the amino acid into which it is converted after ingestion, is a natural component of protein. It is known to have neuroexcitatory properties, and glutamate is a possible neurotransmitter in the nervous system. In 1968, a group of symptoms experienced by some people after eating in Chinese restaurants was traced to MSG in the food. Later, Schaumberg et al. (20) found that sensitive individuals respond to less than 3 g, but that almost everyone responds after a sufficiently high dose. The Chinese restaurant syndrome took its name from the MSG added so generously by many Chinese chefs. Its symptoms include tightness around the face and chest, burning sensations in the upper torso, and headache. Some people also report dizziness, diarrhea, nausea, and stomach cramps. Children also experience the Chinese restaurant syndrome, but a few may display their sensitivity in other ways. For example, some children experience "shudder" attacks, mistaken by clinicians and parents for epilepsy. One report described a child apparently suffering from epilepsy whose attacks stopped after MSG was removed from the diet (21). The amount in food is within the range that will provoke attacks in many people. Schaumburg et al. (20) found 3 g of MSG in a 6-oz serving of soup. The commercial MSG product Accent recommends about 3 g/lb of meat. Schaumburg et al. reported that 5 g (1 teaspoon) can produce symptoms in 30% of tested individuals.

Is MSG harmful? No gross, overt damage in humans has been documented. MSG, however, is not, like glutamate, released slowly in the gut as protein is broken down. With MSG, the individual may receive a sudden load. The question of permanent toxic effects, however, is more pertinent to its previous incorporation in baby food. It was removed in response to findings, originally reported by Olney (22), that MSG administered to infant rats and mice produced brain damage. The damage appeared largely in areas surrounding the inner fluid system, the ventricles, of the brain. Some investigators denied Olney's claims, only to discover later that their histology was incomplete or that they had used a histologic stain, routinely used in pathology, that failed to define the area of destruction (23). Olney's results have also been criticized because he administered the MSG in a single large dose that would be unlikely in normal human consumption. More recently, however, he showed that animals consuming drinking water containing MSG suffered equivalent brain damage (24). Additional studies, moreover, reveal a more subtle effect. The areas destroyed by MSG are important in the production of several important brain hormones. The ability of the brain to produce these hormones is hindered by doses of MSG that do not produce clear structural damage (25). Olney and others assert that such findings should make us even more careful about adding MSG to foods, especially those likely to be consumed by young children. They have warned against the replacement of MSG by protein hydrolysates that contain large amounts of free glutamate and against the widespread adoption of the sweetener aspartame that poses a similar danger. Since the retina of the eye is also at risk, some investigators (26) are concerned by the possibility of subtle damage to the visual system.

SAFETY TESTING PROTOCOLS

Table 5 compares the estimates of daily food color intake calculated by the Nutrition Foundation, the estimates made by my group in our study in California, and the Allowable Daily Intake (ADI) calculated by the Food and Drug Administration from animal toxicity testing. The ADI is the amount that presumably can be consumed by humans without harm. It typically is calculated from animal toxicity data; the highest dose in the diet that produces no adverse effects is divided by a factor of 100 to allow a safety margin for humans. The ADIs calculated in this fashion are at least 50 times greater for food dyes than the amounts causing adverse behavioral effects in some children. This comparison is a compelling argument for including behavioral testing in food additive safety evaluation. It is incongruous to continue conventional toxicity testing with food additives, which are so widely distributed, while we now insist on behavioral testing for commercial chemicals whose distribution is far more restricted. Estimates of additive safety are flawed by other problems as well. The animals subjected to toxic challenge in toxicity protocols are provided with a highly nutritious diet, receive superb medical care, and are challenged by only a single agent. Children often consume a less-than-adequate diet, may receive far less than optimal medical care, and consume an enormous range of additives and environmental contaminants. Large amounts of fiber also are found in the typical rat stock diet. Children often eat a diet containing minimal fiber. Yet, diets low in fiber greatly magnify the toxicity of food colors and other additives (27). Those observations parallel reports that absorption of lead may reach nearly 20% of the lead in the diet when rats eat commercial baby foods, and only 0.44% when they consume a conventional laboratory diet (28).

Table 5.   Estimates of Food Dye Daily Intake (mg/day)

Color	Weiss et al. (15)	Nutrition Foundation	ADI
Blue 1	0.80	0.85	300
Blue 2	0.15	0.46	37
Green 3	0.11	0.04	150
Red 3	0.57	1.66	150
Red 40	13.80	10.45	420
Yellow 5	9.07	7.34	300
Yellow 6	10.70	6.20	300

The most critical component of behavioral testing that needs to be assimilated into food additive hazard evaluation is behavioral teratology. Teratology is the discipline that studies birth deformities. Now we are aware that easily visible morphologic derangements, like the missing limbs induced by the drug thalidomide, may not be the sole consequences to the developing organism of toxic exposure. The deficits may be functional, such as learning disabilities, and may be hidden from view until the child reaches school age. Hence, the term "behavioral teratology." As noted by Stare et al. (17), clinical trials of the Feingold diet and of the impact of food colors suggest that the youngest children are those most at risk. Such a suggestion is buttressed by findings in animals (18, 19). England, France, and Japan now require testing for behavioral teratology. It is illogical for the United States to lag so significantly.

Another important flaw, especially in human trials, is misuse of statistics. Feingold has never asserted that all hyperactive children benefit from the diet. His estimates range from 30—60%; yet, in nearly all the investigations conducted so far, group comparisons were used to evaluate the difference between experimental and control treatments. Such statistics are inappropriate for situations in which only a proportion of the subjects are expected to respond. The largest study so far included 36 subjects (10). A population containing 30% responders would require a sample of 265 subjects to be certain of finding a statistically significant difference 90% of the time, even if the susceptible members of the group, on the whole, responded as much as 1 standard deviation (e.g., 10 IQ points) beyond the control mean. Experimental designs in which subjects are challenged repeatedly would be more cogent. Such single-subject designs have been made popular by investigators in behavior modification.

NUTRITIONAL STRATEGIES AND IMPLICATIONS

This review of food additive safety is not directed toward abstract, academic issues. More frequently than ever before, nutritionists, physicians, and other specialists are questioned intensively by concerned patients and parents, a concern illustrated by the proliferation of allegedly natural foods. Those who are asked for advice cannot hide behind a barrier of scientific skepticism. They are certain to lose their credibility if they advise clients to wait until all the scientific evidence is in. Clients will simply shop elsewhere for answers. Such advice could take the form of a three-part tactic. First, the client should be helped to become an investigator. Parents who are considering the option of the Feingold diet need guidance, not only on how to select nutritious foods that meet the criteria of an elimination diet, but also on how to ask properly the question of whether or not the diet is beneficial to the child. Most parents can comprehend the requirements of evidence. They should be helped to design a protocol for their own use. A second part of the strategy, which most nutritional scientists would welcome, is to wean clients from highly processed food products. Often called junk foods, they contain the most additives and are the least adequate nutritionally. Even apart from the possible toxic impact of food additives, consumers should be educated to these deficiencies and encouraged to adopt more optimal diets. Third, the nutrition and medical community should take a stand on cosmetic as opposed to functional additives. Food colors are cosmetic ingredients and are not added to promote nutritional value or safety. The same is true for most synthetic flavors and for flavor enhancers such as MSG. Few additives are devoid of risk. If the benefit is zero, the risk:benefit ratio becomes infinity.

ACKNOWLEDGMENTS

Preparation of this paper was supported in part by grant ES-01247 from the National Institute of Environmental Health Services, grant MH-11752 from the National Institute of Mental Health, and in part by contract no. DE-AC02-76EV03490 with the U.S. Department of Energy at the University of Rochester, Department of Radiation Biology and Biophysics, and has been assigned report no. UR-3490-2014.

REFERENCES

1. B. Weiss, Food additives. In Committee on Nutrition, ed., *Pediatric Nutrition Handbook*, American Academy of Pediatrics, Evanston, Ill., 1979, p. 454.
2. FASEB Select Committee on GRAS Substances. Evaluation of health aspects of GRAS food ingredients: lessons learned and questions unanswered. *Fed. Proc.* 36, 2525 (1977).
3. B. F. Feingold, *Why Your Child is Hyperactive*, Random House, New York, 1975.
4. B. F. Feingold, *Introduction to Clinical Allergy*, C. C. Thomas, Springfield, Ill., 1973.
5. L. Juhlin, G. Michaelsson, and O. Zetterstrom, Urticaria and asthma induced by food-and-drug additives in patients with aspirin hypersensitivity. *J. Allergy Clin. Immunol.* 50, 92 (1972).
6. G. Michaelsson, L. Pettersson, and L. Juhlin, Purpura caused by food and drug additives. *Arch. Dermatol.* 109, 49 (1974).
7. H. E. Noid, T. W. Schulze, and R. K. Winkelmann, Diet plan for patients with salicylate-induced urticaria. *Arch. Dermatol.* 109, 866 (1974).
8. I. Neuman, R. Elian, H. Nahum, P. Shaked, and D. Creter, The danger of "yellow dyes" (tartrazine) to allergic subjects. *Clin. Allergy* 8, 65 (1978).
9. C. K. Conners, C. H. Goyette, D. A. Southwick, J. M. Lees, and P. A. Andrulonis, Food additives and hyperkinesis: a controlled double-blind experiment. *Pediatrics* 58, 154 (1976).
10. J. P. Harley, R. S. Ray, L. Tomasi, P. L. Eichman, C. G. Matthews, R. Chun, C. S. Cleeland, and E. Traisman, Hyperkinesis

and food additives: Testing the Feingold hypothesis. *Pediatrics* **61**, 818 (1978).

11. B. Weiss, Food additives and environmental chemicals as sources of childhood behavior disorders. *J. Am. Acad. Child Psychiatry*, **21**, 144 (1982).

12. C. H. Goyette, C. K. Conners, T. A. Pettit, and L. E. Curtis, Effects of artificial colors on hyperkinetic children: A double-blind challenge study. *Psychopharmacol. Bull.* **14**, 39 (1978).

13. J. I. Williams, D. M. Cram, F. T. Tausig, and E. Webster, Relative effects of drugs and diet on hyperactive behaviors: An experimental study. *Pediatrics* **61**, 811 (1978).

14. J. M. Swanson and M. Kinsbourne, Food dyes impair performance of hyperactive children in a laboratory learning test. *Science* **207**, 1485 (1980).

15. B. Weiss, J. H. Williams, S. Margen, B. Abrams, B. Caan, L. J. Citron, C. Cox, J. McKibben, D. Ogar, and S. Schultz, Behavioral responses to artificial food colors. *Science* **207**, 1487 (1980).

16. M. A. Lipton, C. B. Nemeroff, and R. B. Mailman, Hyperkinesis and food additives. In R. J. Wurtman and J. J. Wurtman, eds., *Nutrition and the Brain, Vol. 4*, Raven Press, New York, 1979, p. 1.

17. F. J. Stare, E. M. Whelan, and M. Sheridan, Diet and hyperactivity: is there a relationship? *Pediatrics* **66**, 521 (1980).

18. B. A. Shaywitz, J. R. Goldenring, and R. S. Wool, Effects of chronic administration of food colorings on activity levels and cognitive performance in developing rat pups treated with 6-hydroxydopamine. *Neurobehav. Toxicol.* **1**, 41 (1979).

19. J. R. Goldenring, R. S. Wool, B. A. Shaywitz, D. K. Batter, D. J. Cohen, G. J. Young, and M. H. Teicher, Effects of continuous gastric infusion of food dyes on developing rat pups. *Life Sci.* **27**, 1897 (1980).

20. H. H. Schaumburg, R. Byck, R. Gerstl, and J. H. Mashman, Monosodium-L-glutamate: Its pharmacology and role in the Chinese restaurant syndrome. *Science* **163**, 826 (1969).

21. L. Reif-Lehrer and M. G. Stemmermann, Monosodium glutamate intolerance in children. *N. Engl. J. Med.* **293**, 1204 (1975).

22. J. W. Olney, Brain lesions, obesity and other disturbances in mice treated with monosodium glutamate. *Science* **164**, 719 (1969).

23. J. W. Olney, Excitotoxic mechanisms of neurotoxicity. In P. S. Spencer and H. H. Schaumburg, eds., *Experimental and Clinical Neurotoxicology*, Williams & Wilkins, Baltimore, 1980, p. 272.

24. J. W. Olney, J. Labruyere, and T. de Gubareff, Brain damage in

mice from voluntary ingestion of glutamate and aspartate. *Neurobehav. Toxicol.* **2**, 125 (1980).

25. J. S. Kizer, C. B. Nemeroff, and W. W. Youngblood, Neurotoxic amino acid and structurally related analogs. *Pharmacol. Rev.* **29**, 301 (1978).
26. L. Reif-Lehrer, Possible significance of adverse reactions to glutamate in humans. *Fed. Proc.* **35**, 2205 (1976).
27. B. H. Ershoff, Effects of diet on growth and survival of rats fed toxic levels of tartrazine (FD & C Yellow No. 5) and Sunset Yellow FCF (FD & C Yellow No. 6). *J. Nutr.* **107**, 822 (1977).
28. K. Kostial and B. Kello, Bioavailability of lead in rats fed "human" diets. *Bull. Environ. Contam. Toxicol.* **21**, 312 (1979).

ADDITIONAL RECENT REFERENCE

National Institutes of Health Consensus Development Panel, National Institutes of Health consensus development conference statement: defined diets and childhood hyperactivity. *Am. J. Clin. Nutr.* **37**, 161, 1983.

3

Fructose and Health

LEIF SESTOFT, M.D.
Herlev Hospital
Herlev, Denmark

Address correspondence to Leif Sestoft, M.D., Department of Medicine, F 112, Herlev Hospital, 2730 Herlev, Denmark.

ABSTRACT

Fructose is metabolized in the liver via unique pathways that convert fructose to glucose and lactate. The metabolism of fructose induces regulatory changes in carbohydrate, lipid, and nucleotide metabolism. These effects are well elucidated and explain much of the experience with the dietary use of fructose in humans. However, in animals fructose seems to have specific effects with respect to the development of diabetes, diabetic complications, and reduction in growth rate. Fructose cannot be recommended for the dietary use of diabetics, but may perhaps be used as a sweetener by patients with reactive hypoglycemia. It is unknown to what extent fructose is involved in the pathogenesis of disease in humans, apart from its role in hereditary fructose intolerance. The consumption of fructose is increasing and the impact of this increase on public health is uncertain.

Fructose is supplied to humans in the food as a part of sucrose or as the monosaccharide itself. These constituents have been part of the diet through most of human evolution, and humans are equipped to metabolize fructose. It was recognized by Cori in 1926 that fructose is metabolized very rapidly and, 10 years later, that its initial conversion is independent of insulin (1). The latter discovery confirmed a 100-year-old observation that fructose is tolerated better than glucose by diabetics. Fructose is metabolized mainly in the liver (2) via a pathway which, in its initial steps, is different from that of glucose (3). In the 1960s, it was clearly shown that the high rate of metabolism of fructose in the liver may give rise to side effects in nucleotide (energy-rich phosphate compounds) metabolism. Since then, more has been learned about the details of fructose metabolism (for a review, see reference 4), but knowledge about the long-term effects of dietary fructose is still scanty.

The advent of new technology has allowed the production of crystalline fructose on an industrial scale, but this product cannot compete with sucrose in price. This is not the case with corn syrups that have a varying but usually high content of fructose (42–55% or more). Such syrups are isosweet (have the same degree of sweetness) with sucrose, are easy to transport, and are being used increasingly in food technology. Since the nonnutritional sugar substitutes cyclamate and saccharin are suspected carcinogens, the use of fructose in the diet of humans has been an increasingly important issue in recent years (5). In Europe, opinions on the usefulness of fructose as a dietary constituent have been divided along geographic lines. Scientists advocating the use of fructose may be found in Germany and Finland, whereas opposition has arisen in Belgium, the United Kingdom, Denmark, and Switzerland.

The use of fructose as a dietary constituent for humans is, thus, a matter of controversy, where the issue is dominated by practical needs, theoretical reservations, and industrial interests. Since there are no conclusive dietary experiments with respect to most of the the areas of fructose use for humans, the following will be an interpretation of available data.

ABSORPTION OF FRUCTOSE FROM THE INTESTINE

Fructose is absorbed from the jejunum about one-half as quickly as glucose, whether the fructose is in solution or as a component of sucrose (6). The hydrolysis of sucrose (to glucose and fructose) is a process which is independent of the absorption of its constituent monosaccharides, and is not limiting for their rate of absorption. Although the rate of fructose uptake, measured with double lumen tubes placed at various levels of the intestine, is lower than that of glucose, it may well be as fast as that of glucose, when the whole length of the jejunum is working under normal conditions. This may be facilitated by an increased rate of intestinal passage due to a lowered rate of water absorption concomitant with fructose absorption (7).

Jejunal mucosa metabolizes fructose and contains an enzyme (ketohexokinase) which phosphorylates fructose with a high affinity, but in the rat jejunum fructose metabolism is not accompanied by any extraordinary increase in fructose-1-phosphate or decrease in ATP concentration (8). Therefore, fructose is partly converted to glucose and lactate before delivery to the portal vein. This conversion shows a great difference among species (9), but it is believed that in human beings about 80% of absorbed fructose reaches the liver as fructose (10).

During fructose absorption from the gut, concentrations of fructose in peripheral blood remain below 0.5 mM (9mg/dl)[1] (11). Thus, most of the absorbed fructose is eliminated in intestinal mucosa and liver. Since the rate of hepatic uptake of fructose is a linear function of the extracellular fructose concentration at low fructose concentrations (12), it is of great importance to know the portal fructose concentration. After a fructose loading (about 50 g taken orally), the portal concentration of fructose may be as high as about 5 mM (10, 13). Concentrations of fructose in peripheral venous blood have been found to be two times higher after sucrose than after an equivalent loading of fructose plus glucose (11). Thus, the portal concentration of fructose may be increased to levels considerably above 5 mM after a sucrose load.

In conclusion, fructose is absorbed from the gut at a sufficient rate to increase the fructose concentration in the portal venous blood to between 2 and 5 mM. At this concentration, fructose exerts significant metabolic effects on the liver.

FRUCTOSE METABOLISM BY THE LIVER

The liver is the main organ for fructose elimination after fructose (sucrose) administration (see Fig. 1). Fructose metabolism in the liver is remarkably unregulated by other substrates or by hormones, including insulin. After the entrance into the liver, fructose is rapidly phosphorylated by the ketohexokinase reaction and the product, fructose-1-phosphate, accumulates in concentrations that are extraordinarily high for an intermediate metabolite (about 10 mM). In this way, inorganic phosphate is trapped in fructose-1-phosphate, and, because of the rather slow rate of transport of inorganic phosphate across the liver plasma membrane, the intracellular concentration of inorganic phosphate decreases (14). Since inorganic phosphate is an inhibitor of the enzyme AMP deaminase, this enzyme is activated by the fructose-induced lowering of the inorganic phosphate concentration in the cell; and in this way fructose increases the rate of degradation of adenine nucleotides (4). Thus, fructose leaves the liver with a high concentration of fructose-1-phosphate, a low concentration of inorganic phosphate, and a low concentration of the energy-rich phosphate compound ATP (15). The changes in the concentration of regulator metabolites alter the pattern of metabolic response of the liver to demands from peripheral tissues: for example, the handling of lactate, glucose, and FFA. These effects of fructose are strongly dose-

---

[1]One mM of fructose/liter is equivalent to 18 mg/dl.

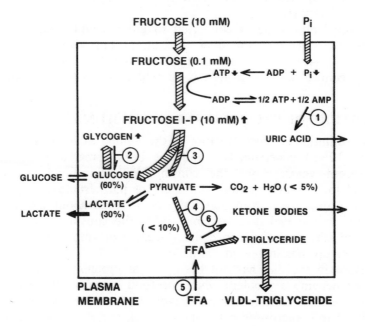

Figure 1. Fructose metabolism in the liver. At physiologic fructose concentrations, the transport of fructose into the cell is rate limiting for fructose metabolism. Once taken up in the cell, fructose is very rapidly converted to fructose-1-phosphate, which accumulates in large amounts. By this process, ATP is converted to ADP, and the liver is depleted of inorganic phosphate (P_i). The low phosphate concentration elicits an activation of the enzyme which degrades AMP to uric acid (1), and uric acid is excreted from the cell. The high concentration of fructose-1-phosphate has several metabolic effects. It inhibits the activity of the glycogen-degrading enzyme phosphorylase a (2). Therefore, fructose metabolism is accompanied by a net glycogen synthesis that may lead to an uptake of glucose from the blood. Further, fructose-1-phosphate activates the enzyme pyruvate kinase (3), and thus facilitates the production of lactate from fructose. About two-thirds of fructose is converted to glucose, which may either accumulate in the liver as glycogen or be released from the liver as glucose. About one-third of the metabolized fructose is released from the liver as lactate. Therefore, the lactate concentration in the blood increases. Only a small percentage of the metabolized fructose is oxidized to carbon dioxide and water. Another minor part goes into lipid synthesis, and this rate increases considerably with an increased supply of substrate to pyruvate, and on activation of the pyruvate-converting enzyme pyruvate dehydrogenase (4). Fructose has no effect upon the uptake of free fatty acids (FFA) in the liver (5), but inhibits the ketone body production markedly (6). Therefore, the FFA that are taken up are mostly converted to triglyceride, which may be excreted from the liver as very-low-density lipoprotein (VLDL) triglyceride. However, since the plasma lactate concentration is increased, and lactate inhibits the supply of FFA to the liver from adipose tissue, even the triglyceride synthesis in the liver may go down.

dependent (16), and they are basic to an understanding of metabolic effects of dietary fructose.

Fructose-1-phosphate is converted to glucose and lactate. Glucose may be released from the liver or accumulated within the liver as glycogen. Lactate is, for the most part, released from the liver. Only a small percentage enters lipogenesis or oxidation to carbon dioxide and water.

MAGNITUDE OF FRUCTOSE INTAKE IN HUMANS

The consumption of pure fructose in the United States has been low, between 10–20 g/person/day, and has been remarkably unchanged until recent years. Since the consumption of refined sugars has increased in the same period, the share of pure fructose in the total intake has decreased from about 4% in 1910 to about 2% in 1970. However, in the two decades since 1955, the consumption of baked goods and soft drinks, which contain sucrose or (more recently) high fructose syrup, has increased dramatically (17, 18). Therefore, the use of fructose in the diet has not been a great problem in the past, but may well become a problem when the food industry replaces glucose and sucrose with corn syrups that have a high content of fructose. On the other hand, sucrose is half fructose, and, therefore, dietary aspects of fructose cannot be covered without a view to sucrose. The average daily intake of this sugar in most countries in the Western world is somewhat above 100 g/person/day, or above 15% of the total daily caloric intake (18, 19). Thus, the daily average intake of fructose (including that present in sucrose) in Western countries is in the range of 60–80 g, with individual extremes above and below this level.

EFFECTS OF DIETARY FRUCTOSE

The whole discussion of this subject has been distorted by the misunderstanding that fructose given orally should be metabolized considerably more slowly than that given intravenously. It is, however, obvious that 50–100 g of fructose taken in a short time (minutes) has significant metabolic effects and that the rate of metabolism in the liver reaches the same values as though fructose were infused at a rate of 1 g/kg body weight/hour (20).

Immediate Effects of a Large Dose of Fructose Taken Orally

Effect on Plasma Uric Acid Concentration. The concentration of circulating uric acid increases (from 4.8–5.3 mg/dl, for example) as a result of the depletion of adenine nucleotides in the liver after a 50–100-g oral fructose load. Probably gouty patients are more susceptible to the hyperuricemic effect of fructose than are other persons (21). The quantitative role of fructose (sucrose) in the development of gout in a larger population is not known, but it must be considered potentially important. It is also unknown whether the continual intake of large amounts of fructose leads to an adaptation with regard to the hyperuricemic effect of fructose.

Effect of Blood Lactate Concentration—The Lactic Acidosis Problem. Even small doses of fructose are accompanied by a significant release of lactate from the liver of feeding animals as well as fasting ones (16). When fructose is taken orally, the plasma lactate and pyruvate concentrations are increased by a factor of two to four in humans (22). When given intravenously to severely ill patients, fructose may elicit lactic acidosis by preventing uptake of lactic acid in the liver and by adding a large net lactic acid production from this organ (for a warning, see reference 23). However, fructose administration always leads to an increased rate of acid production in the body and a small lowering of blood pH (24, 25).

Effects on Blood Glucose Concentration. As mentioned above, fructose is very rapidly metabolized to glucose and lactate in the liver. Glucose originating from fructose may either be released to the bloodstream or may accumulate in the liver as glycogen. The literature on the effect of oral intake of fructose on blood glucose reflects this diversity. In some investigations, fructose leads to a lowering of blood glucose (26), that is, the net rate of glycogen uptake from fructose and from blood glucose is increased because glycogen breakdown is inhibited. In other investigations, fructose taken orally increases the concentration of blood glucose, that is, fructose is not quantitatively converted to glycogen but is, in part, released from the liver as glucose (22, 27). The accumulated fructose-1-phosphate acts as an inhibitor of the glycogen-degrading enzyme phosphorylase, and the same effect is elicited by the low concentration of inorganic phosphate (4). Therefore, fructose facilitates glycogen formation from glucose which may originate from fructose itself and may come from the blood (28, 29). The net uptake of glucose and the block of glycogen breakdown may explain the hypoglycemic tendency that is sometimes seen during a fructose load.

Diabetes mellitus. It is particularly important that one keep these facts in mind when interpreting the clinically important effect of fructose taken orally on blood glucose in diabetics. With such patients it is likely that fructose tolerance, defined as the effect of fructose taken orally on the blood glucose concentration, depends on the state of metabolic regulation of the diabetic; the more pronounced the state of diabetic malregulation, the more the blood glucose concentration is prone to increase after an oral fructose challenge (22, 27). However, this area has not been fully explored, since the existing studies only encompass limited numbers of patients; and the characterization of these patients is insufficient with respect to (1) their classification as type 1 or 2 diabetics, (2) the degree of preservation of endogenous insulin secretion in the type 1 diabetics, (3) their present state of insulin therapy, and (4) their state of starvation at the time of the investigation. Probably fructose will tend to decrease the blood glucose concentration under conditions in which the liver is able to synthesize glycogen at a maximal rate, that is, under conditions with a high circulating glucose concentration, with sufficient insulin in the blood, and with empty or half empty glycogen stores. Under such conditions, fructose will increase the rate of glucose uptake in the liver. On the other hand, if the above mentioned conditions are not present, and especially if hepatic glycogen stores are already filled up, fructose will greatly increase the rate of glucose release from the liver and will raise the peripheral blood glucose concentration. As an example, on the basis of our knowledge of the handling of fructose by the liver, we can predict that a hyperinsulinized diabetic who is given fructose to cope with a hypoglycemic attack will run the risk of an aggravation of the hypoglycemia; whereas the same patient a few days later may get an overt increase in blood glucose after the same amount of fructose, because he or she is now hypoinsulinized, or is well insulinized, but already has maximally filled glycogen stores.

Thus, much of the debate on whether fructose is harmless or harmful for diabetics is tenuous and we lack the hard data to reach a generally accepted resolution.

Effect on Insulin Receptor Number. In humans, fructose (1000 kcal/day), but not glucose in the same amount, caused a 30% decrease in the number of insulin receptors on monocytes in one week (30). The impact of this action on the diabetogenic effect of fructose is unknown.

Effect on Insulin Secretion. In vitro fructose is not able to increase the rate of insulin secretion, but may evoke insulin secretion if the beta cell is preconditioned by a glucose stimulus (31). In contrast to the ingestion of glucose, the ingestion of fructose is not accompanied by any secretion of the gut hormone GIP (gastric inhibitory polypeptide), which enhances insulin secretion after a glucose load (32). Since fructose in normal humans has a limited effect on the level of blood glucose and does not stimulate insulin secretion in itself, substitution of fructose for sucrose (or glucose) in the diet may prevent attacks in patients suffering from reactive hypoglycemia (33).

Effect on the Concentration of Plasma Lipids.   Fructose does not appear to influence the concentration of plasma cholesterol (34). With respect to the effect of fructose on the plasma triglyceride concentration, conflicting reports have appeared in the literature claiming that the serum triglyceride concentration rises, remains unaltered, or decreases (for two reviews, see references 5 and 6).

The results are explainable, however, within the following framework of experimental observations: (1) fructose does not influence the rate of uptake of free fatty acids (FFA) in the liver (35); (2) fructose is strongly antiketogenic and, thus, increases the rate of incorporation of FFA into very-low-density lipoprotein (VLDL) triglyceride in the liver; (3) fructose increases the concentration of lactate in peripheral blood to concentrations that are inhibitory to lipolysis in adipose tissue (36); (4) fructose increases the rate of *de novo* synthesis of FFA in the liver by a factor of 2 or more (37) and provides ample substrate of L-glycerol-3-phosphate for triglyceride synthesis (16). In other words, within the liver the conditions for an increased rate of triglyceride synthesis are present during fructose metabolism, but, because of a significant fall in the supply of FFA from adipose tissue, the net result may be a decreased rate of VLDL secretion and, thus, the VLDL-triglyceride concentration in plasma goes down, as shown in several reports (38).

In the perfused organ, the effects of fructose and of insulin on triglyceride synthesis are additional. Therefore, it is not surprising that sucrose has a more pronounced hypertriglyceridemic effect than does fructose (34), since insulin secretion is stimulated by the glucose moiety. However, there is no explanation as to why sucrose is also more hypertriglyceridemic than are its constituent carbohydrates (39).

It is not known whether fructose intake plays any role in the development of atherosclerotic disease in man.

Effect on Ethanol Elimination Rate.   The rate of ethanol elimination is increased 50% by oral intake of, for example, 30 g fructose in solution (40). This effect has also been found with sucrose. However, the lowering of the blood ethanol concentration is not accompanied by any improvement in the performance of the ethanol-intoxicated subject (41), and treatment of drunken persons with fructose does not cause any relief in hangover symptoms (42). Drivers should be warned against the misunderstanding that fructose intake improves their capacity to drive a car after ethanol intake. The mechanism by which fructose exerts its effect seems in some way to be connected with the fructose-induced rise in hepatic oxygen uptake and with the significant effect of fructose on *de novo* synthesis of FFA in liver. By both mechanisms the rate of removal of oxidizable material is increased.

Physiologic Effects of Fructose. The oral intake of as little as 30 g fructose in solution (in contrast to fructose incorporation in meals; see below) causes abdominal discomfort increasing to severe pain. After taking fructose orally a few patients suffer abdominal symptoms that are so disabling for daily life that it is necessary to treat them with a fructose-free diet (43). Intravenous infusion of fructose also elicits epigastric pain, after which substernal pain ensues. The infusion of fructose is accompanied by a coronary arterial vasodilatation that coincides with the great fructose-induced increase in lactate load to the heart (44). It is unknown whether the symptoms elicited by intravenous and oral fructose are alike, and it is also unknown whether the physiologic mechanism behind these symptoms can be ascribed to (1) the fructose-induced drop in blood pH, (2) the greatly raised concentration of lactate, (3) the drop in plasma inorganic phosphate (22), or (4) some other process that is unknown or difficult to assess.

Long-Term Use in Humans of Fructose Incorporated into the Meals

The existing studies show no measurable side effects in normal humans who are given, for example, 50—100 g fructose as part of their meals for a period of up to several months (34, 45). The measured parameters have been blood lipids, glucose tolerance, parameters of liver function, weight, and uricemia. None of these parameters showed any significant change when fructose was substituted for sucrose or starch. In diabetics, long-term fructose administration in the diet is prone to increase the serum triglyceride concentration slightly (46). Diabetic children can tolerate 1 g fructose/kg body weight/day in their diet without any measurable signs of impairment of control (47).

However, the experiments that have been performed do not give us the answer as to whether (1) fructose has any long-term effects on cardiovascular disease, (2) fructose in the diet leads to any metabolic adaptation which counteracts the processes that are potentially dangerous (e.g., hyperuricemia), or (3) whether the use of fructose in the diet on a large scale will be deleterious for some persons and well tolerated by others.

Effects of Fructose on Selected Groups of People

Newborn Children. In contrast to some animal species, the human newborn infant is able to metabolize fructose. The capacity is low, but after a few weeks the child converts fructose at a high rate (48). Interestingly, the newborn infant is very sensitive to the hypoglycemic effect of fructose. Since this effect is attributed to the accumulation of fructose-1-phosphate, one might suggest that the relatively low capacity for fructose elimination can be attributed to a defect not in the phosphorylating enzyme ketohexokinase, but rather to a low capacity of the next step, the aldolase, as is seen in fructose intolerance.

Persons with Fructose Intolerance. In people with this rather rare inborn error of metabolism, the activity of the enzyme aldolase, which splits fructose to glyceraldehyde and dihydroxyacetone phosphate, is very low (49). Therefore fructose-1-phosphate accumulates to extraordinarily high concentrations and traps the inorganic phosphate from the intracellular fluid as well as from the plasma. The lack of inorganic phosphate leads to a severe decrease in the concentration of ATP, which is necessary for fructose phosphorylation, so that the fructose elimination rate decreases to low values after a short time. Further, fructose-1-phosphate is an inhibitor of glycogen phosphorylase, and the activity of this enzyme is also lowered by lack of one of its substrates, namely inorganic phosphate (4, 49). At the same time there seems to be an enzymatic block of gluconeogenesis from lactate (16). These mechanisms tend to block glucose output from the liver, and fatal hypoglycemia then ensues.

The widespread use of fructose solutions for intravenous infusions has led to tragic and unecessary deaths in those countries which still stick to fructose media for unselected use in wards (50, 51). It is of interest that in patients with fructose intolerance even very small oral doses of fructose give rise to symptoms and signs of severe hepatic injury (52). This rather rare inborn error of metabolism is mentioned here because the overt toxic effects of fructose revealed in these patients can be considered the end stage of a continuum of side effects that are seen to varying degrees in normal persons. In normal people, the effect may depend on their individual activity of fructose-1-phosphate aldolase and of the dose of fructose which reaches their livers.

Long-Term Effect of a High Dietary Fructose in Experimental Animals

Fructose feeding, at levels greater than 50% of calories as fructose, generally inhibits the growth of normal animals (53, 54). In laboratory animals, fructose introduces a variety of pathologic effects that seem to be connected to inherited dispositions, since only a fraction of the animals respond in a pathologic way. In some animals, fructose feeding is accompanied by a significant lowering of the glucose tolerance, with permanent hyperglycemia, hyperinsulinism, and signs of diabetic complications (55, 56). In these animals, the fructose-induced rise in blood glucose is also increased. It has been shown in other experiments that fructose feeding leads to an excess in glycogen storage (glycogenosis), but the glycogen in these livers is mobilized in about 2 days of starvation (57). This observation fits with the observation that liver weight relative to body weight is increased in fructose-fed animals, without any significant change occurring in the liver lipid content (54). Taken together, all these observations suggest to me that some animals develop diabetes-like symptoms after fructose feeding because of an accumulation of glycogen in the liver that inhibits the uptake of glucose, and that these symptoms are based on inherited traits. The engorgement of the liver with glycogen leads in turn to permanent hyperglycemia and an increased blood glucose response to glucose and fructose.

On the other hand, fructose and other monosaccharides may also lead to destruction of pancreatic islets in selected mice, and, by a mechanism which is not well understood, to diabetes (58).

Other Issues of Dietary Fructose

It was claimed that fructose is less cariogenic than sucrose (59), but other studies have failed to confirm this matter (60).

Furthermore, fructose-containing diets have been claimed to favor weight loss. This view was based on the fact that fructose under some conditions has a more sweet taste than does sucrose or glucose. However, in practice a weight-loss regimen cannot rely upon such faint differences in sweetness of taste. Since fructose actually has a rather pleasant sweet taste, its use may actually evoke appetite.

REFERENCES

1. J. N. Davidson, W. O. Kermack, D. M. Mowat, and C. P. Stewart, Fructose metabolism in the intact animal. *Biochem. J.* **30**, 433 (1936).
2. J. L. Bollman and F. C. Mann, The physiology of the liver: The utilization of fructose following complete removal of the liver. *Am. J. Physiol.* **96**, 683 (1931).
3. H. G. Hers, La fructokinase du foie. *Biochim. Biophys. Acta* **8**, 416 (1952).
4. G. van den Berghe, Metabolic effects of fructose in the liver. In B. L. Horecker and E. R. Stadtman, eds., *Current Topics in Cellular Regulation*, Academic Press, New York, 1978, p. 98.
5. J. D. Brunzell, Use of fructose, sorbitol, or xylitol as a sweetener in diabetes mellitus. *Diabetes Care* **1**, 223 (1978).

6. G. M. Gray and F. J. Ingelfinger, Intestinal absorption of sucrose in man: Interrelation of hydrolysis and monosaccharide product absorption. *J. Clin. Invest.* **45**, 388 (1966).
7. C. D. Holdsworth and A. M. Dawson, The absorption of monosaccharides in man. *Clin. Sci.* **27**, 371 (1964).
8. J. M. J. Lamers and W. C. Hülsmann, The effect of fructose on the stores of energy-rich phsophate in rat jejunum *in vivo. Biochim. Biophys. Acta* **313**, 1 (1973).
9. J. Y. Kiyasu and I. L. Chaikoff, On the manner of transport of absorbed fructose. *J. Biol. Chem.* **224**, 935 (1957).
10. G. C. Cook, Absorption products of D(−)fructose in man. *Clin. Sci.* **37**, 675 (1969).
11. I. MacDonald and L. J. Turner, Serum-fructose levels after sucrose or its constituent monosaccharides. *Lancet* **1**, 841 (1968).
12. L. Sestoft and P. Fleron, Determination of the kinetic constants of fructose transport and phosphorylation in the perfused rat liver. *Biochim. Biophys. Acta* **345**, 27 (1974).
13. C. D. Holdsworth and A. M. Dawson, Absorption of fructose in man. *Proc. Soc. Exp. Biol. Med.* **118**, 142 (1965).
14. L. Sestoft and L. Ø. Kristenson, Determination of unidirectional fluxes of phosphate across plasma membrane in isolated perfused rat liver. *Am. J. Physiol.* **236**(5), C202 (1979).
15. J. C. Bode, O. Zelder, H. J. Rumpelt, and U. Wittkamp, Depletion of liver adenosine phosphates and metabolic effects of intravenous infusion of fructose or sorbitol in man and in the rat. *Eur. J. Clin. Invest.* **3**, 436 (1973).
16. L Sestoft, Regulation of fructose metabolism in the perfused rat liver: Interrelation with inorganic phosphate, glucose, ketone body and ethanol metabolism. *Biochim. Biophys. Acta* **343**, 1 (1974).
17. H. L. Sipple and K. W. McNutt, *Sugar in Nutrition*, Academic Press, New York, 1974.
18. C. A. M. Hough, K. J. Parker, and A. J. Vlitos, *Developments in Sweeteners-1*, Applied Science Publishers, London, 1979.
19. C. B. Singleton, Jr., The outlook for isoglucose in the United States, Western Europe and Japan. In F. O. Licht, ed., *International Sugar Report*, Ratzeburg, W. Germany, 1978, p. 7.
20. L. Sestoft, Fructose and the dietary therapy of diabetes mellitus. *Diabetologia* **17**, 1 (1979).
21. F. Stirpe, E. Della Corte, E. Bonetti, A. Abbondanza, A. Abbati, and F. De Stefano, Fructose-induced hyperuricemia. *Lancet* **2**, 1310 (1970).

22. M. Miller, J. W. Craig, W. R. Drucker, and H. Woodward, The metabolism of fructose in man. *Yale J. Biol. Med* 29(I), 335 (1956).
23. H. F. Woods and K. G. M. M. Alberti, Dangers of intravenous fructose. *Lancet* 2, 1354 (1972).
24. O. R. Kruesi, M. F. Goodbody, Jr., T. B. van Ittallie, and J. G. Hilton, Effect of intravenously administered fructose on blood acid-base balance in patients with pre-existing acidosis. *Diabetes* 4, 104 (1955).
25. R. Kaye, M. L. Williams, and G. Barbero, Comparative study of glucose and fructose metabolism in infants with reference to utilization and to the accumulation of glycolytic intermediates. *J. Clin. Invest.* 37, 752 (1958).
26. R. Schwartz, H. Gamsu, P. B. Mulligan, S. H. Reisner, S. H. Wybregt, and M. Cornblath, Transient intolerance to exogenous fructose in the newborn. *J. Clin. Invest* 43, 333 (1964).
27. P. A Crapo, O. G. Kolterman, and J. M. Olefsky, Effects of oral fructose in normal, diabetic, and impaired glucose tolerance subjects. *Diabetes Care* 3, 575 (1980).
28. J. Corvilain and R. Tagnon, Effects of fructose infusion on glucose uptake and circulating insulin-like activity in normal men. *J. Physiol.* 155, 337 (1961).
29. L. H. Nilsson and E. Hultman, Liver and muscle glycogen in man after glucose and fructose infusion. *Scand. J. Clin. Lab. Invest.* 33, 5 (1974).
30. H. Beck-Nielsen, O. Pedersen, and H. O. Lindskov, Impaired cellular insulin binding and insulin sensitivity induced by high-fructose feeding in normal subjects. *Am. J. Clin. Nutr.* 33, 273 (1980).
31. J. R. Lawrence, C. E. Gray, J. S. Grant, J. A. Ford, W. B. McIntosh, and M. G. Dunnigan, The insulin response to intravenous fructose in maturity-onset diabetes mellitus and in normal subjects. *Diabetes* 29, 736 (1980).
32. P. Ganda, J. S. Soeldner, R. E. Gleason, J. G. M. Cleator, and C. Reynolds, Metabolic effects of glucose, mannose, galactose, and fructose in man. *J. Clin. Endocrinol. Metab.* 49, 616 (1979).
33. N. V. Bohannon, J. H. Karam, and P. H. Forsham, Advantages of fructose ingestion over sucrose and glucose in humans. *Diabetes Suppl.* 27, 438 (1978) (abstract).
34. E. A. Nikkilä, Influence of dietary fructose and sucrose on serum triglycerides in hypertriglyceridemia and diabetes. In H. L. Sipple and K. W. McNutt, eds., *Sugars in Nutrition*, Academic Press, New York, 1974, p. 439.

35. D. L. Topping and P. A. Mayes, Comparative effects of fructose and glucose on the lipid and carbohydrate metabolism of perfused rat liver. *Br. J. Nutr.* **36**, 113 (1976).
36. P. Dieterle, C. Dieterle, P. Bottermann, K. Schwarz, and J. Henner, In vitro Versuche zur antilipolytischen Wirkung von Milchsäure. *Diabetologia* **5**, 238 (1969).
37. M. M. Gale and M. A. Crawford, Different rate of incorporation of glucose and fructose into plasma and liver lipids in guinea pigs. *Metabolism* **18**, 1021 (1969).
38. N. A. Kaufmann, J. Kapitulnik, and S. H. Blondheim, Studies in carbohydrate-induced hypertriglyceridemia: Aspects of fructose metabolism. *Isr. J. Med. Sci.* **6**, 80 (1970).
39. R. G. Thompson, J. T. Hayford, and J. A. Hendrix, Triglyceride concentrations: the disaccharide effect. *Science* **206**, 838 (1979).
40. F. Lundquist and H. Wolthers, The influence of fructose on the kinetics of alcohol elimination in man. *Acta Pharmacol. Toxicol.* **14**, 290 (1958).
41. J. Merry and V. Marks, Effect on performance of reducing blood-alcohol with oral fructose. *Lancet* **2**, 1328 (1967).
42. R. H. Ylikahri, T. Leino, M. O. Huttunen, A. R. Pöso, C. J. P. Eriksson, and E. A Nikkilä, Effects of fructose and glucose on ethanol-induced metabolic changes and on the intensity of alcohol intoxication and hangover. *Eur. J. Clin. Invest.* **6**, 93 (1976).
43. D. E. H. Andersson and A. Nygren, Four cases of long-standing diarrhoea and colic pains cured by fructose-free diet: a pathogenic discussion. *Acta Med. Scand.* **203**, 87 (1978).
44. W. C. Elliott, L. S. Cohen, M. D. Klein, F. J. Lane, and R. Gorlin, Effects of rapid fructose infusion in man. *J. Appl. Physiol.* **23**, 865 (1967).
45. J. K. Huttunen, K. K. Mäkinen, and A. Scheinin, Turku sugar studies XI. Effects of sucrose, fructose and xylitol diets on glucose, lipid and urate metabolism. *Acta Odontol. Scand.* **33**, Suppl. 70, 239 (1975).
46. R. Pelkonen, A. Aro, and E. A. Nikkilä, Metabolic effects of dietary fructose in insulin dependent diabetes of adults. *Acta Med. Scand.* Suppl. 542, 187 (1972).
47. H. K. Akerblom, I. Siltanen, and A.-K. Kallio, Does dietary fructose affect the control of diabetes in children? *Acta Med. Scand.* Suppl. 542, 195 (1972).
48. K. Beyriss and M. Rautenbach, Utilization and turnover rate of fructose during continuous intravenous infusion in pre-term and term newborns in dependence on age. *Biol. Neonate* **24**, 330 (1974).

49. E. R. von Froesch, A. Prader, H. P. Wolf, and A. Labhart, Die heriditäre Fructoseintoleranz. *Helv. Paediat. Acta* **14**, 99 (1959).
50. J. M. Hackl, D. Balogh, F. Kunz, E. Dworzak, B. Puschendorf, A. Decristoforo, and F. Maier, Postoperative Fruktoseinfusion bei wahrscheinlich heriditärer Fruktoseintoleranz. *Wien. Klin. Wochenschr.* **90**, 237 (1978).
51. M.-J. Schulte and W. Lenz, Fatal sorbitol infusion in a patient with fructose-sorbitol intolerance. *Lancet* **2**, 188 (1977).
52. F. Adachi, D. T. Yu, and M. J. Phillips, An ultrastructural study of fructose-induced hepatic cell injury. *Virchows Arch.* **10**, 200 (1972).
53. A. R. MacRae, S. J. Slinger, and T. S. Neudoerffer, Studies on carbohydrate digestibility and weight gain response in rats fed dietary sucrose, glucose or fructose. *Nutr. Metabol.* **17**, 37 (1974).
54. C. G. R. Tuovinen and A. E. Bender, Some metabolic effects of prolonged feeding of starch, sucrose, fructose and carbohydrate-free diet in the rat. *Nutr. Metabol.* **19**, 161 (1975).
55. A. M. Cohen, A. Teitelbaum, and E. Rosenman, Diabetes induced by a high fructose diet. *Metabolism* **26**, 17 (1977).
56. R. Boot-Handford and H. Heath, Identification of fructose as the retinopathic agent associated with the ingestion of sucrose-rich diets in the rat. *Metabolism* **29**, 1247 (1980).
57. C. Matthaei, D. Sasse, and U. N. Riede, Die Fruktose-induzierte "Glykogenose". II. Histochemische Untersuchungen zum Glykogenstoffwechsel der Rattenleber nach Fruktosebelastung und bei vergleichbaren Diäten. *Beitr. Pathol.* **157**, 56 (1976).
58. E. H. Leiter, D. L. Coleman, A. B. Eisenstein, and I. Strack, Dietary control of pathogenesis in C57BL/KsJ *db/db* diabetes in mice. *Metabolism*, **30**, 554 (1981).
59. A Scheinin, K. K. Mäkinen, and K. Ylitalo, Turku sugar studies. I. An intermediate report on the effect of sucrose, fructose and xylitol diets on the caries incidence in man. *Acta Odontol. Scand.* **32**, 383 (1974).
60. T. Koulourides, R. Bodden, S. Keller, L. Manson-Hing, J. Lastra, and T. Housch, Cariogenicity of nine sugars tested with an intraoral device in man. *Caries Res.* **10**, 427 (1976).

ADDITIONAL RECENT REFERENCE

W.J. Ravich, T. M. Bayless, and M. Thomas, Fructose: Incomplete intestinal absorption in humans. *Gastroenterology* **84**, 26 (1983).

4
Dietary Sodium and Hypertension

JANET K. GROMMET, Ph.D.

AARON M. ALTSCHUL, Ph.D.

Division of Nutrition
Department of Community and Family Medicine
Georgetown University School of Medicine
Washington, D.C.

Address correspondence to Janet K. Grommet, Ph.D., Weight Control Unit, St. Luke's-Roosevelt Hospital Center, 411 W. 114th Street, Suite 3D, New York, New York 10025.

ABSTRACT

Hypertension or high blood pressure is considered to be a primary risk factor in the development of cardiovascular disease. Control of hypertension can lead to improved management of cardiovascular disease which for years has been the number one cause of death in the American public. Sodium has long been implicated in the etiology or development of hypertension, but in recent years more discerning evidence has clarified the relationship between sodium and blood pressure.

Included in this chapter are updates of biological and consumer issues relevant to sodium and hypertension. The update on sodium-related research concentrates on several mechanisms or modes of action that begin to explain the influence of sodium on blood pressure. These modes of action include some that are primarily constitutional and have a strong genetic component and others that are primarily external or nutritional.

The consumer issues addressed in this chapter center on the dilemma of interpreting sodium labeling of food, including problems in both ingredient and nutritional labeling. Additionally, to assist the consumer in recognizing the sodium content of foods, we have categorized dietary sodium intake in terms of discretionary and nondiscretionary intake. The latter is further reckoned with by the development of general concepts of the sodium content of various groups of food.

The end-result of this chapter is to delineate more clearly the interface of the nutrient sodium and the chronic disease of hypertension and to prepare the consumer to decrease sodium intake as necessary.

Having been used since biblical times, salt is sprinkled through our language as well as through our food supply. We speak of salt of the earth, an old salt, worth one's salt, with a grain of salt, to salt away, a pillar of salt, earning one's salt, and a salty tale. Salt was one of the first intentional food additives. The addition of salt to a food system helps to prevent bacterial growth. Furthermore, salt can act as a functional food ingredient providing specific technical effects during food processing, such as the ripening of cheese and the conditioning of bread dough.

More commonly, however, salt serves as a flavor enhancer. The home cook, the restaurant chef, and the food industry all subscribe to this familiar use of salt. Salt is used to season food during preparation and, similarly, the salt shaker is used at the table to season or enhance the flavor of the food being served. These multiple uses of salt—preservative, functional ingredient, and flavor enhancer—plus the naturally occurring sodium in foodstuffs result in a per capita salt consumption in the United States of approximately 10–12 g/day, the equivalent of 1-1/2 teaspoons each day.

In spite of the fact that for centuries salt has been used in home and commercial food preparation, salt consumption is not risk free. Under certain circumstances, sodium can be an etiologic factor in the development of hypertension or high blood pressure. In simple terms, the rationale relating sodium to hypertension is that excess salt consumption in sodium-sensitive individuals elevates blood pressure. This explanation leaves many questions, but several points of consensus concerning sodium and hypertension are outlined in Table 1.

The general consensus is that the sodium ion, as opposed to the chloride ion, is the component of salt implicated in hypertension; that sodium is found in greater concentration extracellularly than intracellularly; that dietary intake of sodium far exceeds requirements; that the kidneys under the influence of the endocrine system strive to maintain a homeostatic concentration of plasma sodium; that epidemiologic studies suggest a positive correlation between sodium intake and hypertension incidence among cultures; and that the influence of dietary sodium on individual blood pressure is not universal, being influenced by other factors such as genetic predisposition.

Although sodium is recognized as a factor in the etiology of hypertension, its role in the pathogenesis of hypertension is not well understood. The sodium and hypertension research frontier is focused on elucidating the mechanisms whereby sodium influences blood pressure and on deciphering why these mechanisms are evoked in certain persons. This chapter provides an update of several possible modes of action that are being actively investigated. In addition, the current status of sodium labeling on food products is reviewed. And lastly, for individuals who decide to take a prudent approach to dietary sodium intake, practical dietary suggestions for reducing sodium intake are discussed.

Table 1. General Points of Consensus Relating Sodium and Hypertension

---

1. Salt, or sodium chloride, is composed of two elements that are required by the human body. Of the two, only the cation (positive ion) sodium has been implicated in the pathogenesis of hypertension (1, 2).

2. Physiologically, sodium is found in higher concentrations extracellularly than intracellularly, a concentration gradient which is maintained by the sodium pumps located on the cell wall membranes. Sodium is the primary extracellular ion in maintaining osmotic balance (3).

3. The adult human requirement for sodium is less than 1 g salt/day (400 mg. sodium); on the average, adults consume ten to twelve times this amount daily (4–6).

4. Sodium influences fluid or blood volume. To achieve a constant concentration of sodium in the blood, endocrine or hormonal factors influence the resorption of sodium and water from the kidney tubules. Aldosterone, a mineral corticoid hormone of the adrenal cortex, enhances sodium resorption; similarly, the renin-angiotensin system enhances uptake of both sodium and water (7, 8).

5. With few exceptions, cultures that ingest moderate amounts of sodium have a low incidence of hypertension, whereas cultures with a generous intake of sodium are prone to hypertension. In general, cultures with modest sodium intake are developing countries, whereas those with high intakes are industrialized countries (9–11).

6. The effect of sodium intake on individual blood pressure is not universal. Increasing dietary sodium intake in normotensive and hypertensive individuals results in either no change or an increase in pressure; decreasing sodium intake in normotensive and hypertensive individuals results in either no change or a decrease in pressure. The effect of sodium intake on blood pressure is thought to be modified by genetic predilection (12–17).

MODES OF ACTION

A number of genetic and environmental factors are considered to be predisposing to the development of hypertension, including nutritional factors (1). Factors proposed as having primarily a genetic component include race or ethnic background, family history, and variations in endocrine and kidney function. Environmental factors implicated in hypertension include psychogenic stress as well as several nutritional factors, with excess sodium intake being strongly implicated (19). In the following sections, recent findings concerning several genetic and nutritional factors are discussed.

Genetic Factors

The underlying cause of hypertension is probably genetic, with some individuals being more sensitive to, or less efficient in handling, the nutritional and other environmental factors (20). Yet the postulated genetic factors—ethnic background, family history, and endocrine and kidney function—have not resulted in a sufficiently detailed mode of action to establish a genetic basis for hypertension. Recently, however, two avenues of research have been reported: one involving the sodium exchange system and one involving the sodium-potassium pump, both of which suggest that genetic defects in handling sodium may consequently elevate blood pressure. Presumably, dietary sodium intake further exacerbates the situation.

Sodium Exchange Process and Hypertension. Current investigation by Tosteson of the relationship of sodium to hypertension involves the sodium exchange process of cells (21). In the exchange process, a sodium ion can leave a cell at the same time another sodium ion enters. The exchange system, however, is not completely selective, as calcium or lithium ions can be exchanged for sodium and, thus, enter the cell. Tosteson's work indicates that the maximum exchange rate in red blood cells is genetically determined, perhaps indicating a genetic basis for hypertension (22). Individuals with high blood pressure were found to have the highest exchange rates. On the average, those with normal blood pressure reportedly had significantly lower exchange rates, and few with normal blood pressure had a high exchange rate. Some, however, with normal blood pressure who had a family history of hypertension had high exchange rates, suggesting that those individuals were genetically predisposed to the development of hypertension.

Exchange rates have been studied in erythrocytes (red blood cells) because these cells are more readily available than are muscle cells of the arterioles (small blood vessels). Researchers hypothesize that the sodium exchange rate is inherited in the arterioles as well as in the erythrocytes. Individuals with very active exchange rates may develop high blood pressure as a result of excessive amounts of calcium entering the smooth muscle cells of the arterioles causing contraction of the arteriole muscles. This contraction would increase resistance and, thus, elevate blood pressure. One of the particularly optimistic features of this work on the sodium exchange process is that it could possibly be applied as a screening procedure to identify those children who are genetically predisposed to the development of hypertension (23).

Natriuretic Hormone and Hypertension. Another facet of sodium and hypertension research that may have genetic implications is the recently reported work with natriuretic hormone (24, 25). This hormone is distinct from other endocrine factors that are known to influence blood pressure, such as norepinephrine, aldosterone, and the renin-angiotension system (26). It is not a newly discovered hormone, as some investigators have studied natriuretic hormone for years, particularly in cases of expanded blood volume such as in uremia. However, its relationship to hypertension was not recognized until recently (27).

Excess dietary sodium intake results in an expanded blood volume, albeit a transient expansion, that is thought to release natriuretic hormone. The hormone then affects sodium balance at the level of the sodium-potassium (Na-K) pump. Na-K pumps are located on all cell membranes where they maintain an intracellular concentration that is low in sodium and high in potassium. These concentrations are maintained by concurrently pumping sodium out of the cell and potassium into the cell. This is an active, not passive, diffusion, and energy for it is derived from adenosine triphosphate (ATP). The enzyme Na, K-ATPase hydrolyzes ATP to release energy for the cell membrane pumps. Natriuretic hormone apparently works by inhibiting the Na, K-ATPase enzyme and, thus, decreasing pump activity.

As a result of the inhibition of the Na-K pumps, sodium accumulates in the cells, resulting in increased contraction of smooth muscles. In the cells of the arteriole walls, this increased concentration of sodium and the subsequent contraction increases vascular resistance and elevates blood pressure. In the cells of the kidney tubules, however, the increased sodium results in increased secretion of sodium by the distal kidney tubule. This increased secretion of sodium by the kidney, however, does not adequately compensate for the increased resistance and elevated blood pressure. Quite possibly, the sensitivity of natriuretic hormone to dietary sodium varies, accounting for genetic variability in sodium sensitivity.

Nutritional Factors

In addition to the ingestion of excess dietary sodium, nutritional factors that have been implicated in the pathogenesis of hypertension include excess sucrose, excess calories, and limited linoleic acid intake. Sodium has been considered the most detrimental of these various nutritional factors, yet recent work suggests that several of these factors may be interrelated.

Carbohydrate Intake and Hypertension. Several investigators have wrestled with the determination of the relative effect of sodium and carbohydrate (particularly sucrose) intake, on blood pressure (28–30). Recent work, however, indicates that sucrose and sodium are perhaps not independent influences but, rather, are interrelated, with insulin being the connecting link.

In studies involving high levels of simple carbohydrate, both hyperglycemia and hyperinsulinemia occurred. By using infusion systems, however, DeFronzo was able to study three groups of dogs: control, hyperglycemic hyperinsulinemic, and euglycemic (with normal blood sugar) hyperinsulinemic, and, thus, was able to differentiate between high glucose and high insulin levels (31). His work demonstrated that hyperinsulinemia resulted in increased serum sodium levels.

Insulin enhances the renal resorption of sodium as well as the resorption of potassium and phosphate but inhibits calcium resorption. Apparently, a high level of simple carbohydrate intake stimulates insulin release, which increases renal handling of sodium. Quite possibly then, an individual might ingest only a moderate amount of sodium; however, a high intake of simple carbohydrates would stimulate insulin production, causing enhanced renal absorption of sodium and a subsequent rise in blood pressure. High levels of sodium intake would further accentuate the problem. Thus, sodium balance appears to be central, but hormonal influences such as insulin levels may mediate.

Linoleic Acid and Hypertension. Both animal (32) and clinical work (32, 33) from the 1970s suggest that dietary linoleic acid intake lowers blood pressure. Consistent with this work, the Heidelberg, Germany study (35), an epidemiologic survey of 650 healthy men, reported in 1980 that linoleic acid content of adipose tissue was negatively correlated with blood pressure. Since the fatty acid composition of adipose tissue tends to reflect dietary fat intake, these data again suggest a relationship between linoleic acid intake, that is, essential fatty acid intake, and blood pressure. The percentage of linoleic acid also correlated with the percentage of arachidonic acid in adipose tissue.

Arachidonic acid, made in the body primarily from linoleic acid, is unknown to be a precursor in prostaglandin synthesis. Prostaglandins, particularly E_2 which has a natriuretic action, are involved in blood pressure regulation by affecting renal blood flow and the renin-angiotension system. The Heidelberg study noted a positive correlation between dietary linoleic acid intake and urine volume and sodium concentration and a negative correlation with serum sodium concentration, suggesting that linoleic acid might lower blood pressure by increasing urinary sodium excretion.

Obesity and Hypertension. The effect of sodium intake and excess body weight on hypertension has been debated for some time. Dahl et al., for instance, postulated that the effect of obesity on blood pressure was mediated through sodium intake (36). According to these investigators, a higher percentage of obese individuals than normal weight ones are hypertensive, since the obese individuals consume more sodium as a result of increased caloric intake: ↑calories → ↑sodium → ↑blood pressure.

Recent work, however, indicates that one must consider other factors when examining the effect of obesity and sodium intake on blood pressure. Hiramatsu et al. (37) reported changes in endocrine activity in obese individuals that may contribute to the higher incidence of hypertension found in obese persons. Plasma renin activity was inversely correlated with the increase in relative body weight but not with urinary sodium excretion. Despite the decrease in renin activity with increased body weight, serum aldosterone was not influenced by body weight; therefore, the aldosterone-renin activity ratio increased progressively with an increase in relative body weight. This inappropriately high ratio was normalized by (1) thiazide (i.e., diuretic) therapy, (2) reduced caloric intake, and (3) restricted sodium intake. These researchers concluded that the high-sodium intake by obese subjects increased unduly the aldosterone-renin activity ratio. Apparently, aldosterone contributes to the additional retention of sodium. Perhaps Dahl's original algorithm should be revised as follows: ↑calories → ↑sodium → ↑A/R (aldosterone/renin) activity ratio → ↑blood pressure.

Krotkiewski et al. (38) reported yet another metabolic derangement involving sodium balance and obesity. In studying long-term (i.e., 6 months) physical training on body composition in 27 obese women, they reported that blood pressure consistently decreased with training, although there was no significant change in body fat. In order to study metabolic variables, Krotkiewski et al. divided the women into two groups: (1) low serum insulin ($<$ 11 μUnits/ml) and (2) high serum insulin $\geq$ 11 μUnits/ml). With physical training, the high insulin group experienced a more pronounced decrease not only in serum insulin, triglycerides, and blood glucose, but also in blood pressure, particularly diastolic blood pressure.

Krotkiewski's work, as well as other recent work reported by Kolanowski (39), indicates that insulin increases sodium resorption in the distal tubule of the kidney. Thus, the decrease in plasma insulin produced in obese individuals by physical training or by caloric restriction might well be associated with decreased sodium resorption and, therefore, with decreased blood pressure.

We have focused in this section on an update of factors that clarify the relationship between sodium and hypertension. Some of these factors are primarily constitutional and have a strong genetic component, while others are primarily nutritional factors influencing blood pressure. The subsequent sections of this chapter focus on consumer issues relevant to sodium, including sodium labeling of food products and sodium composition of food.

SODIUM LABELING OF FOOD

Package Labeling

Food labeling includes both the labeling of ingredients and of nutritional factors. But for the individual who is concerned about sodium intake, there are unfortunate limitations in both systems, so that it is difficult, if not impossible, for the consumer to determine the sodium content of food.

Ingredient Labeling. Ingredient labeling requires the manufacturer to list the ingredients in descending order by weight, that is, from the ingredient which is present in the greatest quantity by weight to that which is present in the least. The mass or percentage of the ingredients is not required. The ingredient list in Figure 1 is fairly easy to interpret in terms of sodium content, as salt is listed as the primary ingredient. The consumer can conclude that this must be a food of high-sodium content. And it is, as it describes bouillon cubes, which contain 960 mg or approximately 1 gram of sodium per cube.

INGREDIENTS: SALT, HYDROLYZED VEGETABLE PROTEIN, CORN SYRUP SOLIDS, SUGAR, BEEF FAT, MONOSODIUM GLUTAMATE (FLAVOR ENHANCER), DEXTROSE, CORN SUGAR, ONION POWDER, WATER, GARLIC POWDER, CARAMEL COLOR, NATURAL FLAVORINGS, DISODIUM GUANYLATE & DISODIUM INOSINATE, FLAVOR ENHANCERS, PARTIALLY HYDROGENATED VEGETABLE OIL (SOYBEAN OIL AND OR PALM OIL AND OR COTTONSEED OIL), ARTIFICIAL COLOR

NUTRITION INFORMATION PER SERVING
SERVING SIZE: 1 CUBE PROTEIN: LESS THAN 1 GRAM
SERVINGS PER CONTAINER: 25 CARBOHYDRATE: 1 GRAM
CALORIES: 6 FAT: LESS THAN 1 GRAM
PERCENTAGE OF U.S. RECOMMENDED DAILY ALLOWANCES (U.S. RDA)*
*CONTAINS LESS THAN 2 PERCENT OF THE U.S. RDA OF PROTEIN, VITAMIN A, VITAMIN C, THIAMINE, RIBOFLAVIN, NIACIN, CALCIUM, AND IRON.

41258 75117
BEST WHEN USED BY DATE STAMPED ON THE CAP

KEEP IN COOL DRY PLACE
RECIPES ON BACK OF LABEL
CUT ALONG DOTTED LINE

"If it's Borden, it's got to be good!!" WYLER FOODS-C, BORDEN, INC. COLUMBUS, OHIO 43215 U.S.A. PRINTED IN U.S.A. PRODUCT OF U.S.A. ©1978 BORDEN, INC.

DIRECTIONS:
DISSOLVE 1 BOUILLON CUBE IN 1 CUP (8 OUNCES) BOILING WATER.

Figure 1. Food label from bouillon cubes.

INGREDIENTS: POTATOES, VEGETABLE OIL SHORTENING (CONTAINS PALM OIL OR PARTIALLY HYDROGENATED SOYBEAN OIL), SALT, ENRICHED WHEAT FLOUR (FLOUR, NIACIN, IRON, THIAMINE MONONITRATE, RIBOFLAVIN), RICE FLOUR, MONOSODIUM GLUTAMATE, NATURAL FLAVORING, HYDROLYZED VEGETABLE PROTEIN, DEXTROSE, DISODIUM DIHYDROGEN PYROPHOSPHATE (TO RETAIN NATURAL COLOR).

Figure 2. Food label from frozen potato product.

INGREDIENTS: WHOLE GRAIN CORN, VEGETABLE OIL (CONTAINS ONE OR MORE OF THE FOLLOWING: COTTONSEED, PEANUT, SOYBEAN), SALT.

NUTRITION INFORMATION PER SERVING

SERVING SIZE .... 1 OZ
SERVINGS PER CONTAINER 10
CALORIES 150
PROTEIN .... 2 g
CARBOHYDRATE .... 12 g
FAT .... 8 g
CHOLESTEROL
  (0 mg/100 g) .... 0 mg
SODIUM (600 mg/100 g) .... 170 mg

PERCENTAGE OF RECOMMENDED DAILY ALLOWANCE (U.S. RDA)

INGREDIENTS (IN ORDER OF PREDOMINANCE): TOMATOES, TOMATO JUICE, SALT, CALCIUM CHLORIDE AND CITRIC ACID.

NUTRITION INFORMATION
SERVING SIZE 1 CUP
SERVINGS PER CONTAINER 2

CALORIES 50 CARBOHYDRATES 11g
PROTEIN 2g FAT 0

PERCENTAGE OF U.S. RECOMMENDED DAILY ALLOWANCES (U.S. RDA):

PROTEIN 2 NIACIN 10
VITAMIN A 30 CALCIUM 8
VITAMIN C 60 IRON 4
THIAMINE 8 PHOSPHORUS 4
RIBOFLAVIN 2 MAGNESIUM 8

DISTRIBUTED BY GIANT FOOD INC. WASHINGTON, D.C. 20013

PROTEIN .... 2 RIBOFLAVIN .... *
VITAMIN A .... * NIACIN .... *
VITAMIN C .... * CALCIUM 2
THIAMINE .... * IRON .... *

*Contains less than 2% of U.S. RDA of these nutrients.
**Information on fat and cholesterol content is provided for individuals who, on the advice of a physician, are modifying their dietary intake of fat and cholesterol.

Figure 3. Food label from canned tomatoes.

Figure 4. Food label from corn chips.

The ingredient list in Figure 2, however, is more typical of the ambiguity found in ingredient labeling as concerns sodium. An assessment of total sodium content entails an awareness of the ingredient salt as well as an awareness of other sodium compounds. For instance, the label in Figure 2 notes that the product contains salt and the compounds monosodium glutamate and disodium dihydrogen pyrophosphate. Although this frozen potato product contains three sodium ingredients, they occur midway and toward the end of the ingredient list. Without further quantitative information, the consumer would probably be unable to determine whether the product was relatively high or low in sodium content.

Similarly, salt occurs midway in the ingredient list in Figure 3. Again, the consumer has the problem of determining the relative sodium content of the product, but, in this case, the consumer may be unaware of the naturally occurring sodium content. This product, canned tomatoes, is relatively high in sodium, 300 mg/cup, since total sodium includes the naturally occurring sodium in tomatoes plus the salt added during canning. The ingredient list, of course, only notes the ingredients added to the product and does not necessarily reflect the total sodium content of the product.

Nutrition Labeling. Nutrition labeling complements ingredient labeling by noting the serving size; the number of servings per container; the calories per serving; the grams of macronutrients per serving, that is, protein, carbohydrate, and fat; and the percentage of the U.S. Recommended Daily Allowance (U.S. RDA) of protein and of several vitamins and minerals. Nutrition labeling, which was instituted in 1976, is voluntary unless the food manufacturer makes a nutritional claim for the product or enriches it, in which case nutritional labeling is required for documentation. If the manufacturer is interested in presenting any piece of nutrition information, the entire array of information, that is, number of servings, calories, and so on, must be presented in a standard format. Sodium content, however, does not have to be stated; consequently, the majority of products with nutrition labeling do not display sodium content.

The ingredient label in Figure 1, for instance, indicates that salt is the predominant ingredient; yet, the nutrition label contains no information about the nutrient sodium since this is not required information. The label in Figure 4, however, is an example of a product containing the optional sodium information. The sodium content of the corn chips is reported in the upper portion of the nutrition label, following the standard information regarding serving size, number of servings, and macronutrient content.

Point-of-Purchase Labeling

Granted that total sodium content labeling is sketchy, nevertheless many consumers, when informed of the quantitative sodium content of a product, are still uncertain as to whether the product is considered to be relatively low, moderate, or high in sodium content unless other supportive or interpretative information is provided. Recognizing this situation, several retail grocery chains with active consumer affairs departments have instituted in-store or point-of-purchase consumer information programs to supplement food labeling.

Noteworthy programs include those of Giant Food, Inc. in the Washington, D.C., metropolitan area and Schnuck Markets of the St. Louis, Missouri, area. These stores use shelf labels to assist shoppers in locating low-sodium foods. In the Giant Food program, for instance, an item must have less than 100 mg sodium/serving to qualify as a low-sodium food (40). Considering that Americans consume approximately 10 g salt/day (i.e., 4 g or 4000 mg sodium/day), this in-store program alerts shoppers to foods that provide a very small amount of an adult's typical daily sodium intake, a realistic criterion. Such voluntary labeling programs are to be commended and it is hoped that they are the advent of further point-of-purchase consumer education programs.

Proposed Labeling Changes

Hearings in the U.S. House of Representatives in the spring of 1981 focused on dietary sodium content and its relationship to hypertension (41). These hearings were conducted by the Subcommittee on Investigations and Oversight (Chairman Albert Gore, Democrat, from Tenessee) of the House Committee on Science and Technology. Testimony from the Food and Drug Administration (FDA), which is responsible for food labeling regulations, indicated that, because of the growing concern over dietary sodium levels, government action will encourage the food industry voluntarily to reduce sodium in food items and to label sodium content. Perhaps the most noteworthy point of the FDA testimony, however, was that the agency is considering altering food labeling regulations to allow sodium labeling of products without requiring full nutrition labeling.

The FDA testimony has been dubbed the five-point sodium plan and is summarized as follows (41):

1. To encourage food processors voluntarily to reduce sodium content and to encourage more research.

2. To propose new rules to include quantitative sodium declaration, to permit manufacturers to include quantitative sodium labeling without triggering full nutrition labeling, and to define such terms as "low-sodium" and "reduced sodium" when used in labeling.
3. To consider legislative options for including sodium labeling on other products where need is evident.
4. To work with the U.S. Department of Agriculture and other agencies to help consumers make effective use of new labeling and to raise consumer awareness of sodium health effects.
5. To continue monitoring efforts to determine if sodium consumption levels are going down.

SOURCES OF SODIUM INTAKE

Sodium labeling, even in its current imperfect state, does aid the consumer in identifying the presence of salt and other sodium compounds (via ingredient labeling) and in some instances in noting the quantitative amount of sodium (via nutrition labeling). But to reduce sodium intake effectively, the consumer must have a more intimate knowledge of food composition than is generally available on food labels.

Classification of Sodium Intake

Dietary sodium can be classified as either discretionary or nondiscretionary. Discretionary sodium is that which consumers voluntarily add to food, that is, at their own discretion, such as during home food preparation or in seasoning food at the table. The remainder of sodium intake is nondiscretionary. The consumer has limited discretion as to whether to consume sodium, as it is either added by the manufacturer during food processing or is naturally occurring sodium.

Common lore suggests that discretionary sodium is the larger portion of sodium intake. But dietary surveys indicate just the opposite. Most sodium consumed is nondiscretionary, sodium already in the food supply. The most extensive review of the scientific literature on salt is probably that prepared by the Life Sciences Research Office for the Food and Drug Administration as part of the FDA's evaluation of the status of salt on the generally recognized as safe (GRAS) list of food additives (42). This review estimated that only one-third of dietary sodium intake is discretionary, the majority being nondiscretionary.

Thus, if Americans consume approximately 10 g salt/day, approximately 3 g would be from discretionary sources and the remaining 7 g would be from nondiscretionary sources. There are limited data to indicate that daily sodium intake has significantly changed during this century (43). Rather, the significant change has been in a shift from discretionary to nondiscretionary intake. As consumers purchase more convenience-style foods which have already been seasoned, the discretionary use of sodium (during home food preparation and seasoning food at the table) decreases.

Since the majority of sodium intake is nondiscretionary, the reduction of sodium intake is more challenging today. A *Washington Post* food writer assessed this situation by saying, ". . . salt is so ubiquitous . . . it is virtually impossible to restrict salt by merely putting oregano in the salt shaker" (44). The effective reduction of sodium intake requires more than a limitation on the use of the salt shaker; the individual needs some knowledge of food composition to make judicious food choices and, thus, reduce nondiscretionary sodium intake.

In the following section, foods have been classified into familiar groups, for example, grain products, meats, dairy products, fruits, and vegetables, to furnish concepts of the nondiscretionary sodium composition of foods. This conceptual approach is thought to be more useful in understanding sodium composition than would be a listing of the sodium content of an inordinate number of individual food items.

Nondiscretionary Sodium Intake (45)

The definition of low, moderate, and high sodium-containing foods is quite arbitrary. Americans generally consume 10 g salt/day (i.e., 4 g or 4000 mg sodium/day), so that foods that contain less than 100 mg sodium per serving are certainly low-sodium foods; foods with moderate sodium content may be defined as those containing 100–250 mg per serving; and those with more than 250 mg per serving are assuredly high-sodium foods. As categories of foods, grain products, meats, and dairy products have moderate to high-sodium content, whereas vegetables and fruits contain moderate to low amounts.

Grain Products. Many bread and cereal products contain moderate amounts of sodium. A slice of bread or a hard roll, for instance, contains 200 mg. Several compounds may contribute to the sodium content of grain products. For instance, in baked products the sodium content may be due to the use of salt for flavoring, baking soda, or baking powder (i.e., sodium bicarbonate) as a leavening agent, and other sodium compounds such as sodium benzoate as a freshness preservative. Furthermore, in commercially baked products, salt is added as a dough conditioner (46).

Although most grain products individually contain only moderate amounts of sodium, as a category they are the largest contributor of nondiscretionary sodium (24%) in the American diet, as shown in Table 2 (47). One might consume only one or two servings of meat in a day, but multiple servings of grain products are commonly consumed in a day. Thus, grain products are the principal contributor to nondiscretionary sodium, primarily because of the quantity of grain products being consumed and not because they are particularly concentrated sources of sodium.

Table 2. Distribution of Nondiscretionary Sodium in the American Diet (44)

Food or Food Group	% Sodium
Grain products	24
Dairy products	14
Mixed protein dishes	12
Meat	9
Soups	8
Fruits and vegetables	7
Fats and oils	6
Other	20
Total	100

Meat, Poultry, and Shellfish. In general, meat, poultry, fish, and eggs contain moderate amounts of sodium. A 1/4 lb hamburger patty, for instance, contains about 100 mg of sodium. Shellfish, however, including clams, crabs, lobsters, oysters, scallops, and shrimp are high in sodium content. Other high-sodium meats are foods that are processed by canning, curing, smoking or salting (!). This includes bacon; corned beef; ham; luncheon meats such as bologna, frankfurters, and kosher meats; and fish such as caviar and herring. A frankfurter, for instance, typically contains 500 mg or 1/2 g sodium and, thus, is extremely high in sodium.

Dairy Products. Fluid whole milk is not a low-sodium food as might be assumed, but, rather, it contains a moderate amount of sodium at 120 mg/cup. As is the case with other food groups, sodium content tends to increase with processing. Chocolate milk, malted milk, and milk mixes have increased sodium content due to the addition of salt. Cheese and condensed milk are also examples of processing which result in elevated sodium content. These are essentially concentrated milk products and, consequently, the sodium content is also concentrated; furthermore, salt is added during cheese production (46). One oz of cheddar cheese, for instance, contains the same amount of protein as a cup of milk but has 200 mg sodium compared to 120 mg sodium in milk.

Incidentally, human breast milk contains only 5 mg sodium/oz or 40 mg/cup. Thus, the sodium content of breast milk is only one-third that of cow's milk. A breast-fed infant consumes a low-sodium food compared to one who consumes cow's milk.

Fats. Foods such as butter, margarine, and salad dressings which are primarily fat are more accurately classified as a separate group rather than in a traditional food group. Many of the foods in this fat category, however, contain moderate to high amounts of sodium. Butter, for example, is traditionally salted to retard spoilage (46). Commercial salad dressings are in this category and contain moderate amounts of sodium due to sodium compounds used for flavor and preservation. Other foods with relatively high-sodium content include commercial mayonnaise, olives, and (salted) peanuts.

Fruits. Fruits generally contain insignificant amounts of sodium and, thus, the sodium-conscious individual can consume fruits liberally. Apples, apricots, bananas, cherries, grapes, oranges, peaches, and strawberries, for instance, all contain less than 25 mg per serving. Processing, including canning, glazing or candying, and drying all tend to increase the sodium content. For example, the sodium content of equivalent weights of raw, canned, and dried apricots is 4, 5, and 118 mg, respectively. Sodium content of the dried fruit is elevated because the naturally occurring sodium is concentrated as a result of the fruit being dehydrated and because the compound sodium sulfite is used in the drying process (48).

Vegetables. Fresh vegetables, like fresh fruit, contain insignificant amounts of sodium. Exceptions to this, however, include several leafy vegetables such as spinach, beet greens, dandelion greens, and Swiss chard, which edge into the moderate-sodium range. As with other food categories, processing tends to increase sodium content. Freezing, canning, and brining progressively increase the amounts of sodium. A cup of fresh peas, for instance, contains only 2 mg sodium; a cup of frozen peas contains 185 mg; and a cup of canned peas contains 400 mg. Thus, fresh peas are a low-sodium food, but processing, particularly the addition of salt during canning, results in a high sodium-containing food. The indiscriminate consumer may actually add further salt by seasoning canned vegetables in the kitchen or at the table. Canned vegetable juices and vegetable-derived snacks such as potato and corn chips are also high in sodium content.

Discretionary Sodium Intake

As previously noted, discretionary sodium is that which an individual voluntarily adds to foods during home food preparation or in seasoning food at the table. Since the salting of food is largely habit, the first step in reducing discretionary sodium intake might be to remove the salt shaker from the table. Behaviorists call this "removing the cue." Then, each time the salt shaker is needed to season food, the individual is keenly aware of it. Is it worth the inconvenience of getting the salt shaker or can the food be enjoyed as it is? Furthermore, a salt mill might effectively replace a salt shaker. Milling salt is more time-consuming, so less salt is delivered, particularly when compared with a heavy hand on the shaker.

Another approach to curbing discretionary sodium intake is to substitute other seasonings for salt; that is, herbs, spices, and garnishes can be an alternative to salt. This may require some relearning to break the familiar salt and pepper habit. But the end results may be more creative than salt-flavored foods.

Substitutions cannot, however, be made indiscriminately, as several flavoring aids are high in sodium content and would not be effective substitutes. Barbecue sauce, bouillon cubes, catsup, monosodium glutamate, prepared mustard, soy sauce, and Worcestershire sauce are high in sodium content. But the spice cabinet and herb jars present many creative alternatives. For starters, popcorn can be sprinkled with seasoned salt. This does not eliminate sodium but does decrease the sodium content. Scrambled eggs can be sprinkled with ground pepper and chopped chives, which are more visually attractive than salt and pepper. Tomato juice might be acceptable with only a lemon wedge or perhaps a dash of oregano rather than salt. And corn-on-the-cob could be rolled in parsley flakes with or without butter.

A recent study supported by the U.S. Department of Agriculture analyzed salt consumption patterns by using population segmentation techniques, the same techniques used by marketing professionals when designing advertising campaigns (49). The researchers reasoned that segmentation analysis could identify groups or segments of the population that have the most serious problems with sodium consumption; nutrition education resources could then be targeted toward these specific groups. The researchers did not state explicitly that their study focused on discretionary sodium intake, but the study methodology quantified the number of shakes from the salt shaker; thus, discretionary intake and not total intake was primarily represented.

Basing their findings on demographic segmentation, the researchers reported that, by age, the problem population segment encompassed individuals under 25 years of age; on a sex basis, the problem population was men. Race and family income were not significant determinants of discretionary sodium intake. By eating habits, the problem population segments were several overlapping categories including individuals who ate away from home as well as those who patronized fast food restaurants, vending machines, and traditional restaurants four or more times per week. Those who snacked three or more times per day also had a high salt intake.

Lastly, this study noted that the lowest discretionary salt consumption was associated with the highest nutrition IQ scores, as determined by a 14-point nutrition index developed by the researchers, which supports the case for nutrition education.

SODIUM AND HYPERTENSION

Hypertension is the most prevalent and most dangerous precipitating factor in the genesis of cardiovascular disease (50), and cardiovascular disease, in spite of a recent decline in mortality incidence, is the leading cause of death in this country. It outranks deaths due to malignant neoplasms (cancer), accidents; and pneumonia and influenza.

The 1971–1975 Health and Nutrition Examination Survey (HANES) indicates that 18% of adult Americans aged 25–74 years are hypertensive (51). The overwhelming majority, probably 90%, have idiopathic or essential hypertension, meaning that the cause of the elevated blood pressure is unknown (52). Only the minority of cases are nonessential, or secondary, hypertension, meaning that the elevated blood pressure is secondary to a known factor such as chronic renal disease, coarctation of the aorta, primary aldosteronism, or estrogen administration.

A number of factors are considered as being predisposing in the development of essential hypertension; these include both genetic and environmental factors. Isolation of the initiating defect in essential hypertension has been difficult, and separating the cause of the elevated pressure from the effect is at least equally difficult. Very likely, the underlying cause of hypertension is genetic, with some individuals being less efficient in handling the environmental or nutritional factors (20).

Sodium intake is thought to play a strong role in the pathogenesis of essential hypertension. In this chapter, research findings were presented that attempt to elucidate the underlying mechanisms of action whereby sodium influences blood pressure. A synthesis of current literature on the pathogenesis of hypertension indicates that dietary sodium may be involved in the pathogenesis, both from a genetic and an environmental perspective. Mechanisms with a predominantly genetic or inherited basis involving sodium balance include the sodium exchange system and a hormonal inhibitor of the enzyme Na, K-ATPase. Thus, some individuals may, in fact, have a genetic basis for sodium sensitivity, and a generous dietary sodium intake would exacerbate this defect.

Environmental or nutrition-related parameters include not only the ingestion of dietary sodium but also other dietary factors that may influence the body's handling of sodium. For example, the simple sugar content of a diet reportedly acts as a stimulant of insulin, which enhances renal sodium resorption; dietary linoleic acid, a precursor of prostaglandin E_2, has a natriuretic effect and reportedly lowers blood pressure via increased urinary sodium excretion; and excess body weight reportedly results in metabolic variations such as an increased aldosterone-renin ratio that elevates blood pressure. Thus, the absolute amount of sodium ingested may not be an isolated factor, and other dietary factors may influence the physiologic handling of sodium.

In addition to an update of biological research, consumer-related sodium information was reviewed, including the current status of sodium labeling. In ingredient labeling, the consumer must be alert for salt as well as other sodium compounds and must remember that ingredient labeling reflects only the sodium-related ingredients in the product and not the naturally occurring sodium. In nutrition labeling, total sodium content labeling is currently an optional component, but recent testimony from the Food and Drug Administration proposed that food manufacturers be allowed to label the sodium in food without the requisite full nutrition labeling.

Lastly, both the discretionary and nondiscretionary components of total sodium intake were addressed. Of these two components, nondiscretionary intake constitutes the major portion of dietary sodium intake and is the more difficult to limit because sodium is added during food processing and because sodium occurs naturally in foods. The limiting of discretionary or voluntarily added sodium would undoubtedly be helpful in curbing total sodium intake, but to reduce total intake significantly necessitates a decrease in the major component, nondiscretionary intake. Sodium labeling of foods can be an eminent help to consumers in identifying sodium content of food, but not all products have nutrition labeling, and, furthermore, sodium labeling is currently optional. The sodium content of various foods was presented by food categories to encourage a working knowledge of the sodium composition of foods. In general, grain products, meats, and dairy products have moderate to high-sodium content, whereas vegetables and fruits contain moderate to low amounts.

REFERENCES

1. W. L. T. Addison, The use of sodium chloride, potassium chloride, sodium bromide, and potassium bromide in cases of arterial hypertension which are amenable to potassium chloride. *Can. Med. Assoc. J.* **18**, 281–285 (1928).
2. I. McQuarrie, W. H. Thompson, and J. A. Anderson, Effects of excessive ingestion of sodium and potassium salts on carbohydrate metabolism and blood pressure in diabetic children. *J. Nutr.* **11**, 77–101 (1936).
3. A. C. Guyton, *Textbook of Medical Physiology*, Saunders, Philadelphia, 1981, pp. 52–53.
4. L. K. Dahl, Salt intake and salt need. *N. Engl. J. Med.* **258**, 1152–1157 (1958).
5. P. L. Altman and D. S. Dittmer, eds., *Biology Data Book*, 2nd ed., Vol. 3, Federation of American Societies for Experimental Biology, Bethesda, Md., 1974, p. 1496.
6. G. R. Meneely and H. D. Battarbee, Sodium and potassium. *Nutr. Rev.* **34**, 225–235 (1976).
7. A. C. Guyton, *Textbook of Medical Physiology*, Saunders, Philadelphia, 1981, p. 256.
8. H. J. Reineck and J. H. Stein, Renal regulation of extracellular fluid volume. In B. M. Brenner and J. H. Stein, eds., *Contemporary Issues in Nephrology, Vol. 1, Sodium and Water Homeostasis*, Churchill Livingstone, New York, 1978, pp. 24–50.
9. L. K. Dahl, Possible role of chronic excess salt consumption in the pathogenesis of essential hypertension. *Am. J. Cardiol.* **8**, 571–575 (1961).
10. A. M. Altschul, W. R. Ayers, J. K. Grommet, and L. Slotkoff, Salt sensitivity in experimental animals and man. *Int. J. Obesity* **5**, (suppl.), 27–38 (1981).
11. L. K. Dahl and R. A Love, Evidence for relationship between sodium (chloride) intake and human essential hypertension. *Arch. Intern. Med.* **94**, 525–531 (1954).

12. W. M. Kirkendall, W. E. Connor, F. Abboud, S. P. Rastogi, T. A Anderson, and M. Fry, The effect of dietary sodium on the blood pressure of normotensive man. In J. Genest and E. Koiw, eds., Hypertension, Springer-Verlag, New York, 1972, pp. 360–373.

13. J. Parijs, J. V. Joossens, L. Van der Linden, G. Verstreken, and A. K. P. C. Amery, Moderate sodium restriction and diuretics in the treatment of hypertension. Am. Heart J. 85, 22–34 (1973).

14. L. Tobian, Current status of salt in hypertension. In O. Paul, ed., Epidemiology and Control of Hypertension, Stratton Intercontinental Medical Book Corporation, New York, 1974, pp. 131–146.

15. R. H. Murray, F. C. Luft, R. Bloch, and A. E. Weyman, Blood pressure responses to extremes of sodium intake in normal man. Proc. Soc. Exp. Biol. Med. 159, 432–436 (1978).

16. T. Morgan, A. Gillies, G. Morgan, W. Adam, M. Wilson, and S. Carney, Hypertension treated by salt restriction. Lancet 1, 227–230 (1978).

17. A. M. Altschul and J. K. Grommet, Sodium intake and salt sensitivity. Nutr. Rev. 38, 393–402 (1980).

18. N. M. Kaplan, The control of hypertension: A therapeutic breakthrough. Am. Sci. 68, 537–545 (1980).

19. E. D. Freis, Salt, volume, and the prevention of hypertension. Circulation 53, 589–595 (1976).

20. L. Tobian, The relationship of salt to hypertension. Am. J. Clin. Nutr. 32, 2739 (1979).

21. D. C. Tosteson, Cation countertransport and cotransport in human red cells. Fed. Proc. 40, 1429–1433 (1981).

22. M. Canessa, N. Adrangan, H. S. Solomon, T. M. Connolly, and D. C. Tosteson, Increased sodium–lithium countertransport in red cells of patients with essential hypertension. N. Engl. J. Med. 302, 772–776 (1980).

23. M. Canessa, N. Adrangan, H. S. Solomon, T. M. Connolly, and D. C. Tosteson, Sodium transport as diagnostic tool for secondary hypertension. J. Am. Med. Assoc. 245, 1404 (1981).

24. H. E. de Wardener and G. A MacGregor, Hypothesis: further observations on Dahl's hypothesis that a saluretic substance may be responsible for a sustained rise in arterial pressure; its possible role in essential hypertension. Kidney Int. 18, 1 (1980).

25. L. Poston, R. B. Sewell, S. P. Wilkinson, P. J. Richardson, R. Williams, E. M. Clarkson, G. A. MacGregor, and H. E. de Wardener, Evidence for a circulating sodium transport inhibitor in essential hypertension. Br. Med. J. 282, 847–849 (1981).

26. R. Fraser, J. J. Brown, A. F. Lever, J. J. Morton, and J. I. S. Robertson, The renin–angiotensin system and aldosterone in hypertension: A brief review of some aspects. *Int. J. Obesity* 5 (suppl.), 115–123 (1981).

27. J. L. Marx, Natriuretic hormone linked to hypertension. *Science* **212**, 1255 (1981).

28. C. G. Beebe, R. Schemmel, and O. Mickelsen, Blood pressure as affected by diet and concentration of NaCl in drinking water. *Proc. Soc. Exp. Biol. Med.* **151**, 395–399 (1976).

29. R. A. Ahrens, P. DeMuth, M. K. Lee, and J. W. Majkowski, Moderate sucrose ingestion and blood pressure in the rat. *J. Nutr.* **110**, 725–731 (1980).

30. M. B. Preuss and H. G. Preuss, The effects of sucrose and sodium on blood pressure in various substrains of Wistar rats. *Lab. Invest.* **43**, 101–107 (1980).

31. R. A. DeFronzo, Insulin and renal sodium handling: clinical implications. *Int. J. Obesity* 5 (suppl.), 93–104 (1981).

32. G. Triebe, H. U. Block, and W. Förster, On the blood pressure response of salt-loaded rats under different content of linoleic acid in the food. *Acta Biol. Med. Ger.* **35**, 1223–1224 (1976).

33. H. U. Comberg, S. Heyden, C. G. Hames, A. J. Vergroesen, and A. I. Fleischman, Hypotensive effect of dietary prostaglandin precursor in hypertensive man. *Prostaglandins* **15**, 193–197 (1978).

34. J. M. Iacono, M. W. Marshall, R. M. Dougherty, M. A. Wheeler, J. F. Mackin, and J. J. Canary, Reduction in blood pressure associated with high polyunsaturated fat diets that reduce cholesterol in man. *Prev. Med.* **4**, 426–443 (1975).

35. P. Oster, L. Arab, B. Schellenberg, M. Kohlmeier, and G. Schlierf, Linoleic acid and blood pressure. *Prog. Food Nutr. Sci.* **4**, 39–40 (1980).

36. L. K. Dahl, L. Silver, and R. W. Christie, The role of salt in the fall of blood pressure accompanying reduction in obesity. *N. Engl. J. Med.* **258**, 1186–1192 (1958).

37. K. Hiramatsu, T. Yamada, K. Ichikawa, T. Izumiyama, and H. Nagata, Changes in endocrine activities relative to obesity in patients with essential hypertension. *J. Am. Geriat. Soc.* **29**, 25–30 (1981).

38. M. Krotkiewski, K. Mandroukas, L. Sjöström, L. Sullivan, H. Wetterqvist, and P. Björntorp, Effects of long-term physical training on body fat, metabolism, and blood pressure in obesity. *Metabolism* **28**, 650–658 (1979).

39. J. Kolanowski, Influence of insulin and glucagon on sodium balance in obese subjects during fasting and refeeding. *Int. J. Obesity* 5 (suppl.), 105–114 (1981).

40. Special alert diet. Giant Food, Inc., Landover, Maryland, 1981.

41. U.S. Congress, House of Representatives. Committee on Science and Technology. Sodium in food and high blood pressure. Hearings before the Subcommittee on Investigations and Oversight. Ninety-seventh Congress, first session. April 13–14, 1981.

42. Federation of American Societies for Experimental Biology. Life Science Research Office. Evaluation of the health aspects of sodium chloride and potassium chloride as food ingredients (SCOGS-102), Food and Drug Administration, Washington, D.C., 1979.

43. W. E. Dickinson, Salt sources and markets. In M. J. Kare, M. J. Fregly, and R. A. Bernard, eds., *Biological and Behavioral Aspects of Salt Intake*, Academic Press, New York, 1980, p. 52.

44. S. Rovner, Healthtalk: a salty story, *The Washington Post*, 1981 March 6; Sect. C:5.

45. American Dietetic Association. *Handbook of Clinical Dietetics*, Yale University Press, New Haven, Conn., 1981, pp. G3–G16.

46. R. H. Forsythe and R. A. Miller, Salt in processed foods. In M. R. Kare, M. J. Fregly, and R. A. Bernard, eds., *Biological and Behavioral Aspects of Salt Intake*, Academic Press, New York, 1980, p. 226.

47. U.S. Department of Health, Education, and Welfare. National Center for Health Statistics. Fats, cholesterol, and sodium intake in the diet of persons 1–74 years: United States. Advance Data (no. 54); December 17, 1979.

48. G. E. Vail, R. M. Griswold, M. M. Justin, and L. O. Rust, Food: *An Introductory College Course*, Houghton Mifflin, Boston, 1967, p. 615.

49. J. Goodman, J. Goodman, H. Schutz, M. Grainer, and E. Megna, *An Investigation of Added Sugar and Salt Consumption Patterns, 1981 Agriculture Outlook*, U.S. Government Printing Office, Washington, D.C., January 1981.

50. The Pooling Project Research Group. Relationship of blood pressure, serum cholesterol, smoking habit, relative weight and ECG abnormalities to incidence of major coronary events: final report of the Pooling Project. *J. Chronic Dis.* 31, 201–306 (1978).

51. U.S. Department of Health and Human Services. National Center for Health Statistics. Hypertension in adults 25–74 years of age, United States, 1971–1975. Vital and Health Statistics (series 11, no. 221, DHHS no. PHS 81-1671), U.S. Government Printing

Office, Washington, D.C., April 1981.

52. J. L. Marx, Hypertension: a complex disease with complex causes. *Science* **194**: 821 (1976).

ADDITIONAL RECENT REFERENCES

National Kidney Foundation; U.S. Department of Health and Human Services, and International Life Sciences Institute, Proceedings of Nutrition and Blood Pressure Control: Current Status of Dietary Factors and Hypertension. Arlington, Virginia, September 13–15, 1982.

Anon., The case for moderating sodium consumption. *FDA Consumer* **15**: 8–13 (1981).

Sodium Labeling. *Fed. Register.* June 18, 1982.

M. Bertino, G. K. Beauchamp, and K. Engelman, Long-term reduction in dietary sodium alters the taste of salt. *Am. J. Clin. Nutr.* **36**, 1134–1144 (1982).

J. Wylie-Rossett, Spices to the rescue. *The Professional Nutritionist* **14**, 4–6 (1982).

5
Nutrition and Alcohol
A CLINICAL PERSPECTIVE

SPENCER SHAW, M.D.

CHARLES S. LIEBER, M.D.

VA Medical Center and Mount Sinai School of Medicine (CUNY)
New York, New York

Address correspondence to Charles S. Lieber, M.D., Alcohol Research & Treatment Center, VA Medical Center, 130 West Kingsbridge Road, New York, New York 10468.

ABSTRACT

The relationship between nutrition and alcohol is complex, stemming from many levels of interaction. Alcoholic beverages are themselves nutrients, and they displace required nutrients in the diet. Ethanol has multiple actions on almost every level of the gastrointestinal tract, especially the liver, and, thus, profoundly affects the storage, mobilization, activation, and metabolism of many nutrients.

While alcohol is directly toxic to many bodily tissues, the synergism of malnutrition and alcohol in this regard remains to be fully clarified. Nevertheless, with the increase in alcoholism, the extent of related physical damage in our society has dramatically increased. The resulting pathologic alterations require complex nutritional therapy; also, alcoholism remains one of the major causes of nutritional deficiency syndromes in the United States. Nutritional therapy in the alcoholic is often difficult and may be a balance between maximizing recovery and avoiding iatrogenic (physician-induced) complications.

NUTRITIONAL VALUE OF ALCOHOL

Alcoholic beverages differ little in nutritive value except for carbohydrate content (which varies considerably), trace amounts of B vitamins (especially niacin and thiamin), and iron content (1). The significance of congeners in beverages remains largely unexplored except for occasional instances in which harmful amounts of iron, lead, or cobalt may be present. The estimated contribution of alcohol to the average American diet is 4.5% of total calories, based on national consumption figures (2). The share of dietary calories is much greater in heavy drinkers, generally estimated to be more than one-half of their daily caloric intake.

Alcoholic beverages provide little nutritive value aside from calories; as such, alcohol is not as adequate as equivalent carbohydrate. Calorimetrically, the combustion of ethanol liberates 7.1 kcal/g, but ethanol does not provide food value equivalent to carbohydrates. Isocaloric substitution of ethanol for carbohydrate as 50% of total calories in a balanced diet results in a decline in body weight (Fig. 1).

80

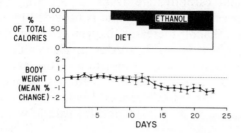

Figure 1. Body weight changes after isocaloric substitution of carbohydrate by ethanol in 11 subjects (means ±standard errors). Dotted line, mean change in weight in control period (Pirola, R. C.; Lieber, C. S. Pharmacology 7: 185; 1972).

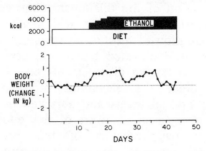

Figure 2. Effect on body weight of adding 2000 kcal/day as ethanol to diet of one subject. Dotted line, mean change during control period (Pirola, R. C.; Lieber, C. S. Pharmacology 7: 185; 1972).

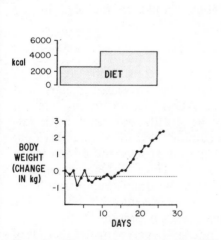

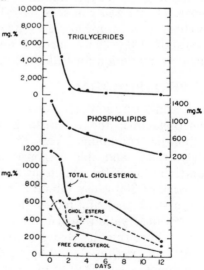

Figure 3. Effect on body weight of adding 2000 kcal/day as chocolate to diet of same subject as shown in Figure 2. Dotted line, mean change during control period (Pirola, R. C.; Lieber, C. S. Pharmacoloy 7: 185; 1972).

Figure 4. Changes in plasma lipid fractions of a patient during recovery from alcoholic hyperlipemia (Losowsky, M.S.; Jones, D. P.; Davidson, C. S.; et al. Am. J. Med. 35: 794; 1963).

When given as additional calories, ethanol causes less weight gain than calorically equivalent carbohydrate (Figs. 2, 3). Support for the view that ethanol increases the metabolic rate is provided by the observation that ingestion of ethanol increases oxygen consumption in normal subjects, and this effect is much greater in alcoholics (3). Oxidation without phosphorylation through stimulation of the microsomal ethanol oxidizing system or other catabolic pathways remains a possible explanation for the observed differences. Evidence for interference with digestion or absorption as an explanation for caloric value differences is lacking.

ALCOHOL AND GOUT (URIC ACID)

The clinical observation of the relationship between alcohol and gout has stimulated investigations of uric acid metabolism in alcoholism. Short-term administration of alcohol given orally or intravenously has been shown to produce elevated blood uric acid (hyperuricemia) in patients who have no known disorders of renal function or uric acid metabolism (4). Since the elevations of serum uric acid were significantly above normal levels and persisted in some instances for several days (4), a physician unaware of this effect of ethanol might inadvertently treat hyperuricemia of this secondary type. The mechanism by which hyperuricemia occurs appears most clearly related to decreased urinary excretion of uric acid secondary to elevated serum lactate. Acute gouty attacks have been observed in patients in relation to changes in serum uric acid associated with alcohol administration or starvation (5). Thus, alcohol restriction should be included in the dietary prescription for patients with gout.

HYPERLIPIDEMIAS

The administration of ethanol to humans consistently results in hyperlipidemia; the response is modified by associated dietary and pathologic conditions. The major elevation occurs in the serum triglycerides, and this response may be greatly enhanced by a fat-containing meal (6). When alcohol is administered for several weeks at a dosage of 300 g/day (about 378 ml) the initial severalfold increase in triglycerides gradually returns to normal (7) (Fig. 4). One explanation for this observation is that continued ethanol administration results in hepatic impairment. Hyperlipemia is usually absent with severe liver injury (e.g., cirrhosis), and hypolipemia is usually present (8, 9).

A characteristic feature of alcohol-induced hyperlipemia is that all of the lipoprotein fractions are increased, although to a variable degree. Alcoholic hyperlipemia is usually classified as type IV according to the

International Classification of Hyperlipidemias and Hyperlipoprotein-emias; the increased particulate fat behaves predominantly as very low density lipoproteins (VLDLs). In an additional 8%, Chylomicrons or chylomicronlike particles can be increased even in the fasting state (10). These patients are classified as type V. Furthermore, 6% of alcoholics have hypercholesterolemia due to hyper-β-lipoproteinemia (type II). Alcohol-induced hyperlipemia may change rapidly, with clearance of triglycerides being most rapid and cholesterol and phospholipids slower; thus, it is difficult to place alcoholic hyperlipemia in a single group (fig. 4).

Some patients may demonstrate a marked sensitivity to the hyperlipidemic effects of alcohol. This may be observed in patients with type IV familial or carbohydrate-induced hyperlipidemia (11). Thus, alcohol consumption should be considered in the diagnosis of any hyperlipidemia.

Recently, moderate ethanol consumption has been observed to increase high density lipoprotein (HDL) levels, and this may possibly act as a beneficial factor against the development of coronary artery disease in such drinkers (12).

CARBOHYDRATES

Glucose homeostasis is impaired in alcoholic liver disease. With severe decompensation and with prolonged fasting following heavy drinking, symptomatic hypoglycemia that may require intravenous glucose administration may occur. Autonomic dysfunction, impaired gluconeogenesis, glycogen depletion, and endocrine effects may be contributory. On the other hand, alcoholics with fatty liver or cirrhosis have impaired glucose tolerance, elevated insulin levels, and abnormal responses to glucagon (13). Alcohol has a priming effect on glucose-mediated insulin release (14) and directly causes glucose intolerance itself (15).

WATER-SOLUBLE VITAMINS

General

Vitamin metabolism demonstrates the many levels at which alcohol may impair nutrition. Abnormalities of ingestion and absorption have been observed. Decreased hepatic stores of folacin, niacin, vitamin B-6, and vitamin B-12 have been described (16), and decreased hepatic affinity, as measured by displacement studies, has been demonstrated for folacin (17) as well as decreased storage and enterohepatic circulation (18). Impaired utilization of folacin, thiamin, and vitamin

B-6 have been reported (19–23). Pyridoxine is normally converted by the liver to pyridoxal phosphate, which is the active coenzyme form of the vitamin. Evidence has been presented that decreased activation of pyridoxine is due to displacement of pyridoxal phosphate from hepatic cytosol binding proteins by acetaldehyde produced by ethanol metabolism. This facilitates hydrolysis by pyridoxal phosphatase and results in a net decrease in activation (23). Mitchell et al. (24) observed increased clearance of serum pyridoxal phosphate in cirrhosis. Circulating levels of vitamins reveal abnormalities in 40% of chronic, malnourished alcoholics with folacin and pyridoxine being most often depressed (25). Clinical correlations are greatest with megaloblastic and sideroblastic anemias and with neurologic syndromes related to thiamin deficiency. Although vitamins are clearly important in such cellular processes as DNA synthesis, the significance of mild deficiencies and massive vitamin therapy in altering recovery from liver injury remains unclear. Vitamin deficiencies have been proposed as causes of alcoholism; and vitamin therapy, as a cure (26). The animal evidence used for these studies, however, is subject to many serious criticisms (27). Since trace elements such as zinc and magnesium play a role in the function of some water-soluble vitamins, alcohol-related deficiencies of these elements may further exacerbate borderline insufficiencies. Increased requirements for vitamins have not been established in alcoholism, except perhaps for folacin.

Associated diseases

Alcoholics remain one of the few groups of patients in the United States with nutritional deficiency syndromes, most commonly presenting with neurologic and hematologic manifestations. The interaction of diet and alcohol in producing these deficiencies, however, remains to be explored. Hypovitaminoses of the B vitamins remain the most well delineated of the deficiency states.

Neurological Diseases

Administration of carbohydrates such as glucose administered intravenously to a marginally vitamin-depleted alcoholic may precipitate a florid neurologic syndrome if supplementary vitamins are not provided. Although dramatically responsive to replacement therapy and pathogenetically fascinating, the neurologic deficiency syndromes are relatively rare, constituting only 1–3% of alcohol-related neurologic admissions (28). Neurologic disorders in the alcoholic that have been related to B vitamin deficiencies include polyneuropathy, Wernicke–Korsakoff syndrome, nutritional amblyopia (partial loss of vision), and pellagra. The role of nutritional factors in central pontine myelenosis (a spinal cord inflammation), Marchiafava-Bignami syndrome, alcoholic cerebellar degeneration, and other rarer syndromes remains speculative. The response of cerebellar degeneration to massive thiamine administration has been reported (29). Vitamin B complex administration in any alcohol-related neurologic state seems prudent.

Hematologic Considerations

Hematologic abnormalities are among the most frequent pathologic alterations resulting from an interaction of alcohol and diet. The frequency and nature of observed abnormalities are highly dependent on the population selected. Small amounts of pyridoxine and folacin in the diet may prevent megaloblastic and sideroblastic anemias. In some selected patients admitted for alcoholism, a high percentage have anemia or bone marrow abnormalities. This is not the case in middle- and upper-class alcoholics whose folacin levels are generally normal (30). Small amounts of folacin (250 μg orally) prevent megaloblastic changes, and 1 mg pyridoxine/day prevents sideroblastic changes during ethanol administration. However, pharmacologic doses of folacin do not prevent vacuolization of erythroid elements in patients fed alcohol with an adequate diet (31). Thus, alcohol has a direct toxic effect on the bone marrow. The timing of a bone marrow examination is important in establishing a diagnosis, since improvement of bone marrow abnormalities may be rapid.

Anemia, low serum folate, and megaloblastic marrow with or without sideroblasts may be used to diagnose folacin- and pyridoxine-related blood abnormalities. Therapy includes vitamin supplementation and abstinence from alcohol. Smaller doses may be adequate, but usually many times the daily requirement of folacin and pyridoxine are administered. Although vitamin B-12 absorption may be affected by acute alcohol administration (32), vitamin B-12 deficiency anemia is not very common among alcoholics.

FAT-SOLUBLE VITAMINS

Fat-soluble vitamins are usually not deficient in the alcoholic, but marginal nutrition, severe steatorrhea, altered gastrointestinal flora, and hepatocellular injury may act synergically to cause deficiencies. The major vitamins to be considered are vitamin K and vitamin D.

Vitamin A

Vitamin A is absorbed and stored within the liver as retinol but must be oxidized to its active form, retinal, within target organs by alcohol dehydrogenase. It is necessary for dark adaptation and spermatogenesis, both of which may be impaired in the alcoholic (33, 34). Alcoholics may have impaired metabolism of vitamin A at several levels, including decreased absorption, steatorrhea, impaired hepatic storage, and diminished activation by retinol dehydrogenase. The latter might occur through competition of retinol and ethanol for the dehydrogenase in the liver, retina (35), and testes (36). Alcoholics were found to have very low hepatic levels of vitamin A, even in the absence of dietary deficiencies and at the early stages of reversible liver involvement, with still normal blood levels of vitamin A and retinol-binding protein (37). Also, coexistent zinc deficiency may potentiate or produce deficiencies, presumably through decreased activity of the dehydrogenase.

Vitamin D

Vitamin D metabolism in conjunction with calcium metabolism is of special interest in the alcoholic. Alcoholic populations have been observed to have decreased bone density (38), increased susceptibility to fractures (39), and increased frequency of osteonecrosis (bone death) (40), compared with other populations. Vitamin D metabolism may be affected at many levels in the alcoholic. In addition to decreased dietary intake, decreased absorption may occur due to pancreatic insufficiency and bile salt abnormalities or by a direct effect of ethanol. Similarly, calcium absorption may be impaired. Patients with alcoholic cirrhosis have been found to have decreased clearance of plasma cholecalciferol and decreased urinary glucuronide conjugates (41). The liver is the first site of hydroxylation of vitamin D_3 (cholecalciferol), which is necessary for its activation. Hepatocellular injury may result in deficient activation of dietary vitamin D and resistance to parenteral vitamin D therapy (42), although debate exists as to the frequency of this observation even in patients with cirrhosis. Other postulated mechanisms of possible alterations in vitamin D metabolism include increased degradation of activated vitamin D by the cytochrome p-450 system (which may be stimulated by alcohol) and decreased storage depots of fat and muscle (42). The increased urinary losses of calcium induced by alcohol, ethanol-induced hypercorticism, and parathyroid stimulation secondary to calcium-binding proteins in cirrhosis are other mechanisms by which bone metabolism may be altered. The extent to which altered vitamin D metabolism specifically contributes to clinical musculoskeletal diseases in alcoholic populations and the site or sites of the abnormalities involved remain to be clarified.

Vitamin K

Vitamin K deficiency may result from dietary deficiency, malabsorption, or decreased synthesis by intestinal flora. Failure of clotting factor synthesis due to alcoholic liver injury may result in prolongation of the prothrombin time. Although deficiency-related abnormalities are uncommon in the alcoholic, vitamin K may correct a prolonged prothrombin time resulting from interaction of the above factors (43). Generally, vitamin K is given intramuscularly (10 mg/day) for 3 consecutive days. Failure to correct the prothrombin time indicates severe parenchymal injury.

MINERALS AND ELECTROLYTES

Pathogenesis

Alcoholics with chronic liver disease may have disorders of water and electrolyte metabolism. Sodium and water retention may be the most common abnormalities that present clinically as ascites, edema, and portal hypertension, hypoalbuminemia, altered renal hemodynamics, endocrine abnormalities, and changes in lymph flow (44). Dietary regime is adjusted according to the severity of salt and water retention. Severe symptoms and refractory cases may require rigid sodium restriction (250 mg/day). Restriction at this level is advocated even if mild hyponatremia (low blood sodium) is present, that is, if the serum sodium level is 125–130 mEq/liter (45). Symptomatic hyponatremia with serum sodium below this level may require intervention with hypertonic saline and rigid water restriction. Fluid restriction of 1500–2000 ml/day (including all liquids taken with medications) is recommended, especially if hyponatremia is present. With less severe retention, sodium restriction of 500–2000 mg/day may be tried. Daily weights and serum electrolytes are necessary to guide therapy. Summerskill et al. (44) recommend not exceeding a weight loss of 5 kg/week by dietary or diuretic therapy.

In refractory cases, especially with symptoms such as severe dyspnea (respiratory distress), paracentesis (fluid removal) may be necessary. Two liters/24 hours has been recommended as a safe rate of removal; more vigorous therapy may cause acute depletion of albumin, salt, and water and may result in cardiovascular collapse. Replacement therapy with intravenous albumin and saline may be required during such therapy. Diuretics may be used, with attention to the possible development of hyponatremia. Following restriction, diuresis and improved handling of dietary sodium may result. A ceiling of 2500 mg of sodium in the diet has been suggested (46).

Patients with chronic liver disease may have difficulty in handling fluid loads. A daily total volume of 1500–2000 ml is recommended, and the patient should be monitored for adequate urine output, weight gain, and hyponatremia.

Low body potassium stores are common in alcoholics with advanced liver disease and may not be reflected by the serum potassium (47). Low potassium may result from vomiting and diarrhea or as a result of hyperaldosteronism, muscle wasting, renal tubular acidosis, and diuretic therapy. Depletion of potassium may be especially significant because of consequent increased renal vein ammonia and worsening of hepatic coma (48). Hypokalemia (low blood potassium) increases renal vein ammonia via a direct effect of increased renal ammonia production and possibly through the increased back diffusion of ammonia from alkaline urine (48). Parenteral or oral potassium may be given in a dosage of approximately 100–200 mEq/day until deficits are corrected, provided normal renal function is present.

Trace Elements

Alcoholics may have decreased plasma levels of zinc, calcium, and magnesium resulting from ethanol-induced renal losses and decreased dietary intake (49–51). The similarity of the neuromuscular excitability of hypomagnesemia and acute alcoholic withdrawal has aroused considerable interest; however, as with other trace elements, clinical correlations have not been significant, and florid deficiency states remain exceedingly rare (52). Abnormalities of other trace elements, such as manganese and copper, in chronic liver disease have been discussed by Prasad et al. (51). Such abnormalities remain chiefly of investigational interest at present.

The combination of small quantities of cobalt combined with heavy ethanol abuse produces a fulminant cardiomyopathy in beer drinkers (53). However, cobalt or ethanol alone taken in amounts comparable to those ingested by patients who develop cobalt-beer-drinker's heart does not produce this disorder. The practice of using cobalt as an additive to beer has been discontinued.

Iron

Iron and the Liver. The question of the metabolism of iron in the alcoholic is particularly relevant because of the association of hepatic injury with excess iron. Acute alcohol administration may increase iron absorption, possibly through stimulation of gastric acid secretion, resulting in increased solubility of the ferric ion in the small intestine (54). Alcoholics may receive excessive dietary iron from the beverages they drink, such as certain wines, or through inadvertent treatment with iron-containing vitamin preparations. In addition, anemias unrelated to iron deficiency may be incorrectly treated with iron. Pancreatic insufficiency, folate deficiency, portosystemic shunting, and cirrhosis may increase iron absorption (55). The potential for excess iron to produce tissue injury and the finding of increased iron stores in a significant percentage of patients with alcoholic cirrhosis make this an important area for future investigation.

Iron Deficiency Anemia. Iron deficiency anemia is uncommon in alcoholics unless factors such as gastrointestinal bleeding from varices (dilated veins), ulcers and gastritis, repeated phlebotomies, dietary extremes, and chronic infections are present (20). However, as discussed above, alcoholics have a propensity to develop increased iron stores that may potentiate tissue injury in the liver and other organs. Transfusions and iron therapy should be used with caution and only to the point of correcting deficiencies. Routine iron supplements are not indicated.

SMALL INTESTINE AND STOMACH

Alcohol has been shown to be directly injurious to the small intestine and stomach, but the nutritional impact of such changes remains to be established. Short-term administration of ethanol (1 g/kg of body weight, taken orally) results in endoscopic and morphologic lesions in the duodenum (56), which experimentally are related to the concentration of ethanol used, with the greatest damage resulting from those solutions with the highest concentration of ethanol (57). Short-term administration of ethanol may impair the absorption of many nutrients and experimentally results in alterations in mucosal enzymes (27, 57, 58). Studies with orally and intravenously administered alcohol have revealed an inhibition of type I (impeding) waves in the jejunum and an increase in type III (propulsive) waves in the ileum (59). These changes have been proposed as one possible mechanism of the diarrhea observed in binge drinkers. Depressed levels of intestinal lactase and lactose intolerance have been observed in apparently well-nourished chronic alcoholics, with recovery following withdrawal from alcohol (60) (Fig. 5). In this latter study, black alcoholics were more susceptible to this injurious effect of ethanol. Thus, in patients with alcoholic gastritis or in alcoholics with peptic ulcer disease, milk products with lactose present must be prescribed for the diet with caution.

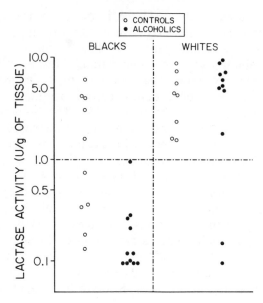

Figure 5. Effects of chronic alcohol consumption on intestinal lactase activity. Black alcoholics were found to be especially sensitive to the effects of ethanol in lowering intestinal lactase activity (Perlow W. E.; Baraona, E.; Lieber, C. S. Gastroenterology 72: 680; 1977).

The effect of chronic ethanol consumption on intestinal function is complicated by the concomitant effects of nutrition. Indeed, malnutrition itself may lead to intestinal malabsorption (61, 62), and folacin depletion, which is common in alcoholics, has been especially implicated in this regard (63–66) in the absence of other malnutrition.

Chronic ethanol administration along with an adequate diet results in impairment of vitamin B-12 absorption in well-nourished volunteers, despite supplementary pancreatin and intrinsic factor (67).

The acute and chronic effects of alcohol upon small intestinal function may be potentiated by concomitant alterations in pancreatic function, bile salts, and small intestinal flora. However, in patients with cirrhosis, steatorrhea (fecal fat greater than 30 g/24 h on a 100 g fat/day diet) is relatively uncommon and in one series was present in only 9% of cases (68). Furthermore, creatorrhea or excess excretion of fecal nitrogen is only rarely reported in the alcoholic (69). Portal hypertension has also been postulated as a cause of malabsorption (70). Finally, specific therapeutic interventions, such as neomycin, may themselves cause malabsorption (71).

LIPOTROPIC FACTORS (METHYL-PRODUCING COMPOUNDS)

The question of the significance of and requirements for lipotropic factors in alcoholism is beset by confusion because of inappropriate extrapolations from animal models. Though in growing rats, deficiencies in dietary protein and lipotropic factors (choline and methionine) can produce fatty liver, primates are far less susceptible to protein and lipotropic deficiency (72). Clinically, treatment with choline of patients suffering from alcoholic liver injury has been found to be ineffective in the presence of continued alcohol intake (73) and, experimentally, massive supplementation of choline has failed to prevent fatty liver produced by alcohol in volunteers (74). This is not surprising, since there is no evidence that a diet deficient in choline is deleterious to adult humans. Unlike rat liver, human liver contains very little choline oxidase activity, which may explain the species difference with regard to choline deficiency. The phospholipid content of the liver represents another key difference between the ethanol and choline-deficiency fatty liver. After the administration of ethanol, hepatic phospholipids increase (75), whereas in the fatty liver produced by choline deficiency, they decrease. Thus, hepatic injury induced by choline deficiency appears to be primarily an experimental disease of rats with little if any relevance to human alcoholic liver injury. Even in the rats, massive choline supplementation failed to prevent fully the ethanol-induced lesion, whether alcohol was administered on a short-term or long-term basis (76). Although excess lipotropes are of no proven value in recovery from liver injury, they may prove harmful by providing excess nitrogen load (77).

LIVER INJURY

Pathogenesis: Respective Roles of Alcohol and Malnutrition

The role of nutrition in the pathogenesis of alcoholic liver injury, the major medical complication of alcoholism, is very significant in terms of prevention and therapy. The role of faulty nutrition in the genesis of alcoholic liver injury has also been implicated by analogy: the fatty liver of kwashiorkor, the frequency of cirrhosis in underdeveloped countries where malnutrition is common, and fatty liver and possible progression to cirrhosis after intestinal bypass (78).

The studies that demonstrated no adverse effects of ethanol in the presence of adequate nutrition generally can be criticized because of the use of amounts of alcohol much below those taken by heavy drinkers. Experimental models of nutritional injury may not be relevant to humans especially with regard to lipotropes. Epidemiologic studies have not borne out a relationship between cirrhosis and malnutrition in underdeveloped countries (79), and liver biopsies of severely malnourished prison camp victims of World War II revealed only minimal abnormalities (80). By contrast, a direct relationship between alcohol consumption and frequency of cirrhosis has been demonstrated in studies dealing with prohibition in the United States and during the rationing of alcoholic beverages during World War II (81, 82). Furthermore, the studies of Lelbach (83) and Péquignot (84) showed a linear relationship between the incidence of cirrhosis in an alcoholic population and amount of alcohol intake, whereas no role for dietary deficiency was revealed.

In addition to showing that even diets relatively rich in protein do not preclude the development of alcoholic cirrhosis, the studies of Péquignot (84) also revealed that the incidence of cirrhosis increased markedly when the daily intake of alcohol reached 160 g. This was interpreted by some to indicate a threshold of toxicity of alcohol at that level. However, more recent studies by Péquignot et al. (85, 86) have also shown that daily intake of alcohol as low as 40 g in men and 20 g in women resulted in a statistically significant increase of the incidence of cirrhosis in well-nourished persons. Obviously, because of individual variations, the exact toxic level for a given subject is usually unknown. However, the public should be made aware of the fact that, even with adequate diets, amounts of alcohol considered before as innocuous may indeed harm the liver. This is particularly pertinent in the case of women, whose increased susceptibility was also indicated by a higher incidence of cirrhosis for a given intake; indeed, Wilkinson et al. (87) found women to be more susceptible than men to the development of alcoholic cirrhosis.

Furthermore, alcohol has been shown to be directly hepatotoxic histologically (light and electron microscope) and biochemically in both alcoholics and nonalcoholics, regardless of dietary variations in fat, protein, vitamins, and lipotropes (74, 75, 88–90). Recently, fatty liver and cirrhosis have been produced in a primate given alcohol in the presence of an adequate diet (91–93).

Ethanol and nutrition may interact with respect to their effects on the liver (94–97). The role of nutrition in the recovery from alcoholic liver injury has been alluded to before and will be discussed subsequently. Erenoglu et al. (98) pointed out that alcoholics are unable to drink in moderation; therefore, in spite of their data that limited consumption was not harmful, they recommended abstinence.

The evidence for the direct toxicity of ethanol makes such advice especially warranted.

Treatment

Since the work of Patek and Post (99), little has been added to the dietary armamentarium for specific therapy of alcoholic liver disease. Advances have been made in the understanding and avoidance of iatrogenic problems and in the therapy of associated conditions, such as sodium and water retention and encephalopathy. The basic diet of normal protein and fat content with vitamin supplements remains the mainstay of therapy.

Prevention

Ethanol consumed in large amounts has been shown to be directly hepatotoxic despite adequate nutrition, including high-protein, low-fat, vitamin-enriched, and lipotrope-supplemented diets. Problem drinkers are generally felt to be unable to drink in moderation. There is no established prophylactic regime except abstinence. Liver injury is time- and dose-related. Although a moderate level of consumption may be safe in a number of individuals, a no-effect dose level has not been established clinically.

Fatty Liver and Alcoholic Hepatitis

Therapy for fatty liver includes abstinence and a regular diet. Specific nutritional deficiencies or clinical problems are treated if present. Patients who are acutely ill with fever, nausea, vomiting, and encephalopathy may require fluid and electrolyte replacement and parenteral alimentation. Specific nutritional therapy is as listed below.

Protein. Finding the optimal dietary protein level is one of the most difficult aspects of nutritional therapy in patients with alcoholic liver injury; protein intake must be adequate to prevent nitrogen wasting but not so great as to precipitate hepatic coma.

In general, the nitrogen requirement in cirrhosis has been reported as normal (100), and some studies have suggested increased nitrogen retention (101). Furthermore, the tolerance to dietary protein may be related to the amino acid content of the protein administered. Blood is less well tolerated than isonitrogenous protein in the form of casein (102). Meat protein is less well tolerated than is isonitrogenous milk (103) or casein (104). These differences have been attributed to the increased content of aromatic amino acids present in meat and blood proteins. These findings have led to the suggestion that in such patients, dietary branched-chain amino acids should be increased while levels of phenylalanine, tyrosine, tryptophan, and methionine should be decreased (105), but the therapeutic benefit of such proteins or mixtures has not been determined.

Initially, 0.5 g/kg/day high quality protein may be tried (approximately 30–35 g/day), unless encephalopathy is present. This amount may be increased in increments of 10–15 g/day every 5–7 days until a level of approximately 70 g/day is reached. Benefit from dietary protein above this level has not been established, and the risk of encephalopathy is increased. A zero-protein regimen, which may be indicated initially when hepatic encephalopathy is present, should not be continued for more than a few days to minimize resultant endogenous protein catabolism. If a minimum of 20–35 g/day is not tolerated, neomycin or lactulose should be employed.

Experimentally, ethanol has a complex effect on nitrogen balance, depending upon dietary conditions. Given as supplementary calories, ethanol may be nitrogen sparing; but given as an isocaloric substitute for carbohydrate, it increases urea excretion (106, 107).

When ethanol is consumed along with adequate dietary protein, essential amino acids are generally normal or increased in the plasma (108). Therefore, as judged by plasma amino acids, ethanol does not have a major impact on dietary requirements for amino acids.

Amino Acids and Hyperalimentation in Patients with Hepatic Insufficiency. Patients with hepatic insufficiency have decreased tolerance to dietary protein, and it has been postulated that they have an increased need for branched-chain amino acids and a decreased requirement for aromatic amino acids. This has led to the development of specific mixtures of amino acids for parenteral therapy that seek to maximize nitrogen balance and recovery from encephalopathy while, at the same time, providing a minimal nitrogen load. These mixtures are rich in branched-chain amino acids and poor in aromatic amino acids. In patients with severe liver disease and hepatic insufficiency, these mixtures have thus far been shown to be of only limited short-term value (105, 109). Clinical trials are currently underway to evaluate the benefits of this therapy. The expense and manpower required for such treatment should be weighed against the long-term benefits provided.

Maddrey et al. (110) used keto analogs of essential amino acids in an effort to provide essential amino acids without administering a nitrogen load. The theoretical basis for this therapy is that, by combining with amino group donors, keto analogs of amino acids yield essential amino acids, provide no nitrogen load, and may reduce hyperammonemia. Mixtures of keto analogs of valine, leucine, isoleucine, methionine, and phenylalanine were given parenterally or orally to patients with severe liver disease and encephalopathy. Administration resulted in significant improvement in the ratio of essential to nonessential amino acids in the plasma of these patients along with a decrease in the levels of plasma glutamine. Clinical improvement in mental status was noted, but no improvement in nitrogen balance was observed. Therapy with keto analogs requires great expense and the load of calcium and/or sodium that must be administered along with the keto analogs may become a problem in patients with severe liver disease and disordered metabolism of electrolytes.

Calories. Calories must be provided in sufficient quantity to allow regeneration and to maximize nitrogen sparing. Estimates for a reasonable minimum are 25 kcal/kg or approximately 1600 kcal/day (46). A level of approximately 2600 kcal, depending on activity and associated problems, is desired. Intravenous glucose may be necessary to supplement dietary calories if nausea, vomiting, and anorexia persist for a long period of time. The nitrogen-sparing effect of calories prevents endogenous protein catabolism.

Fat. Low-fat diets, although of theoretical interest, are not advocated because of the lack of palatability of such regimes, especially in an already anorectic patient (111). Resulting inadequate caloric intake promotes protein catabolism. Fat is generally not restricted unless gastrointestinal intolerance develops because of jaundice, pancreatic insufficiency, or other causes of steatorrhea.

Vitamins. Specific deficiencies should be corrected immediately (often with parenteral administration). Usually, patients are treated with B vitamins. Suggested amounts are approximately five times the recommended allowances, although several times these amounts are commonly given without apparent harm or proven efficacy. Generally, fat-soluble vitamins are not deficient. Vitamin K may be administered intramuscularly (10 mg/day for 3 days) if the prothrombin time is prolonged. Failure to correct a prolonged prothrombin time indicates severe hepatocellular injury.

Miscellaneous. Small infrequent feedings may be useful in maintaining an adequate diet. Value of lipotrope therapy has not been established, and such therapy may be harmful in excess. Trace elements remain of theoretical interest except in extreme deficiency states.

NUTRITIONAL STATUS OF ALCOHOLICS

The nutritional status of alcoholics is generally considered to be very poor. Iber (112) estimated that 20,000 alcoholics suffer major illnesses due to malnutrition requiring hospitalization each year and accounting for 7-1/2 million hospital days. The spread of alcoholism to various socioeconomic classes, and possibly the greater availability and enrichment of foods, have modified the traditional nutritional view of the alcoholic. Neville et al. (113) found no evidence of marked change in nutritional status in the alcoholic and the nonalcoholic who were matched for socioeconomic and health history. The impact of drinking patterns on dietary intake was studied by Bebb et al. (114), who found little significant impact on nutrition as a result of moderate ethanol consumption. However, heavier consumption of alcohol may lead to a decrease in food intake, and the caloric load of alcohol has been postulated as a cause of appetite suppression (2). Other factors that may limit intake in the alcoholic include gastritis and depressed consciousness. Sample selection may have accounted for stereotyped past impressions: also, there is often a lack of correlation among biochemical, dietary, and clinical data. In a recent epidemiologic study, hospitalized alcoholics with liver disease were found to have poor dietary protein intakes (115). Such studies, however, fail to take into account cause and effect, since liver disease and its complications such as encephalopathy and ascites may lead to poor dietary protein intake. Although the stereotype of the malnourished alcoholic may be unfounded as it applies to the millions of alcoholics in the United States, alcohol remains one of the few causes of florid nutritional deficiency in our society. The impact of more subtle nutritional alterations produced by alcohol, as they relate to ethanol-induced and other disease states, remains to be elucidated. Alcohol-related diseases requiring hospital and outpatient dietary therapy have become one of the largest health care problems in the United States. The theory of nutritional deficiency as a cause of alcoholism has not proven valid, and nutritional therapy as a cure for alcoholism has not been successful (27). Alcoholism affects all tissues of the body; the diversity of its pathologic effects and the complexity of the interaction of the toxicity of ethanol with nutritional deficiencies are discussed in detail in a recent monograph (116).

REFERENCES

1. C. S. Leake and M. Silverman, The chemistry of alcoholic beverages. In B. Kissin and H. Begleiter, eds., *Biology of Alcoholism,* Vol. I, Plenum Press, New York, 1974, p. 575.
2. W. W. Westerfeld and M. P. Schulman, Metabolism and caloric value of alcohol. *J. Am. Med. Assoc.* **170**, 197 (1959).
3. J. Trémolière and L. Carré, Études sur les modalités d'oxydation de l'alcool chez l'homme normal et alcoolique. *Rev. Alcoolisme* **7**, 202 (1961).

4. C. S. Lieber, D. P. Jones, M. S. Losowsky, and C. S. Davidson, Interrelation of uric acid and ethanol metabolism in man. *J. Clin. Invest.* **41**, 1986 (1962).

5. M. J. MacLachlan and G. P. Rodnan, Effects of fast food and alcohol on serum uric acid and acute attacks of gout. *Am. J. Med.* **42**, 38 (1967).

6. D. E. Wilson, P. H. Schreibman, A. C. Brewster, and R. A. Arky, The enhancement of alimentary lipemia by ethanol in man. *J. Lab. Clin. Med.* **75**, 264 (1970).

7. C. S. Lieber, D. P. Jones, J. Mendelson, and L. M. DeCarli, Fatty liver, hyperlipemia and hyperuricemia produced by prolonged alcohol consumption, despite adequate dietary intake. *Trans. Assoc. Am. Physicians* **76**, 289 (1963).

8. D. Guisard, J. P. Gonand, J. Laurent, and G. Debry, Étude de l'épuration plasmatique des lipides chez les cirrhotiques. *Nutr. Metab.* **13**, 222 (1971).

9. A. Marzo, P. Ghirardi, P. Sardini, and A. Albertini, Serum lipids and total fatty acids in chronic alcoholic liver disease at different stages of cell damage. *Klin. Wochenschr.* **48**, 947 (1970).

10. A. Chait, W. February, M. Mancine, and B. Lewis, Clinical and metabolic study of alcoholic hyperlipidaemia. *Lancet* **2**, 62 (1972).

11. H. Ginsberg, J. Olefsky, and J. W. Farquhar, Moderate ethanol ingestion and plasma triglyceride levels: A study in normal and hypertriglyceridemic persons. *Ann. Intern. Med.* **80**, 143 (1974).

12. J. J. Barboriak, A. A. Rimm, A. J. Anderson, M. Schmidhoffer, and F. E. Tristani, Coronary artery occlusion and alcohol intake. *Br. Heart J.* **39**, 289 (1977).

13. J. F. Rehfeld, E. Juhl, and M. Hilden, Carbohydrate metabolism in alcohol-induced fatty liver (evidence for an abnormal insulin response to glucagon in alcoholic liver disease). *Gastroenterology* **64**, 445 (1973).

14. R. Metz, S. Berger, and M. Mako, Potentiation of the plasma insulin response to glucose by prior administration of alcohol. *Diabetes* **8**, 517 (1969).

15. C. B. Phillips and H. F Safrit, Alcoholic diabetes: induction of glucose intolerance with alcohol. *J. Am. Med. Assoc.* **217**, 1513 (1971).

16. C. M. Leevy, A. Thompson, and H. Baker, Vitamins and liver injury. *Am. J. Clin. Nutr.* **23**, 493 (1970).

17. G. R. Cherrick, H. Baker, O. Frank, and C. M. Leevy, Observations on hepatic avidity for folate in Laennec's cirrhosis. *J. Lab. Clin. Med.* **66**, 446 (1965).

18. S. E. Steinberg, C. L. Campbell, and R. S. Hillman, Effect of alcohol on hepatic secretion of methylfolate ($CH_3H_4PteGlu_1$) into bile. *Biochem. Pharm.* **30**, 96 (1981).

19. M. Cole, A. Turner, O. Frank, H. Baker, and C. M. Leevy, Extraocular palsy and thiamine therapy in Wernicke's encephalopathy. *Am. J. Clin. Nutr.* **22**, 44 (1969).

20. E. R. Eichner and R. S. Hillman, The evolution of anemia in alcoholic patients. *Am. J. Med.* **50**, 218 (1971).

21. J. D. Hines, Altered phosphorylation of vitamin B_6 in alcoholic patients induced by oral administration of alcohol. *J. Lab. Clin. Med.* **74**, 883 (1969).

22. L. W. Sullivan and V. Herbert, Suppression of hematopoiesis by ethanol. *J. Clin. Invest.* **43**, 2048 (1964).

23. R. L. Veitch, L. Lumeng, and T. K. Li, The effect of ethanol and acetaldehyde on vitamin B_6 metabolism in liver. *Gastroenterology* **66**, 868 (1974).

24. D. Mitchell, C. Wagner, W. J. Stone, G. R. Wilkinson, and S. Schenker, Abnormal regulation of plasma pyridoxas 5-phosphate in patients with liver disease. *Gastroenterology* **71**, 1043 (1976).

25. C. M. Leevy, H. Baker, W. tenHove, O. Frank, and G. Cherrick, B-complex vitamins in liver disease of the alcoholic. *Am. J. Clin. Nutr.* **16**, 339 (1965).

26. R. J. Williams, *Alcoholism — The Nutritional Approach*, University of Texas Press, Austin, Tex., 1954, p. 211.

27. R. W. Hillman, Alcoholism and malnutrition. In B. Kissin and H. Begleiter, eds., *Biology of Alcoholism*, Vol. III, Plenum Press, New York, 1974, p. 513.

28. P. M. Dreyfus, Diseases of nervous system in chronic alcoholics. In B. Kissin and H. Begleiter, eds., *Biology of Alcoholism*, Vol. III, Plenum Press, New York, 1974, p. 265.

29. J. R. Graham, P. Woodhouse, and F. H. Read, Massive thiamine dosage in an alcoholic with cerebellar cortical degeneration. *Lancet* **2**, 107 (1971).

30. E. R. Eichner, B. Buchanan, J. W. Smith, and R. S. Hillman, Variations in the hematologic and medical status of alcoholics. *Am. J. Med. Sci.* **263**, 35 (1972).

31. J. Lindenbaum and C. S. Lieber, Hematologic effects of alcohol in man in absence of nutritional deficiency. *N. Engl. J. Med.* **281**, 333 (1969).

32. J. Lindenbaum and C. S. Lieber, Alcohol-induced malabsorption of vitamin B_{12} in man. *Nature* **224**, 806 (1969).

33. A. J. Patek and C. Haig, The occurrence of abnormal dark adaptation and its relation to vitamin A metabolism in patients with cirrhosis of the liver. *J. Clin. Invest.* **18**, 609 (1939).
34. D. H. VanThiel, J. Gavaler, and R. Lester, Ethanol inhibition of vitamin A metabolism in the testes: Possible mechanism for sterility in alcoholics. *Science* **196**, 941 (1974).
35. E. Mezey and P. R. Holt, The inhibitory effect of ethanol on retinol oxidation by human liver and cattle retina. *Exp. Mol. Pathol.* **15**, 148 (1971).
36. D. H. VanThiel and R. Lester, Alcoholism: Its effect on hypothalamic pituitary gonadal function. *Gastroenterology* **71**, 318 (1976).
37. M. A. Leo and C. S. Lieber, Hepatic vitamin A depletion in alcoholic liver injury. *N. Engl. J. Med.* **307**, 597 (1982).
38. P. D. Saville, Changes in bone mass with age and alcoholism. *J. Bone Joint Surg. Am. Vol.* **47**, 492 (1965).
39. B. E. Nilsson, Conditions contributing to fracture of the femoral neck. *Acta Chir. Scand.* **136**, 383 (1970).
40. L. Solomon, Drug induced arthropathy and necrosis on the femoral head. *J. Bone Joint Surg. Br. Vol.* **55**, 246 (1973).
41. L. V. Avoli, S. W. Lee, J. E. McDonald, J. Lund, and H. F. DeLuca, Metabolism of $D_3^{-3}H$ in human subjects: distribution in blood, bile, feces and urine. *J. Clin. Invest.* **46**, 983 (1967).
42. L. V. Avioli and J. G. Haddad, Vitamin D: current concepts. *Metabolism* **22**, 507 (1973).
43. H. R. Roberts and A. I. Cederbaum, The liver and blood coagulation: physiology and pathology. *Gastroenterology* **63**, 297 (1972).
44. W. H. J. Summerskill, D. E. Barnardo, and W. P. Baldus, Disorders of water and electrolyte metabolism in liver disease. *Am. J. Clin. Nutr.* **23**, 499 (1970).
45. G. J. Gabuzda, Cirrhosis, ascites and edema: clinical course related to management. *Gastroenterology* **58**, 546 (1970).
46. G. J. Gabuzda, Nutrition and liver disease. *Med. Clin. North Am.* **54**, 1455 (1970).
47. N. G. Soler, S. Jain, H. James, and A. Paton, Potassium status of patients with cirrhosis. *Gut* **17**, 152 (1976).
48. L. Shear and G. J. Gabuzda, Potassium deficiency and endogenous ammonium overload from kidney. *Am. J. Clin. Nutr.* **23**, 614 (1970).
49. T. Markkanen and V. Nanto, The effect of ethanol infusion on the calcium-phosphorus balance in man. *Experientia* **22**, 753 (1966).

50. R. J. McCollister, E. B. Flink, and M. D. Lewis, Urinary excretion of magnesium in man following the ingestion of ethanol. *Am. J. Clin. Nutr.* **12**, 415 (1963).

51. A. S. Prasad, D. Oberleas, and G. Rajasekaran, Essential micronutrient elements: biochemistry and changes in liver disorders. *Am. J. Clin. Nutr.* **12**, 415 (1963).

52. F. W. Heaton, L. N. Pyrah, C. C. Beresford, and R. W. Bryson, Hypomagnesaemia in chronic alcoholism. *Lancet* **2**, 802 (1962).

53. Y. Morin and F. Daniel, Quebec beer-drinkers cardiomyopathy: Etiological considerations. *Can. Med. Assoc. J.* **97**, 926 (1967).

54. R. W. Charlton, P. Jacobs, H. Seftel, and T. H. Bothwell, Effect of alcohol on iron absorption. *Br. Med. J.* **2**, 1427 (1964).

55. N. D. Grace and L. W. Powell, Iron storage disorders of the liver. *Gastroenterology* **67**, 1257 (1974).

56. E. Gottfried, M. A. Korsten, and C. S. Lieber, Gastritis and duodenitis induced by alcohol: an endoscopic and histologic assessment. *Am. J. Gastroenterol.* **70**, 587 (1978).

57. E. Baraona, R. C. Pirola, and C. S. Lieber, Small intestinal damage and changes in cell populations produced by ethanol ingestion in the rat. *Gastroenterology* **66**, 226 (1974).

58. Y. Israel, J. E. Valenzuela, I. Salazar, and G. Ugarte, Alcohol and amino acid transport in the human small intestine. *J. Nutr.* **98**, 222 (1969).

59. E. A. Robles, E. Mezey, C. H. Halsted, and M. M. Schuster, Effect of ethanol on motility of the small intestine. *Johns Hopkins Med. J.* **135**, 17 (1974).

60. W. Perlow, E. Baraona, and C. S. Lieber, Symptomatic intestinal disaccharidase deficiencies in alcoholism. *Gastroenterology* **72**, 680 (1977).

61. W. P. T. James, Intestinal absorption in protein—calorie malnutrition. *Lancet* **1**, 333 (1968).

62. L. G. Mayoral, K. Tripathy, F. T. Garcia, S. Klahr, O. Bolanos, and J. Ghites, Malabsorption in the tropics: A second look. I. The role of protein malnutrition. *Am. J. Clin. Nutr.* **20**, 866 (1967).

63. C. H. Halsted, E. A. Robles, and E. Mezey, Decreased jejunal uptake of labeled folic acid (^{3}H-PGA) in alcoholic patients: Role of alcohol and nutrition. *N. Engl. J. Med.* **285**, 701 (1971).

64. C. H. Halsted, E. A. Robles, and E. Mezey, Intestinal malabsorption in folate-deficient alcoholics. *Gastroenterology* **64**, 526 (1973).

65. J. A. Hermos, W. H. Adamas, Y. K. Liu, L. W. Sullivan, and J. S. Trier, Mucosa of the small intestine in folate-deficient alcoholics.

Ann. Intern. Med. **76**, 957 (1972).

66. S. J. Winawer, L. W. Sullivan, V. Herbert, and N. Zanechek, The jejunal mucosa in patients with nutritional folate deficiency and megaloblastic anemia. *N. Engl. J. Med.* **272**, 892 (1965).
67. J. Lindenbaum and C. S. Lieber, Effects of chronic ethanol administration on intestinal absorption in man in the absence of nutritional deficiency. *Ann. N.Y. Acad. Sci.* **252**, 228 (1975).
68. W. G. Linscheer, Malabsorption in cirrhosis. *Am. J. Clin. Nutr.* **23**, 488 (1970).
69. W. O. Atwater and F. G. Benedict, An experimental inquiry regarding the nutritive value of alcohol. *Proc. Natl. Acad. Sci. USA* **8**, 231 (1896).
70. M. S. Losowsky and B. E. Walker, Liver disease and malabsorption. *Gastroenterology* **56**, 589 (1969).
71. W. W. Faloon, Metabolic effects of nonabsorbable antibacterial agents. *Am. J. Clin. Nutr.* **23**, 645 (1970).
72. F. W. Hoffbauer and F. G. Zaki, Choline deficiency in baboon and rat compared. *Arch. Pathol.* **79**, 364 (1965).
73. R. E. Olson, Nutrition and alcoholism. In M. G. Wohl and R. S. Goodhart, eds., *Modern Nutrition in Health and Disease*, Lea and Febiger, Philadelphia, 1964.
74. E. Rubin and C. S. Lieber, Alcohol-induced hepatic injury in non-alcoholic volunteers. *N. Engl. J. Med.* **278**, 869 (1968).
75. C. S. Lieber, D. P. Jones, and L. M. DeCarli, Effects of prolonged ethanol intake: production of fatty liver despite adequate diets. *J. Clin. Invest.* **44**, 1009 (1965).
76. C. S. Lieber and L. M. DeCarli, Study of agents for the prevention of the fatty liver produced by prolonged alcohol intake. *Gastroenterology* **50**, 316 (1966).
77. E. A. Phear, B. Ruebner, S. A. Sherlock, and W. H. J. Summerskill, Methionine toxicity in liver disease and its prevention by chlortetracycline. *Clin. Sci.* **15**, 93 (1956).
78. D. B. McGill, S. R. Humphreys, A. H. Baggenstoss, and E. R. Dickson, Cirrhosis and death after jejunoileal shunt. *Gastroenterology* **63**, 972 (1972).
79. C. S. Davidson, Nutrition, geography and liver diseases. *Am. J. Clin. Nutr.* **23**, 427 (1970).
80. F. L. Siegel, M. K. Roach, and L. R. Pomeroy, Plasma amino acid patterns in alcoholism: the effects of ethanol loading. *Proc. Natl. Acad. Sci. USA* **51**, 605 (1964).
81. S. Lederman, Alcohol, Alcoholisme, alcoholisation. Paris, France: Institut national d'études démographiques, Travaux et

Documents, Cahier No. 41, Presses Universitaires de France, 1964.

82. U.S. Bureau of the Census: Vital statistics rates in the United States, 1900–1940, U.S. Government Printing Office, Washington, D.C., 1943.

83. W. K. Lelbach, Cirrhosis in the alcoholic and its relation to the volume of alcohol abuse. *Ann. N.Y. Acad. Sci.* **252**, 85 (1975).

84. G. Péquignot, Die Rolle des Alkohols bei der Atiologie von Leberzirrhosis in Frankreich. *Munchen Med. Wohenschr.* **103**, 1464 (1962).

85. G. Péquignot, C. Chabert, H. Eydoux, and M. A. ˙Courcoul, Augmentation du risque de cirrhose en fonction de la ration d'alcool. *Rev. Alcohol.* **20**, 191 (1974).

86. G. A. Péquignot, A. J. Tuyns, and J. L. Berta, Ascitic cirrhosis in relation to alcohol consumption. *Internat. J. Epidemiol.* **7**, 113 (1978).

87. P. Wilkinson, J. N. Santamaria, and J. G. Rankin, Epidemiology of alcoholic cirrhosis. *Australas. Ann. Med.* **18**, 222 (1969).

88. B. P. Lane and C. S. Lieber, Ultrastructural alterations in human hepatocytes following ingestion of ethanol with adequate diets. *Am. J. Pathol.* **49**, 593 (1966).

89. C. S. Lieber and E. Rubin, Alcoholic fatty liver in man on a high protein and low fat diet. *Am. J. Med.* **44**, 200 (1968).

90. E. Rubin and C. S. Lieber, Experimental alcoholic hepatic injury in man: Ultrastructural changes. *Fed. Proc.* **26**, 1458 (1967).

91. C. S. Lieber and L. M. DeCarli, An experimental model of alcohol feeding and liver injury in the baboon. *J. Med. Primatol.* **3**, 153 (1974).

92. C. S. Lieber, L. M. DeCarli, and E. Rubin, Sequential production of fatty liver, hepatitis and cirrhosis in sub-human primates fed ethanol with adequate diets. *Proc. Natl. Acad. Sci. USA,* **72**, 437 (1975).

93. H. Popper and C. S. Lieber, Histogenesis of alcoholic fibrosis and cirrhosis in the baboon. *Am. J. Pathol.* **98**, 695 (1980).

94. E. Klatskin, W. A. Krehl, and H. O. Conn, The effect of alcohol on the choline requirement I: Changes in the rat's liver following prolonged ingestion of alcohol. *J. Exp. Med.* **100**, 605 (1954).

95. C. S. Lieber and L. M. DeCarli, Quantitative relationship between the amount of dietary fat and the severity of the alcoholic fatty liver. *Am. J. Clin. Nutr.* **23**, 474 (1970).

96. C. S. Lieber and N. Spritz, Effects of prolonged ethanol intake in man: role of dietary, adipose, and endogenously synthesized fatty

acids in the pathogenesis of the alcoholic fatty liver. *J. Clin. Invest.* **45**, 1400 (1966).

97. C. S. Lieber, N. Spritz, and L. M. DeCarli, Fatty liver produced by dietary deficiencies: its pathogenesis and potentiation by ethanol. *J. Lipid Res.* **10**, 283 (1969).

98. E. Erenoglu, J. G. Edreira, and A. J. Patek, Jr., Observations on patients with Laennec's cirrhosis receiving alcohol while on controlled diets. *Ann. Intern. Med.* **60**, 814 (1964).

99. A. M. Patek and J. Post, Treatment of cirrhosis of the liver by a nutritious diet and supplements rich in vitamin B complex. *J. Clin. Invest.* **20**, 481 (1941).

100. G. J. Gabuzda and L. Shear, Metabolism of dietary protein in hepatic cirrhosis. *Am. J. Clin. Nutr.* **23**, 479 (1970).

101. D. Rudman, S. Akgun, and J. T. Galambos, Observations of the nitrogen metabolism of patients with portal cirrhosis. *Am. J. Clin. Nutr.* **23**, 1203 (1970).

102. A. N. Bessman and G. S. Mirick, Blood ammonia levels following the ingestion of casein and whole blood. *J. Clin. Invest.* **37**, 990 (1958).

103. J. C. B. Fenton, E. J. Knight, and P. L. Humpherson, Milk and cheese diet in portal systemic encephalopathy. *Lancet* **1**, 164 (1966).

104. N. J. Greenberger, J. Carley, S. Schenker, I. Bettinger, C. Stamnes, and P. Beyer, Effect of vegetable and animal protein diets in chronic hepatic encephalopathy. *Am. J. Dig. Dis.* **22**, 845 (1977).

105. J. E. Fischer, J. M. Funovics, A. Aguirre, J. H. James, M. Keane, R. I. C. Wesdrop, N. Yoshimira, and T. Westman, The role of plasma amino acids in hepatic encephalopathy. *Surgery* **78**, 276 (1975).

106. G. Klatskin, The effect of ethyl alcohol on nitrogen excretion in the rat (abstr). *Yale J. Biol. Med.* **34**, 124 (1961).

107. C. Rodrigo, C. Antezana, and E. Baraona, Fat and nitrogen balances in rats with alcohol-induced fatty liver. *J. Nutr.* **101**, 1307 (1971).

108. S. Shaw and C. S. Lieber, Plasma amino acid abnormalities in the alcoholic: respective role of alcohol, nutrition, and liver injury. *Gastroenterology* **74**, 677 (1978).

109. J. E. Fischer, A. M. Ebeid, H. M. Rosen, J. H. James, J. M. Keane, and P. B. Soeters, Improvement in hepatic encephalopathy by "normalization of plasma amino acid patients." *Gastroenterology* **70**, 981 (1976).

110. W. C. Maddrey, F. L. Weber, A. W. Coulter, C. M. Chura, N. P. Chapanis, and M. Wulser, Effects of keto analogues of essential amino acids in portal-systemic encephalopathy. *Gastroenterology* **71**, 190 (1976).

111. R. H. Crews and W. W. Faloon, The fallacy of a low-fat diet in liver disease. *J. Am. Med. Assoc.* **181**, 754 (1962).

112. F. L. Iber, In alcoholism, the liver sets the pace. *Nutr. Today* **6**, 2 (1971).

113. J. N. Neville, J. A. Eagles, G. Samson, and R. E. Olson, Nutritional status of alcoholics. *Am. J. Clin. Nutr.* **21**, 1329 (1968).

114. H. T. Bebb, H. B. Houser, J. C. Witschi, A. S. Littell, and R. K. Fuller, Calorie and nutrient contribution of alcoholic beverages to the usual diets of 155 adults. *Am. J. Clin. Nutr.* **24**, 1042 (1971).

115. A. J. Patek, E. G. Toth, M. G. Saunder, G. A. M. Castro, and J. J. Engel, Alcohol and dietary factors in cirrhosis. *Arch. Intern. Med.* **135**, 1053 (1975).

116. C. S. Lieber, *Medical Disorders of Alcoholism: Pathogenesis and Treatment*, W. B. Saunders Co., Philadelphia, 1982.

6

Hazards in the Food Supply

LEAD, AFLATOXINS, AND
MUTAGENS PRODUCED BY COOKING

L. F. BJELDANES, Ph.D.
University of California, Berkeley

Address correspondence to L.F. Bjeldanes, Ph.D., Associate Professor, Department of Nutritional Sciences, University of California, Berkeley, CA 94720.

ABSTRACT

The term "hazard," in the present context, refers to a toxic substance present in the food supply in quantities large enough to cause harm to persons who consume average diets. Recent findings are discussed concerning the presence in the diet of lead and aflatoxins, and of mutagens and carcinogens from the cooking of food.

Children are more susceptible than are adults to lead poisoning, and nutritional deficiencies increase the toxicity of ingested lead. Results of recent studies show that performance of children on standard psychologic examinations decreases as lead exposure increases. Also, certain personality traits such as distractibility and impulsivity become more pronounced as lead exposure increases. These adverse effects are observed at lead exposure levels near those which begin to produce detectable biochemical changes in blood. These levels are well below levels which produce acute symptoms of classical lead poisoning.

The aflatoxins are a series of substances of varying carcinogenic potency produced by the common molds *Aspergillus flavus* and *A. parasiticus*. Recent severe outbreaks of aflatoxin contamination have occurred in corn crops in Iowa and in the southeastern United States. Aflatoxin contamination in corn reached as high as 94% of ears tested in Georgia in 1978. Cottonseed meal used for dairy feed was heavily contaminated with aflatoxins in 1977 in the southwestern United States and resulted in unacceptably high levels of aflatoxin M_1 in milk samples. Although results of metabolism studies suggest that humans may be a species resistant to aflatoxin carcinogenesis, epidemiologic evidence suggests that human liver cancer rates correlate with aflatoxin levels in the diet, even when these levels are very low.

Mutagens and carcinogens produced in foods as a result of cooking procedures are polycyclic neutral or basic compounds. The neutral compounds (such as benzo(a)pyrene) are produced by the high temperature heat treatment of broiling. These substances undergo a series of metabolic transformations to form an active metabolite that reacts chemically with DNA. The basic compounds (polycyclic amines) are a recently discovered group of substances that are produced during normal frying and roasting of high protein foods. The amounts of basic

106

compounds in the food depend on the type of food and the time and temperature of cooking. These basic substances are potent bacterial mutagens and their potential hazard to humans is under extensive study.

HAZARDS IN THE FOOD SUPPLY

To gain an overall perspective of problems of safety of the food supply, one should keep in mind the distinction between the terms toxin and hazard. Since a toxin is a substance that causes a harmful effect on an organism, any substance may be considered a toxin. Thus, even the most innocuous substance can be administered in sufficiently high doses to cause a toxic effect and, therefore, can be termed a toxin. The term hazard refers to the degree of danger resulting from exposure to a substance under usual conditions. Thus, whereas all foods contain many substances that would cause toxic effects at high doses, the actual levels of these substances in most foods is low with a low or nonexistent degree of hazard.

The degree of hazard presented by the vast majority of substances in our food supply appears to be very low. Indeed, a major health problem related to the food supply in the United States is overconsumption of calories. However, to evaluate further the degree of hazard of substances in food, one must consider that the term toxin includes substances that may be called acute toxins and those that may be termed chronic toxins. Acute toxins (all chemicals) produce a toxic effect within a fairly short period (days) following administration. Any acute toxin can be consumed in a dose small enough to be nontoxic. During human evolution, most foods that presented a significant hazard because of acute toxicity were gradually excluded from the diet. However, over the years and especially in recent times, special methods of preparation have been developed to reduce toxicity. For example, special procedures are used today in efforts to remove hydrogen cyanide from cassava preparations. Certain chronic toxins produce their toxic effects only after a considerable period (years) has elapsed following ingestion. Until relatively recently, people have not been able to associate consumption of a certain food with a toxic effect (e.g., cancer) that occurred years later. Evidence accumulated recently from several sources suggests that many chronic toxins may exist in food. The apparent wide occurrence of these substances and the experimental difficulty of establishing safe levels have led many investigators to suggest that chronic toxins may be the most hazardous substances in foods.

The following discussion will consider recent findings concerning lead and aflatoxins and the mutagens and carcinogens produced by cooking.

LEAD

Lead is widespread in the environment and occurs at various levels in air, water, and foods (1). The principal source of lead in the environment is industrial manufacture. Procedures for purification and use of lead in industry are centuries old. Industry in the United States currently consumes over one million tons of lead each year in products such as batteries, solders, and antiknock agents for gasoline. Nearly one-half of the total lead consumed is estimated to be released, in one form or another, into the atmosphere. Much of this lead eventually contaminates the water and food supply. Whereas this general lead contamination of food and water is usually low in comparison to contamination levels in products well known to produce the clinical signs of lead poisoning, recent findings suggest that safe levels of lead exposure may be lower than previously thought.

The acute effects of lead poisoning are well known and include in the most severe cases encephalopathy, abdominal colic, anemia, and death. Documented cases of classical acute lead poisoning have resulted from consumption of lead-based paint, juices stored improperly in glazed pottery, and illicit whisky distilled through lead pipes (2, 3). In these cases, the toxic substances contained over 100 ppm lead and resulted in blood lead levels of over 100 μg/dl. Biochemical effects of lead exposure begin to appear at blood levels of 25–30 μg/dl. At these levels lead has an inhibitory effect on enzymes such as δ-aminolevulinic acid dehydratase and brain adenglycyclase (4). Free erythrocyte protoporphyrin levels are elevated in children at blood lead levels as low as 15 μg/dl (5).

Age and nutritional status are reported to influence an individual's susceptibility to acute and chronic lead poisoning. Under usual conditions of dietary exposure (0.2–2 mg lead/day), adults reportedly absorb only about 5–10% of ingested lead. Absorbed lead enters the blood stream and is deposited primarily in bone and liver. Evidence from studies of children (3 mo.–8 yr.) indicates that over 50% of the ingested lead is absorbed (5). Studies with young rats showed similar results. In rats up to 20 days of age, 80% of the administered lead dose was absorbed. Rats older than 22 days of age began to show absorption characteristics of adult animals (6). Certain nutritional inadequacies have been reported to increase the acute and chronic toxic effects of lead (7). Iron deficiency in rats results in increased lead retention in liver, kidney, and bones, and increased urinary lead and δ-aminolevulenic acid excretion as compared to normal controls (5). Protein-deficient diets are reported to result in a 40–73% lead retention in liver, spleen, and bone of rats compared to protein-supplemented animals. Deficiencies of dietary calcium, phosphorus, or vitamin D are reported to result in increased lead absorption and deposition in soft tissue and bone.

Although the range of lead exposures that causes certain biochemical changes or gross toxic effects under chronic conditions is fairly well understood, recent findings suggest that certain neurologic disorders in children may result from exposures to low levels of lead previously thought to be without effect. In a study of over 2000 first and second grade children, lead levels in deciduous teeth were found to be directly related to behavioral and intellectual problems in the children (8). Performance on standard intelligence, language-skill, and auditory tests decreased as lead levels in teeth increased. Characteristics such as distractibility, impulsivity, and inability to follow directions increased with level of lead in the teeth. Blood lead levels in the high lead group averaged 35 μg/dl, very near the minimal levels that produce detectable biochemical changes in blood and well below levels that produce symptoms severe enough to be diagnosed clinically.

A recent National Academy of Sciences report titled *Lead in the Human Environment* concluded, in part, after a review of the available evidence, that "every member of the general population of the U.S. is exposed to elevated levels of lead in air, drinking water and foods" and that a growing body of evidence "suggests that commonplace exposure to lead in urban environments may be associated with detrimental effects on the intellectual development and behavior of children."

Lead pollution may be a major problem of industrialized societies. However, current information is suggestive and not conclusive. Certainly, removal of lead from our individual environments (lead plumbing, lead-containing cooking utensils and cans, and lead-based paints) is justified. Efforts by governmental agencies to remove lead from our collective environment should be supported.

AFLATOXINS

The aflatoxins and the mold that produces them, *Aspergillus flavus*, have been studied extensively since the discovery of their role in the loss of thousands of young turkeys in England in 1960. Many aspects of this work have been the subject of several excellent reviews (9–12).

The aflatoxins (Af) are a series of polycyclic compounds with varying degrees of carcinogenic potency produced by the molds *A. flavus* and *A.*

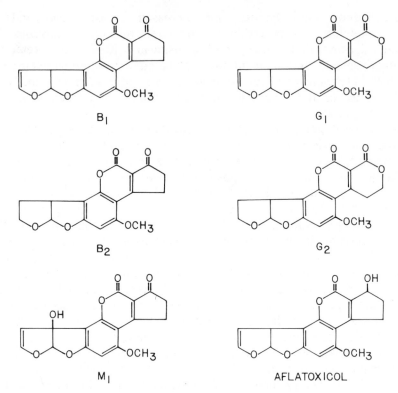

Figure 1. Chemical structures of mold products—aflatoxin B_1, B_2, G_1, and G_2; and mammalian metabolites—aflatoxin M_1 and aflatoxicol (Afl).

parasiticus. The primary compounds appear to be AfB_1 and AfB_2 with AfG_1 and AfG_2 occurring in the fungi as oxidation products of the former compounds (Fig. 1). Many other aflatoxin derivatives are derived from these four natural products via oxidative pathways in various organisms. Some of these compounds will be discussed subsequently.

Aspergillus flavus is a common soil fungus that can produce large amounts of aflatoxins under optimal conditions. The fungus is an established contaminant of peanuts, pistachios and other nuts, rice, wheat, sorghum, oats, sweet potato, grapes, soybean, corn, and other crops. In most cases, aflatoxin levels in these crops are quite low. Early assays of peanut samples in the United States showed AfB_1 levels varied between 0—40 ppb with one of 78 samples containing 91 ppb AfB_1 (13). Aflatoxin contamination of some imported pistachio samples was reported to be as high as 2000 ppb (14). Aflatoxin contamination of most other food crops is infrequent and at low levels, even in some cases when *A. flavus* growth is heavy (15).

Crops of increasing concern with regard to aflatoxin contamination are corn and cotton. *A. flavus* growth and aflatoxin contamination of corn and cotton are generally low in most years. However, at certain times when, for example, there is abnormally heavy rainfall, contamination can be very high. Thus in 1975 analyses of the corn crop in Iowa showed that some corn on plants contained aflatoxins at levels averaging 430 ppb before harvest (16). The 1978 corn crop in the southeastern United States also experienced relatively high contamination with aflatoxins. Aflatoxin contamination in corn ears was 94% and 76% in July and September surveys, respectively (17). Samples of cottonseed meal used for feed in milk production have been found that were heavily contaminated with *A. flavus* and aflatoxins. Some samples of cottonseed meal produced in the southwestern United States in 1977 were heavily contaminated with aflatoxins and resulted in AfM_1 levels in some milk samples of 2—5 ppb, considerably higher than the level allowed by the Food and Drug Administration (0.5 ppb). In most years aflatoxin contamination of milk is very low. For example, analyses of milk samples produced in California in 1979 indicated that none contained higher than 1.0 ppb AfM_1; 8% contained levels between 0.5—1.0 ppb; and 20% between 0.1—0.5 ppb. Of the remaining samples, 72% contained less than 0.1 ppb AfM_1 (D. Hsieh, personal communication).

The metabolism of aflatoxins has been studied extensively in several species in an effort to determine the biochemical mechanisms underlying the range of sensitivity of various species to aflatoxin carcinogenesis. Mice, guinea pigs, and monkeys are resistant to aflatoxin carcinogenesis; and trout, turkeys, ducks, and rats are highly susceptible. A major metabolite of aflatoxin B_1 in liver preparations of some susceptible species is aflatoxicol (Afl). Level of production of Afl in vitro appears to be positively correlated with species susceptibility to both acute and chronic effects of AfB_1 (18). Afl is a reversible bioreduction product which has been suggested to prolong AfB_1 exposure in the cell and increase AfB_1 toxicity (18). Human liver preparations produce low levels of Afl, which suggests that humans may be a species resistant to aflatoxin toxicity.

Epidemiologic evidence relating aflatoxin consumption to human liver cancer appears to support a positive association (19). The results of six studies were reported over a period of 7 years, which, when considered together, show that the rate of liver cancer in various areas in Africa increases with increasing aflatoxin intake above 3.5 ng/kg/body wt/day. Of course, an association does not prove cause. Other mycotoxins, plant products, or nutritional factors may be involved in the incidence of liver cancer. Nevertheless, the association appears strong enough to justify efforts to improve harvesting and storage techniques to reduce *A. flavus* growth and aflatoxin contamination of food and feed crops in these high-incidence areas.

Aflatoxin contamination of foods in the United States is very low as a result of improved food production and monitoring procedures. The principal cause for concern about aflatoxins in U.S. foods may be about foods produced and stored under unstandardized and unmonitored conditions.

MUTAGENS AND CARCINOGENS PRODUCED BY COOKING FOODS

Mutagens and carcinogens[1] may be introduced into food by their synthesis during normal cooking procedures. The chemical class of compounds produced depends on the method of cooking and the type of food. High-protein foods (primarily meats) appear to be the major sources of mutagens from cooked foods. The types of mutagens and carcinogens encountered in cooked uncured foods are generally of two chemical classes, polycyclic aromatic hydrocarbons and polycyclic aromatic amines (see Fig. 2).

Of the polycyclic aromatic hydrocarbons that occur in cooked foods benzo(a)pyrene[2] has been studied most extensively. Benzo(a)pyrene is a product of incomplete combustion of various fuels, and is widely distributed as an environmental contaminant (20). In addition, relatively high levels of benzo(a)pyrene have been reported to occur in certain food products such as plant oils (e.g., 44 ppb in coconut oil) and fresh vegetables (3−24 ppb). The source of benzo(a)pyrene in these latter cases appears to be from biosynthesis in the plants and not from environmental pollution (21). Thus, benzo(a)pyrene appears to be a natural component of certain foods.

---

[1]Mutagens may be defined as substances that cause a heritable change in the cell. Carcinogens may be defined as substances that cause the rapid, uncontrolled division of cells in an organism.

[2]The (a) designation in benzo(a)pyrene refers to the addition of the benzene sustituent to the "a" (alpha) face of pyrene.

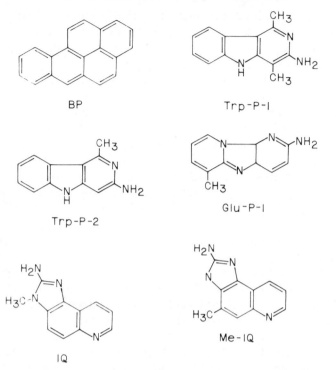

Figure 2. Chemical structures of mutagens and carcinogens produced by heat treatment of food or food components: BP, benzo(a)pyrene, from broiled meats (a polycyclic aromatic hydrocarbon); Trp–P–1, Trp–P–2, and Glu–P–1 from heated amino acids; and IQ and Me–IQ from from fried food (examples of polycyclic aromatic amines).

Benzo(a)pyrene is considered to be a moderately potent carcinogen which shows species selectivity for its toxic effects. Rodents are generally sensitive to carcinogenesis by benzo(a)pyrene administered by topical application, subcutaneous injection, or oral intubation (22). Nevertheless levels of benzo(a)pyrene in the diet higher than 10 ppm were required to produce tumors in mice (23). Rhesus monkeys and other primates generally considered to be good human models are relatively resistant (24).

Introduction of benzo(a)pyrene into foods by cooking (broiling) is well documented (25, 26). The level of this polycyclic aromatic hydrocarbon increases with the fat content of the meat and the degree to which the meat is cooked. Benzo(a)pyrene is formed by heat-induced chemical reactions of fat dripping onto the hot coals. Smoke, which contains benzo(a)pyrene, rises from the coals and is deposited on the meat. Therefore, total polycyclic aromatic hydrocarbons and benzo(a)pyrene levels are minimized by the slow cooking of lean meat under conditions that reduce smoke production. Beef steaks that were charcoal broiled by methods that reduce contact with smoke showed a considerable reduction in benzo(a)pyrene content (0.05–4.5 ppb) compared to meat broiled in a smoky flame (12.6–86.4 ppb) (27).

Recent studies of benzo(a)pyrene toxicity have concentrated on the molecular basis of benzo(a)pyrene carcinogenic activity. Benzo(a)pyrene, inert as a mutagen by itself, is converted by a series of enzymatic reactions to a highly mutagenic dihydrodiol epoxide that reacts with the 2-amino group of guanine residues in nucleic acids (28). This diol epoxide is by far the most potent mutagen of the possible benzo(a)pyrene metabolites tested and is considered to be the ultimate carcinogenic metabolite of benzo(a)pyrene.

Although the occurrence in foods of carcinogenic polycyclic aromatic hydrocarbons has been known for many years, the presence in cooked foods of another class of mutagenic and carcinogenic substances has been established only relatively recently. Proteins and several amino acids yield highly mutagenic polycyclic aromatic amines when heated at temperatures above 300°C (29–31). Similar temperatures were reported necessary to generate appreciable mutagenicity in heated food samples (32). When heated under high-temperature conditions, carbohydrates and lipid components and foods rich in these substances tended to be less mutagenic than the more protein- or amino-acid-rich samples. More recently, however, evidence compiled by several research groups indicates that mutagenic activity is induced in certain foods cooked under more normal conditions of food preparation (33–36). As was observed for samples heated at high temperatures, most cooked protein-rich food (i.e., beef, pork, chicken, and others) is more mutagenic than cooked carbohydrate-rich food (37). The active substances are again polycyclic aromatic amines.

A large-scale survey of the dependence of mutagen production in protein-rich food on cooking methods has been completed in my laboratory. In general, cooking methods that use temperatures near 100°C result in low or undetectable activity. Thus, processes such as stewing, boiling, poaching, and deep-frying near 100°C result in, at most, low activity, regardless of which food is cooked. Cooking methods such as oven roasting and baking, which heat food by an indirect convection process, appear to produce low to intermediate levels of mutagenic activity in most foods cooked by these methods.

Frying and broiling, cooking procedures that heat foods by conductive and radiative processes, tend to be associated with the highest levels of mutagenicity. Thus, rates of mutagen production in the foods tested become appreciable at temperatures of greater than 100°C and are greatly increased by cooking methods that use direct, high-temperature processes. Microwave cooking does not introduce mutagenic substances into cooked foods.

The results of the survey also showed that some classes of cooked foods tend to be more mutagenic than other foods cooked to similar extents. The most severely treated samples of milk, cheese, tofu, rock cod, and several varieties of beans, although charred and considered inedible, were only weakly mutagenic. Less severely treated samples were not active. In contrast, the first signs of charring on samples of chicken, eggs, beef, and pork were accompanied by production of relatively high levels of mutagenic activity as tested in bacteria. Meat patties fried at 200°C for 6 minutes on each side had a dark brown crust and were considered very well done. Moderate levels of mutagenicity (approximately 6000 revertants[3]/patty) were detected in these samples. Meat patties fried at 150°C for 6 minutes on each side had light brown-gray crusts and were considered rare to medium well done. These samples had much lower mutagenic activity (approximately 400 revertants/patty). Thus, use of frying temperatures in this lower range (150–180°C) would be an effective means of reducing mutagen content of fried meats.

The identity of mutagens produced by pyrolytic and normal cooking conditions has been established in some cases, and initial toxicology studies have begun. Examples of mutagens isolated from high temperature heat treatment of amino acids are tryptophan product 1 (Trp-P-1) and tryptophan product 2 (Trp-P-2) from tryptophan pyrolysis and glutamic acid product 1 (Glu-P-1) from glutamic acid pyrolysis (38, 39).

Trp-P-1 and Trp-P-2 have been tested for carcinogenicity by subcutaneous injection into Syrian golden hamsters and rats. Within 10 months Trp-P-1, but not Trp-P-2, induced the formation of transplantable sarcomas in both species (40). Trp-P-1 and Trp-P-2 have been detected in trace amounts in broiled fish but not in pan-fried meats (41).

The major mutagens in broiled fish are an imidazoquinoline (IQ) and methylimidazoquinoline (Me-IQ) (42). IQ is also reported to be a major

---

[3]Revertant as used here refers to an observable change in a bacterial cell used in the mutagenesis assay.

mutagen in fried beef but there appear to be several others as well (43). IQ and Me-IQ are the two most potent bacterial mutagens tested, with activities of 200,000 and 400,000 revertants/μg, respectively (44). Beef extracts, which contain both compounds, are metabolically converted to the active mutagens by liver tissues from several animal species and humans (45 and J. Felton, personal communication).

The estimation of human hazard of these types of mutagens and carcinogens in cooked foods is the goal of extensive, ongoing research. Until we have a better idea as to whether these substances may be harmful to humans, it would appear to be prudent to reduce our intake of heavily cooked and charred meats.

REFERENCES

1. R. A. Kenhoe, Pharmacology and toxicology of heavy metals: lead. *Pharmacol. Ther. Part A* **1**, 161 (1976).
2. S. Piomelli, Lead poisoning: Its detection and treatment. *Drug Therapy Rev. (HOSP)*, p. 19, September (1977).
3. R. W. Henderson, D. Andrews, and G. R. Lightsey, Leaching of lead from ceramics. *Bull. Environ. Contam. Toxicol.* **21**, 102 (1979).
4. F. W. Oehme, *Toxicity of Heavy Metals in the Environment,* Parts 1 and 2, Marcel Dekker, New York, 1979.
5. J. S. Lin-Fu, Vulnerability of children to lead exposure and toxicity. Parts 1 and 2. *N. Engl. J. Med.* **289**, 1229, 1289 (1973).
6. G. B. Forbes and J. C. Reina, Effect of age on gastrointestinal absorption (Fe, Sr, Pb) in the rat. *J. Nutr.* **102**, 647 (1972).
7. O. A. Levander, Lead toxicity and nutritional deficiencies. *Environ. Health Perspect.* **29**, 115 (1979).
8. H. L. Needleman, C. Gunnoe, A. Leviton, R. Reed, H. Peresie, C. Maher, and P. Barrett, Deficits in psychologic and classroom performance of children with elevated dentine lead levels, *N. Engl. J. Med.* **300**, 689 (1979).
9. R. W. Detroy, E. B. Lillehoj, and A. Ciegler, *Microb. Toxins* **6**, 13 (1971).
10. R. Schoental, Carcinogens in plants and microorganisms. In *Chemical Carcinogens,* C. E. Searle, ed., American Chemical Society, Washington, D.C., 1976, p. 626.
11. C. T. Campbell and J. R. Hayes, The role of aflatoxin metabolism in its toxic lesion. *Toxicol. Appl. Pharmacol.* **35**, 199 (1976).

12. D. K. Salunkhe, M. T. Wu, J. Y. Do, and M. R. Maas, Mycotoxins in foods and feeds. In H. D. Graham, ed., *Safety of Foods*, 2nd ed., Avi, Westport, Conn., 1980, p. 202.

13. R. A. Taber and H. W. Schroeder, Aflatoxin producing potential of isolates of the *Aspergillus flavus–oryzae* group from peanuts (*Arachis hypohaea*). *Appl. Microbiol.* 15, 140 (1967).

14. J. W. Dickens and R. E. Welty, Fluorescence in pistachio nuts contaminated with aflatoxin. *J. Am. Oil Chem. Soc.* 52, 448 (1975).

15. O. L. Shotwell, C. W. Hesseltine, M. L. Goulden, and E. E. Vandergraft, Survey of corn for aflatoxin, zearalenone and ochratoxin. *Cereal Chem.* 47, 700 (1970).

16. E. B. Lillehoj, D. I. Fennell, and W. F. Kwolek, *Aspergillus flavus* and aflatoxin in Iowa corn before harvest. *Science* 193, 495 (1976).

17. W. W. McMillian, D. M. Wilson, N. W. Widstrom, and R. C. Gueldner, Incidence and level of aflatoxin in preharvest corn in south Georgia in 1978. *Cereal Chem.* 57, 83 (1980).

18. Z. A. Wong and D. P. H. Hsieh, The comparative metabolism and toxicokinetics of aflatoxin B_1 in the monkey, rat, and mouse. *Toxicol. Appl. Pharmacol.* 55, 115 (1980).

19. C. A. Linsell and F. G. Peers, Aflatoxin and liver cell cancer. *Trans. R. Soc. Trop. Med. Hyg.* 71, 471 (1977).

20. M. Blumer, Benzpyrenes in soil. *Science* 134, 474 (1961).

21. J. Borneff, F. Selenka, H. Kunte, and A. Maximos, Experimental studies on the formation of polycyclic aromatic hydrocarbons in plants. *Environ. Res.* 2, 22 (1968).

22. J. C. Arcos and M. F. Argus, Molecular geometry and carcinogenic activity of aromatic compounds: New perspectives. *Adv. Cancer Res.* 11, 305 (1968).

23. J. Neal and R. H. Rigdon, Gastric tumors in mice fed benzo(a)pyrene: A quantitative study. *Tex. Rep. Biol. Med.* 25, 553 (1967).

24. J. H. Weisburger, Chemical Carcinogenesis. In L. J. Casarett and J. Doull, eds., *Toxicology, the Basic Science of Poisons*, Macmillan, New York, 1975, p. 333.

25. W. Lijinsky and A. E. Ross, Production of carcinogenic polynuclear hydrocarbons in the cooking of foods. *Food Cosmet. Toxicol.* 5, 343 (1967).

26. C. Lintas, M. C. DeMatthaesis, and F. Merli, Determination of benzo(a)pyrene in smoked, cooked, and toasted food products. *Food Cosmet. Toxicol.* 17, 325 (1979).

27. W. Lijinsky and P. Shubik, Benzo(a)pyrene and other polynuclear hydrocarbons in charcoal-broiled meat, *Science* 145, 53 (1964).

28. S. Neidle, Carcinogens and DNA. *Nature* **283**, 135 (1980).
29. T. Matsumoto, D. Yoshida, S. Mizusaki, and H. Okamoto, Mutagenic activity of amino acid pyrolysates in *Salmonella typhimurimn* TA98, *Mutat. Res.* **48**, 279 (1977).
30. T. Matsumoto, S. Yoshida, S. Mizusaki, and H. Okamoto, Mutagenicities of the pyrolysates of peptides and proteins, *Mutat. Res.* **56**, 281 (1978).
31. M. Nagao, M. Honda, Y. Scino, T. Yahagi, T. Kawachi, and T. Sugimura, Mutagenicities of protein pyrolysates. *Cancer Lett.* 7, 335 (1977).
32. M. Uyeta, T. Kanada, M. Mazaki, and S. Taue, Studies on mutagenicity of food. I. Mutagenicity of food pyrolysates, *J. Food Hyg. Soc. Jpn.* **19**, 216 (1978).
33. B. Commoner, A. J. Uithayathil, P. Dolara, S. Nair, P. Madyastha, and G. C. Cuca, Formation of mutagens in beef and beef extract during cooking, *Science* **201**, 913 (1978).
34. M. W. Pariza, S. H. Ashoor, F. S. Chu, and D. B. Lund, Effect of temperature and time on mutagen formation in pan-fried hamburger. *Cancer Lett.* 7, 63 (1979).
35. J. Felton, S. Healy, D. Stuermer, C. Berry, H. Timourian, H. T. Hatch, M. Morris, and L. F. Bjeldanes, Mutagens from the cooking of food. I. Improved isolation and characterization of mutagenic fractions from cooked ground beef. *Mutat. Res.* **88**, 33 (1981).
36. N. E. Spingarn and J. H. Weisburger, Formation of mutagens in cooked foods: I. Beef. *Cancer Lett.* 7, 259 (1979).
37. N. E. Spingarn, L. A. Slocum, and J. H. Weisburger, Formation of mutagens in cooked foods. II. Foods with high starch content. *Cancer Lett.* **9**, 7 (1980).
38. T. Matsumoto, D. Yoshida, S. Mizusaki, and H. Okamoto, Mutagenicities of the pyrolysates of peptides and proteins. *Mutat. Res.* **56**, 281 (1978).
39. T. Kosuge, K. Tsuji, K. Wakabayashi, T. Okamoto, K. Shudo, Y. Iitaka, A. Itai, T. Sugimura, T. Kawachi, M. Nagao, T. Yahagi, and Y. Seino, Isolation and structure studies of mutagenic principles in amino acid pyrolysates. *Chem. Pharm. Bull (Tokyo)* **26**, 611 (1978).
40. T. Ishikawa, S. Takayama, T. Kitagawa, T. Kawachi, M. Kinebuchi, N. Matsukura, E. Uchida, and T. Sugimura, *In vivo* experiments on tryptophan pyrolysis products. In E. C. Miller et al., eds., *Naturally Occurring Carcinogen-Mutagens and Modulators of Carcinogenesis*, Japan Science Society Press, Tokyo University, Park Press, Baltimore, 1979, pp. 159–167.

41. Z. Yamaizumi, T. Shiomi, H. Kasai, S. Nishimura, Y. Takahashi, M. Nagao, and T. Sugimura, Detection of potent mutagens, Trp-P-1 and Trp-P-2, in broiled fish. *Cancer Lett.* **9**, 75 (1980).
42. H. Kasai, S. Nishimura, M. Nagao, Y. Takahashi, and T. Sugimura, Fractionation of a mutagenic principle from broiled fish by high-pressure liquid chromatography. *Cancer Lett.* **7**, 353 (1979).
43. N. E. Spingarn, H. Kasai, L. L. Vuolo, S. Nishimura, Z. Yamaizumi, T. Sugimura, T. Matsushima, and J. H. Weisburger, Formation of mutagens in cooked foods. III. Isolation of a potent mutagen from beef. *Cancer Lett.* **9**, 177 (1980).
44. H. Kasai, S. Nishimura, K. Wakabayashi, M. Nagao, and T. Sugimura, Chemical synthesis of 2-amino-3-methylimidazo[4,5-f]quinoline (IQ), a potent mutagen isolated from broiled fish. *Proc. Jpn. Acad. Ser. B* **56**, 382 (1980).
45. P. Dolara, R. Barole, S. Mazzoli, and D. Benetti, Activation of the mutagens of beef extract *in vitro* and *in vivo*. *Mutat. Res.* **79**, 213 (1980).

ADDITIONAL RECENT REFERENCES

K. R. Mahaffey, Nutritional factors in lead poisoning. *Nutr. Rev.* **39**, 353 (1981).
B. G. Niranjan, N. K. Bhat, and N. G. Avadhani, Preferential attack of mitochondrial DNA by aflatoxin B_1 during hepatocarcinogenesis. *Science* **215**, 73 (1982).
L. F. Bjeldanes, M. M. Morris, J. S. Felton, S. Healy, D. Stuermer, P. Berry, H. Timourian, and F. T. Hatch. Mutagens from the cooking of food II. Survey of mutagen formation in the major protein-rich foods of the North American diet. *J. Food Chem. Toxicol.* **20**, 357 (1982).
L. F. Bjeldanes, M. M. Morris, J. S. Felton, S. Healy, D. Stuermer, P. Berry, H. Timourian, and F. T. Hatch. Mutagens from the cooking of food III. Secondary sources of cooked dietary protein. *J. Food Chem. Toxicol.* **20**, 365 (1982).

SECTION TWO

Update on Nutrients

7

Recent Progress in Zinc Nutrition Research

NOEL W. SOLOMONS, M.D.
Massachusetts Institute of Technology, Cambridge
and
Instituto de Nutrición de Centro America y Panamá (INCAP)
Guatemala, Central America

Address correspondence to Noel W. Solomons, M.D., International Nutrition Programs, Massachusetts Institute of Technology, Room 20A-222, 18 Vassar Street, Cambridge, Massachusetts 02139.

ABSTRACT

The importance of zinc as an essential nutrient in human nutrition has been emphasized by recent developments in research. Food consumption surveys reveal that hardly any age group in the United States consistently ingests the Recommended Dietary Allowances for zinc. The intestine, however, has specialized mechanisms to facilitate zinc uptake and to adjust its absorption to the nutritional requirements of the body. Moreover, a number of substances in foods reduce the biological availability of zinc. When individuals are exclusively dependent on intravenous feeding for their nutrition, specific quantities of zinc must be added to the nutrient solutions. Zinc has important interactions with other nutrients including iron, copper, essential fatty acids, vitamin C, and vitamin A. Zinc also plays a role in the immune defense systems of the body. A major deficiency in our present technology is a lack of suitable clinical indices for the accurate assessment of zinc nutriture in humans.

Eighteen abstracts relating to zinc nutrition were presented in 1970 at the meetings of the Federation of American Societies for Experimental Biology. In 1980, that number had increased to 66. With such burgeoning developments in zinc research, it is challenging to present a comprehensive update of the field. Thus, this review will concentrate on six areas in which substantive insights and conceptual advances have recently emerged: (1) customary consumption of dietary zinc by humans; (2) the intestinal regulation of zinc absorption; (3) interactions of zinc with other nutrients; (4) zinc requirements during total parenteral nutrition; (5) the clinical diagnostic assessment of zinc status in humans; and (6) the role of zinc in host defense and immune function.

CUSTOMARY CONSUMPTION OF DIETARY ZINC BY HUMANS

Since 1974, Recommended Dietary Allowances (RDAs) (1) have been established for zinc (Table 1). Reports from the United States, Finland,

and Chile have recently provided quantitative data on the content of zinc in human milk. Picciano and Guthrie (2) found a range of zinc content in 350 milk samples taken from 50 North American women between the 6th and 12th week postpartum to be 0.14–3.95 mg/liter, with a mean of 1.6 mg/liter. Vuori and Kuitunen (3) noted in Finnish women a decrease in zinc concentration from 4.0 mg/liter during the 2nd week of lactation to 0.48 mg/liter after 9 months of breast-feeding. Ruz et al. (4) in Chile found a mean concentration at 4, 8, and 12 weeks postpartum in 25 adequately nourished women to be 2.65, 1.66, and 1.60 mg/liter, respectively. There is substantial agreement among the three locations. If one uses a mean figure of 800 ml of breast milk as an estimate of daily intake, the various daily intakes by the infant who is exclusively breast-fed can be calculated. As shown in Table 2, except for the first month of life, the zinc intakes fall well short of the RDA recommendation. Stated another way, the density of zinc in human milk is generally insufficient to provide the recommended allowances of the mineral to infants. However, as the RDA for zinc is calculated on the basis of infant formulas, and, as zinc in breast milk may be more absorbable, breast milk still might provide sufficient zinc to meet the needs of infants.

Table 1. Recommended Dietary Allowances for Zinc (1)

Population	Age (yr)	Allowance (mg)
Infants	0.0–0.5	3
	0.5–1.0	5
Children	1–10	10
Males	11+	15
Females	11+	15
Pregnant	–	20
Lactating	–	25

In well-nourished Finnish women, Vuori et al. (5) found no correlation between customary intake of zinc and the zinc concentration in breast milk. A statistically significant reduction of zinc content was found in the milk of undernourished Chilean women at 3 months, compared with that of adequately nourished women (4). Whether or

6

126   NUTRITION UPDATE

Table 2. Daily Intakes of Zinc from Breast Milk at Various Ages[a]

Weeks of Lactation	Ruz et al. (4), Chile	Vuori and Kuitunen (3), Finland	Picciano and Guthrie (2), USA
2	–	3.00	–
4	1.99	1.58	–
6	–	1.88	↑
8	1.24	0.98	1.22[b]
12	1.20	0.66	↓
24	–	0.37	–
36	–	0.36	–

[a]Mg per day, assuming a daily intake of breast milk of 750 ml.
[b]Data from 6–12 weeks of lactation, all in one pool.

Table 3. Daily Intakes of Zinc from Customary Diets in Adults

Subject Population	Zinc Intake (mg)	RDA (%)	Description of Study
Diets for adults (5 diets, 15 meals)	9.4	63	Klevay et al. (7): various hospital diets in North Dakota
Adults, N = 22	8.6	57	Holden et al. (8): self-selected diets of middle-class adults in Maryland
Elderly adult males, N = 31	8.0	53	Greger (9): institutionalized elderly in Indiana
Elderly adult females, N = 34	8.6	57	
Elderly white males, N = 23	9.8	65	Greger & Sciscoe (10): elderly persons in an urban feeding program in Indiana
Elderly black males, N = 21	10.4	69	
Elderly white females, N = 26	9.9	66	
Elderly black females, N = 18	10.2	68	
Pregnant women, N = 29	11.0	55	Krebs et al. (11): middle-income women in Colorado
Pregnant women, 1st and 2nd trimester, N = 344	9.4	47	Hunt et al. (12): low-income Mexican-American women in California
Pregnant women, 2nd trimester, N = 279	10.0	50	
Lactating women, N = 40	11.4	46	Krebs et al. (11): middle-income women in Colorado

not dietary zinc supplementation to nursing mothers would substantially increase zinc output in breast milk has not been satisfactorily established. In contrast to the zinc content in breast milk, that of commercial infant formulas fed to children in Utah was 10.4 mg, exceeding the RDA (6).

Information on zinc consumption by adults has recently been available. Daily zinc intakes for various groups in various localities are presented in Table 3. Once again, it seems to be a question of zinc density in the diets. For lactating women to consume the requisite RDA intake of 25 mg of zinc daily from their accustomed diets, the subjects studied by Krebs et al. (11) in Colorado and those of Vuori et al. (5) in Finland would have had to eat a more zinc-dense diet (ingest 5000 kcal). Hence, based on the available survey data, a reasonable argument for dietary enrichment with zinc can be substantiated. This has been corroborated by evidence from Denver, Colorado, that dietary supplementation of infant formulas (13) and breakfast cereals (14) with zinc improved the zinc nutriture even of children from well-to-do middle-class homes.

REGULATION OF ZINC ABSORPTION

The intestinal absorption of calcium, magnesium, and iron appears to be regulated homeostatically; that is, raising of the dietary content reduces efficiency of absorption; on the other hand, at low dietary intakes, intestinal uptake is increased. Evidence in recent years has suggested that similar regulatory features are operative for zinc, and that specialized mechanisms govern the absorption of dietary zinc.

The Zinc-Binding Ligand

Over a decade ago, several investigators noted that zinc in the intestine was associated with a low-molecular-weight zinc-binding ligand (ZBL). The same ZBL was found in pancreatic secretions from dogs (15). Since it was also observed that pancreatic ligation of rats decreased the absorption of ^{65}Zn, Evans et al. (15) proposed that the ZBL might be a physiologically important factor in the normal absorption of dietary zinc in mammals. Over the ensuing years, a number of chemical entities have been proposed as candidates for the mammalian ZBL. It has been thought by different investigators to consist of amino acids (16), NNN'-trimethyl-1,2-ethanediamine (17), prostaglandin E_2 (18, 19), or a polypeptide (20). Recently, picolinic acid, a derivative of tryptophan metabolism, and citric acid have received the greatest attention.

A team of investigators led by Dr. Gary Evans at the United States Department of Agriculture laboratory in Grand Forks, North Dakota, has supported the notion that picolinic acid is the primary, functional ZBL in the intestinal lumen (21, 22). On the other hand, Hurley, Lönnerdal, and Stanislowski at the University of California have suggested that citrate is the chemical species physiologically important in intraluminal zinc-binding and uptake into mucosal cells (23, 24). A vigorous debate has raged between these two groups, hinging on disputes over the nature of chromatographic separation techniques and chemical analyses. In truth, among all of the compounds mentioned to date, none has unequivocally been shown to be the ZBL. Perhaps the perspective of Cousins and Smith (25) from Rutgers represents the most reasonable position. They have manipulated the zinc content by adding zinc to a sample of breast milk. They found that most of this added zinc was bound by substances of low molecular weight. This suggested to them that it was the lower content of proteins in breast milk that forced the zinc in human milk into an association with smaller molecules. They also submitted that the "spill-over" zinc combines with a heterogeneous variety of low-molecular-weight species that happens to be present in the fluid. Thus, a unique substance, responsible for 100% of the ZBL activity in the intestine or in breast milk, is unlikely to be found. Nonetheless, whether only one chemical or many constitute the ZBL will continue to be a question attracting the attention of investigators in mammalian biology for years to come.

The Role of Zinc-Binding Ligands in Breast Milk

Zinc-binding ligands secreted by the human mammary gland in breast milk appear to play a role in facilitating the absorption of dietary zinc by breast-fed infants. Johnson and Evans (26) demonstrated in the young rat that the zinc content of breast milk, among all human infant foods tested, had the highest biological availability, 46%. This report accompanies a number of other recent reports identifying a ZBL in human milk (23, 24, 27–31). Apparently, cow's milk has a lesser portion of its bound zinc associated with a ZBL fraction (29). As discussed above, the nature of the chemical identity of this ligand is still in dispute.

That the zinc from human breast milk is superior in insuring an adequate zinc nutriture in infants is suggested by observations in infants from middle-class families in Denver, Colorado, as reported by Hambidge et al. (32). He and his colleagues compared the plasma zinc concentration of three cohorts of infants at 6 months of age. One group had been fed a commercial formula with about 2 mg of zinc/liter; a second group, the same formula supplemented to about 6 mg of zinc/liter; and a third group was exclusively breast-fed. From the data presented in an earlier section, I would estimate the average zinc concentration in the breast milk over the course of the 6-month period to have been about 1.2 mg/liter. Nonetheless, the respective plasma zinc concentrations of the three groups of infants at 6 months of age were 70.7 ± 1.8, 76.0 ± 2.9, and 81.9 ± 6.6 μg/dl (mean $\pm$ SEM).

The Role of Zinc-Binding Ligands in Acrodermatitis Enteropathica

A great deal has been learned about the behavior of zinc in human metabolism since the demonstration by Moynahan (33) that the clinical manifestations of acrodermatitis enteropathica (AE) (a severe skin and intestinal disorder in infants due to a metabolic error) were related to zinc deficiency, and by Lombeck et al. (34) that the pathogenesis of this zinc depletion in AE was zinc malabsorption. However, prior to the emergence of these insights, it has been noted that infants did not manifest this disorder while they were being breast-fed, and that a diet of breast milk could ameliorate the signs and symptoms of this disorder. With the detection of a ZBL in breast milk, an hypothesis was formulated that the etiology of zinc malabsorption in this disease might represent a defect in the endogenous ZBL system (22).

Workers in Denver, Colorado, aspirated samples of intestinal secretions from patients with AE and from healthy individuals. These fluids apparently did not exhibit a reduction in the amount of total binding ligand (35), but the affinity of the ZBL for binding zinc in the secretions of patients appeared to have been significantly diminished (36). As discussed, Evans has presented evidence for a ZBL role for picolinic acid. Krieger and Evans (37) studied a young child with AE who, prior to definitive diagnosis, had undergone an empirical therapeutic trial with pancreatic extract (Viokase). She responded to the Viokase, but was subsequently maintained on 60 mg of oral zinc daily. Chemical analysis of the pancreatic extract revealed a picolinic acid content of 3.4 μmoles (123 μg) per gram. This patient is now being maintained on a daily intake of 10 mg of zinc, 5 mg being provided from the diet and 5 mg being provided by a physiologic dose of zinc dipicolinate (38). Although this case study substantiates a high biologic availability for zinc from the picolinic acid salt, it does not prove unequivocally that picolinate is the endogenous ZBL defective in patients with AE.

Intracellular Transport and Regulation

As noted above, the entry of zinc into the body appears to be regulated at the level of the intestine. Using an isolated, perfused rat intestine, Smith and Cousins (39) have shown a marked difference in the transfer of zinc from the lumen of the intestine to the blood, based on the previous diet of the animals. Intestines from rats on zinc-deficient diets took up more zinc than did those from zinc-supplemented animals. The subcellular mechanism for this regulation has also been partially elucidated by the group at Rutgers. Cousins and colleagues have shown that some of the zinc from an oral dose is bound to an intramucosal protein called metallothionein, and the zinc status of a rat or the amount of zinc in its diet appears to govern the induction of this protein (40, 41). This suggests a mucosal block theory, in which the zinc not required for the body's metabolism is trapped in the intestinal cells and denied passage into the bloodstream.

An interesting observation in human subjects tends to support the notion of regulation of zinc uptake by intestinal mechanisms under the influence of the diet. Dr. Freeland-Graves and coworkers at the University of Texas (42) performed zinc absorption tests in seven women who had been eating a mixed diet containing meat. She then placed these subjects for 3 weeks on a strict vegetarian diet with a high content of phytic acid. A repeat of the zinc absorption study after the period on the vegetarian regimen revealed a more avid uptake of zinc. This has been interpreted as suggesting that the intestinal mucosa of these women had made an adjustment to capture more of the zinc from the high phytate diet in which the bioavailability of the zinc would otherwise be greatly reduced.

The metallothionein proteins, however, may not only serve to reduce zinc absorption but also, under certain conditions, facilitate its absorption. This perspective comes from recent experiments published by Starcher et al. (43) in which they confirm the observations of Cousins on high intestinal concentrations of metallothioneins. Starcher and coworkers also demonstrated that, at the other end of the spectrum, that is, low intramucosal metallothionein contents, these proteins appear to favor the absorption of zinc. Thus, the fine control of mucosal transfer of dietary zinc, the full extent of participation by metallothionein, and the operation of this regulatory system in humans still await more detailed description.

INTERACTION OF ZINC WITH OTHER NUTRIENTS

It has been recognized for some time that a series of dietary binding or chelating agents—dietary fiber, phytates, inorganic phosphates, and tannins—will reduce the intestinal absorption of zinc. Recent research has extended our understanding of the interaction of zinc with other nutrients, not only in the intestine but also at the tissue level.

In terms of intestinal interaction, competition between zinc and iron and zinc and copper has recently been described. Investigators in Ontario, Canada, have shown that ratios of iron to zinc of from 2.5:1 to 10:1 will decrease the absorption of zinc in mice (44, 45). In the human intestine, a ratio of 2:1 or 3:1 of inorganic (nonheme) iron to zinc reduces the uptake of zinc (46). Heme iron, as would be derived from dietary consumption of meat and blood sausages, had no effect on zinc absorption in humans.

In short-term balance studies involving 12 elderly adults, an increase of dietary zinc consumption from 7.8 to 23.3 mg daily significantly reduced the retention of dietary copper (47). Fischer et al. (48) have localized the level of the zinc-copper interaction to competitive binding for a common intramucosal binding-protein of the metallothionein class. In their experiments with rats, a high-zinc diet reduced uptake and transfer of stable copper into inverted intestinal sacs in vitro.

Studies by Solomons et al. (49) failed to demonstrate either an inhibitory or a promoting effect of a range of doses of ascorbic acid from 0.5 to 2.0 g on the absorption of zinc in human subjects. McDonald and Margen (50) provided long-term balance data suggesting that the congeners of red wine enhance the absorption of zinc from the diet. In experimental animals, oxalates, which are potent inhibitors of iron absorption, did not affect the absorption of zinc (51).

At the tissue level, zinc interacts with a number of vitamins and other nutrients. Keltz et al. (52) found that the increment in dietary zinc from 11.0 to 19.5 mg daily produced a significant rise in urinary excretion of vitamin C and metabolites in young adult subjects. The nutritional significance of this finding remains to be elucidated. An interaction between zinc and vitamin A at two distinct anatomic levels has been identified. First, the enzyme responsible for the catalysis of the interconversion of vitamin A alcohol (retinol) to the vitamin A aldehyde (retinal) is an alcohol dehydrogenase. Mammalian alcohol dehydrogenases are zinc metalloenzymes, and the form of this enzyme found in the retinas of rats is zinc-dependent. Its activity can be reduced substantially by experimental zinc deficiency (53). In addition, zinc deficiency interferes with the transport of vitamin A out of the liver (54, 55). The major transport protein for hepatic vitamin A, retinol-binding protein, is thought to be sensitive to the zinc status of the organism (56). However, as protein deficiency and energy restriction can also reduce the synthesis or release of retinol-binding protein, the degree of influence exerted by zinc nutriture, per se, cannot be precisely determined.

Deficiencies of both zinc and essential fatty acids (EFA) result in impaired growth and scaly skin rashes. In rats, the combined deficiency of zinc and EFA had a synergistic effect, aggravating the cutaneous signs and producing growth retardation (57). Feeding of an EFA-deficient ration to chicks reduced the manifestations of zinc deficiency (58). In both rats and chicks, the combined deficiency of zinc was associated with a high proportion of arachidonic acid in the fatty acids of the skin.

ZINC REQUIREMENTS DURING TOTAL PARENTERAL NUTRITION

The solution used for total parenteral nutrition (TPN) has a variable content of zinc, ranging from 0.02–4 mg/liter (59). In patients followed prospectively during TPN, an average decline in circulating zinc concentration of 4.9–6.6 μg/dl/week has been seen (60, 61). Clinical symptoms of zinc deficiency, including alopecia, skin lesions, diarrhea, immune deficiencies, behavioral disturbances, impaired taste acuity, and impaired wound healing, have developed during TPN in patients who were not receiving supplementation with zinc. The clinical manifestations responded to the administration of zinc.

Zinc balance studies recently conducted at the University of Toronto in 24 patients undergoing TPN treatment, reported by Wolman and colleagues (62), have contributed to our understanding of the nutritional requirements for zinc during TPN. Patients (three to four in each group) were assigned to receive amounts of parenteral zinc of 0.1, 2.5, 4.0, 7.0, 13.0, and 24.0 mg/day for each of three 1-week balance periods. In patients without diarrhea or small-bowel drainage, positive zinc balance was generally achieved with 2.5 mg zinc/day. In patients with gastrointestinal fluid loss, positive zinc balance required a daily infusion of 12.0 mg of zinc. Plasma zinc levels were positively correlated with the amount of zinc infused. During periods in which a patient was in positive zinc balance, nitrogen retention and insulin secretion were improved.

Based on an improved understanding of zinc metabolism and requirements, recommendations for parenteral administration of zinc during TPN have been made (63). The human fetus accumulates zinc at the rate of 250 μg/kg/day in the final trimester of pregnancy (64). An expert committee of the American Medical Association recommended that the premature infant receive a parenteral zinc dosage of 300 μg/kg/day (63), although, due to the variability of urinary excretion of zinc, many premature infants may require a larger dosage (65). For the full-term infant and for children up to 5 years of age, the parenteral zinc requirement has been estimated to be 100 μg/kg/day. For stable individuals over 5 years of age, from 2.5 to 4.0 mg of zinc should be supplied daily during TPN. If the patient is in an acute catabolic state, zinc dosage should be increased to 4.5 to 6.0 mg. If TPN is indicated in a patient with substantial intestinal fluid loss, zinc requirements are greatly increased (62). In addition to the maintenance dose, 12.2 mg of zinc should be given to replace each liter of small-bowel fluid lost; 17.1 mg of zinc should be added for each kg of liquid stool or ileostomy fluid lost (Table 4).

Table 4. Recommended Daily Delivery of Zinc
for Individuals Receiving Total Parenteral Nutrition

Population	Amount Recommended
Premature infants	300 μg/kg/day
Pediatric patients	100 μg/kg/day
Stable adults	2.5-4.0 mg/day
Adults in acute catabolic states	4.5-6.0 mg/day
Stable adults with intestinal losses	Add 12.2 mg for each liter of small bowel fluid and 17.1 mg for each liter of stool or ileostomy output

Until recently, no commercial preparation of sterile, pyrogen-free zinc was available. Zinc had to be prepared and added to solutions by individual hospital pharmacists. The FDA, however, has recently approved the marketing of such solutions of trace minerals, and zinc for TPN can now be purchased in ampules. Two biochemical determinations apparently assist the monitoring of zinc status during TPN. First, if one has a baseline concentration of circulating zinc, serial determinations serve as an index of the adequacy of the infused dosage. Moreover, a number of investigators report that a decline in the serum alkaline phosphatase often heralds the onset of zinc deficiency during TPN (66, 67). Excessively rapid administration of parenteral zinc can cause hypothermia, sweating, and blurred vision (68). Accidental administration of 22.7 mg of zinc/liter of infusion caused asymptomatic rises in serum amylase in seven patients (69).

ASSESSMENT OF ZINC STATUS

Hindering our understanding of zinc nutrition in humans is the lack of an unequivocal tool for the clinical assessment of total body zinc nutriture. An impressive array of tests and procedures has been used clinically or investigationally to determine zinc status (Table 5). The instruments include (1) measurements of zinc concentration in tissues and body fluids, (2) determination of zinc metalloenzymes or zinc-dependent proteins, (3) functional parameters, and (4) turnover and balance. The potential and pitfalls have been reviewed in detail elsewhere (59, 70).

The most widely used index of zinc status is the concentration of zinc, either in the serum or plasma. Under certain circumstances, for example, serial determinations made during TPN or in experimental zinc depletion, circulating zinc levels do reflect dynamic changes in zinc status. However, a number of factors, listed in Table 6, affect the validity of plasma or serum levels to determine zinc nutriture. Zinc determinations are subject to external contamination during extraction, transfer, storage and handling. Plastic syringes and zinc-free tubes should be used. As red cells contain 10 times the amount of zinc as does serum, hemolysis produces artifacts in zinc concentration. Ligation of the arms with a tourniquet while blood samples are being extracted raises zinc concentration (71). Prolonged fasting raises serum zinc (72). Endogenous or exogenous corticosteroids or estrogen hormones lower zinc concentration. Leukocytic endogenous mediator(s) (LEM), produced by phagocytic cells during inflammation or infection, mediates an internal redistribution of zinc from circulation to liver, transiently lowering zinc levels. Zinc concentration falls progressively following a meal; thus, blood samples taken while the individual is fasting are preferred. The absolute concentration of albumin can be a determinant of circulating zinc. Moreover, altered affinity of albumin for zinc can, in part, explain the depression of serum zinc levels of alcoholic cirrhotic patients (73). This altered affinity may also explain the rare instances of abnormal elevations in concentrations of circulating zinc, which may be related to changes in the affinity of serum proteins for zinc (74, 75). Zinc levels in hair have been used in an attempt to determine the average zinc status over a given interval. Normally, hair grows at the rate of about 1 cm/month. Traditional analytical methods for measuring hair zinc involve the digestion of the most proximal 1 to 2 cm of a whole *tuft* of hair cut close to the scalp. Hair zinc concentration varies with age. Moreover,

Table 5.   Laboratory and Clinical Determinations Employed in the Assessment of Zinc Nutriture in Humans

Measurement of zinc concentration
  In plasma
  In red cells
  In white cells
  In hair
  In saliva
  In sweat
  In skin
  In fingernails
  In urine (24-hr excretion)

Measurement of zinc metalloenzymes or zinc-dependent proteins
  Serum alkaline phosphatase
  Red cell carbonic anhydrase
  Serum ribonuclease
  Serum retinol-binding protein
  Salivary gustin

Functional parameters
  Dark adaptation of retina
  Taste acuity threshold
  White cell chemotaxis
  Red cell ^{65}Zn uptake

Turnover and balance
  Zinc balance (intake/output)
  Zinc turnover and pool size
    (measured with radio- or stable isotopes)

shampoos, hair dyes, and rinses can contaminate hair with exogenous zinc. Various washing/rinsing procedures have been used among the various laboratories, but results obtained with different procedures are not comparable. Recently, nondestructive techniques involving anatomically and spatially oriented analyses have been developed in which proton-induced or electron-induced X-ray emission spectroscopy was used. In addition to zinc, these techniques can often provide simultaneous quantification of 20 to 50 elements in hair, and cross-sectional analysis of hair is also possible.

Table 6.   Factors Affecting the Reliability and Validity of Circulating Zinc Determinations to Reflect Zinc Nutriture

Condition	Type of Error
External contamination	False increase
Hemolysis of red cells	False increase
Use of a tourniquet during blood sampling	False increase
Prolonged fasting	False increase
High estrogen levels or use of oral contraceptives	False decrease
Use of corticosteroid hormones such as cortisone	False decrease
Infectious diseases or inflammatory conditions	False decrease
Sampling after a meal	False decrease

An exciting area of zinc status assessment is that of functional (physiologic) tests. Two sensory functions, taste acuity and dark adaptation, have been used to determine zinc status. A decade ago, zinc supplementation was reported to improve the taste acuity of individuals with hypogeusia (impaired taste-acuity thresholds) (76, 77). Taste acuity assessment has been used in a number of recent studies to assess zinc status or monitor the effects of zinc supplementation (78–82). Conclusions about its clinical diagnostic utility have been variable. As suggested by Bartoshuk (83), other parameters of gustatory function, such as taste preference or taste intensity scaling, may prove to be more sensitive and specific functional indices of zinc nutriture.

As noted earlier, zinc is a component of the retinol dehydrogenase enzyme of the retina of the eye. Both Morrison et al. (84) in Baltimore and McClain et al. (85) in Minneapolis have demonstrated a zinc-responsive night blindness in zinc-deficient alcoholic cirrhotic patients. This formal dark-adaptation testing holds promise as a functional index of zinc nutriture. Studies are currently underway to evaluate this procedure in our laboratories.

Ideally, zinc nutriture could be measured by determining the total-body exchangeable pool by isotopic dilution techniques. Unfortunately, the available radioisotopes of zinc are either too long-lived, as ^{65}Zn, or too short-lived, as ^{69m}Zn, to be of significant application in humans.

Advances in analytical methodology, however, portend a real possibility that stable, nonradioactive isotopes of zinc may soon become practical tools for the routine determination of pool size in the human body.

THE ROLE OF ZINC IN IMMUNE FUNCTION AND HOST DEFENSE

Zinc is also involved in the immune response. Several aspects of the role of zinc in immunity have been described. Gross et al. (86) found that rats that were fed zinc-deficient diets had depressed transformation of lymphocytes from the spleen, thymus, and peripheral blood in cell culture. The effects of zinc on other components of the cell-mediated immune response have been investigated. In rats (87) and mice (88, 89), T-cell helper function is depressed by ingestion of a zinc-deficient diet. In addition, zinc depletion of mice produced a significant increase in natural killer-cell activity of splenic cells (87).

Human zinc deficiency associated with acrodermatitis (90) or Down's syndrome (91) reduces the ability of the phagocytic white blood cells to move purposefully. The transformation of stimulated lymphocytes in cell culture and the ability of an individual to have a positive skin-test reaction are indices of cellular immunity. Zinc-deficient patients on TPN (92), with Down's syndrome (91), undergoing improper tube-feeding with a zinc-poor liquid formula (93) and with protein-energy malnutrition (94) showed a defect in one or both of these clinical measures of cell-mediated immunity. Zinc deficiency appears to have little effect on humoral immunity, that is, on antibodies. Zinc does seem to be involved, however, in the acute phase response to injury, a component of the host defense system by which the liver synthesizes acute phase proteins, such as ceruloplasmin and haptoglobin, at the onset of fever, infection, or inflammation. Part of the acute phase response entails the redistribution of zinc from the circulation to the liver. It has been suggested that this uptake of zinc in the liver facilitates the synthesis of these new proteins (95). The effects of a preexisting zinc deficiency on the acute phase response have not received concerted investigative attention.

CONCLUSIONS

The essentiality of zinc and its role in mammalian metabolism has moved to the forefront of nutritionists' consciousness in the past decade. RDA allowances have been set, but surveys have revealed that intakes generally fall below these levels; the biologic availability of zinc from certain foods is reduced; and its interaction with other minerals may limit its absorption under certain circumstances. On the other hand, intestinal mechanisms to regulate zinc absorption, possibly honing it to the nutritional needs of the body, appear to be operative.

Zinc depletion does occur, usually in the face of disease or with improper administration of total parenteral nutrition, and the clinician should be alert to the implications of taste abnormalities, night blindness, and immune system dysfunction. Many more clinical consequences of zinc deficiency in humans may yet be recognized in the ensuing years.

The prevalent nutritional status of the majority of individuals in the United States and around the world is difficult to estimate. This stems, in part, from inadequacies in the traditional approach to diagnostic assessment of zinc nutriture, which relies heavily on determination of zinc levels in tissue and body fluids. Contemporary strategies aim at defining the physiologic and functional consequences of marginal zinc deficiency. A promising approach to nutritional assessment may be realized in the determination of total-body pool size by the use of stable isotopes of zinc.

REFERENCES

1. Committee on Dietary Allowances, Food and Nutrition Board, National Research Council. *Recommended Dietary Allowances*, 9th ed., National Academy of Sciences, Washington, D.C., 1980.
2. M. F. Picciano and H. A. Guthrie, Copper, iron and zinc contents of mature human milk. *Am. J. Clin. Nutr.* **29**, 242–254 (1976).
3. E. Vuori and P. Kuitunen, The concentrations of copper and zinc in human milk: a longitudinal study. *Acta Paediatr. Scand.* **68**, 33–37 (1979).
4. M. Ruz, E. Atulah, P. Bustos, and J. Araya, Hierro, cobre y zinc en la leche materna: influencia del estado nutritional de la nodriza. V Congresso Latinoamericano de Nutrición, Puebla, Mexico (abstract), **83** (1980).
5. E. Vuori, S. Mäkinen, R. Kara, and P. Kuitunen, The effects of the dietary intakes of copper, iron, manganese and zinc on trace element content of human milk. *Am. J. Clin. Nutr.* **33**, 227–231 (1980).
6. R. R. Butrum, A. W. Sorenson, and W. R. Wolf, Dietary intake of zinc and copper of American infants (abstract). *Fed. Proc.* **38**, 449 (1979).
7. L. M. Klevay, S. J. Reck, and D. F. Barcome, Evidence of dietary copper and zinc deficiency. *J. Am. Med. Assoc.* **241**, 1916–1918 (1979).

8. J. M. Holden, W. R. Wolf, and W. Mertz, Zinc and copper in self-selected diets. *J. Am. Diet. Assoc.* **75**, 23–28 (1979).
9. J. L. Greger, Dietary intake and nutritional status in regard to zinc of institutionalized aged. *J. Gerontol.* **32**, 549–553 (1977).
10. J. L. Greger and B. S. Sciscoe, Zinc nutriture of elderly participants in an urban feeding program. *J. Am. Diet. Assoc.* **70**, 37–41 (1977).
11. N. F. Krebs, K. M. Hambidge, C. C. Lyle, S. F. Freeland, P. Chanmugan, and C. E. Casey, Dietary intake of zinc in pregnancy and lactation by middle-income women. Program, Western Hemisphere Nutrition Congress VI, Los Angeles, California (abstract), **82** (1980).
12. I. F. Hunt, N. J. Murphy, J. Gomez, and J. C. Smith, Jr., Dietary zinc intake of low-income pregnant women of Mexican descent. *Am. J. Clin. Nutr.* **32**, 1511–1518 (1979).
13. P. A. Walravens and K. M. Hambidge, Growth of infants fed a zinc supplemented formula. *Am. J. Clin. Nutr.* **29**, 1114–1121 (1976).
14. K. M. Hambidge, M. N. Chavez, R. M. Brown, and P. A. Walravens, Zinc nutritional status of young middle-income children and effects of consuming zinc-fortified breakfast cereals. *Am. J. Clin. Nutr.* **32**, 2532–2539 (1979).
15. G. W. Evans, C. I. Grace, and H. J. Votava, A proposed mechanism for zinc absorption in the rat. *Am. J. Physiol.* **228**, 501–505 (1975).
16. C. J. Hahn and G. W. Evans, Identification of a low-molecular-weight ^{65}Zn complex in rat intestine. *Proc. Soc. Exp. Biol. Med.* **144**, 793–801 (1973).
17. C. J. Hahn, M. L. Severson, and G. W. Evans, Structure of a zinc ligand isolated from duodenum (abstract). *Fed. Proc.* **35**, 863 (1976).
18. G. W. Evans and P. E. Johnson, Defective prostaglandin synthesis in acrodermatitis enteropathica (letter to the editor). *Lancet* **1**, 52 (1977).
19. M. K. Song and N. F. Adham, Role of prostaglandin E_2 in zinc absorption in the rat. *Am. J. Physiol.* **234**, E99–E105 (1978).
20. B. R. Schricker and R. M. Forbes, Studies on the chemical nature of a low molecular weight zinc binding ligand in rat intestine. *Nutr. Rep. Int.* **18**, 159–166 (1978).
21. G. W. Evans, Normal and abnormal zinc absorption in man and animals: The tryptophan connection. *Nutr. Rev.* **38**, 137–141 (1980).
22. G. W. Evans and E. C. Johnson, Zinc absorption in rats fed a low protein diet and a low protein diet supplemented with tryptophan or

picolinic acid. *J. Nutr.* **110**, 1076–1080 (1980).

23. L. S. Hurley, B. Lönnerdal, and A. G. Stanislowski, Zinc citrate, human milk and acrodermatitis enteropathica. *Lancet* 1, 677–678 (1979).

24. B. Lönnerdal, A. G. Stanislowski, and L. S. Hurley, Isolation of a low-molecular-weight zinc-binding ligand from human milk. *J. Inorg. Biochem.* **12**, 71–77 (1980).

25. R. J. Cousins and K. T. Smith, Zinc-binding properties of bovine and human milk in vitro: influences of change in zinc content. *Am. J. Clin. Nutr.* **33**, 1083–1087 (1980).

26. P. E. Johnson and G. W. Evans, Relative zinc availability in human breast milk, infant formulas, and cow's milk. *Am. J. Clin. Nutr.* **31**, 416–421 (1978).

27. C. D. Eckhert, M. V. Sloan, J. R. Duncan, and L. S. Hurley, Zinc binding: a difference between human and bovine milk. *Science* **195**, 789–790 (1977).

28. L. S. Hurley, J. R. Duncan, M. V. Sloan, and C. D. Eckhert, Zinc-binding ligands in milk and intestine: A role in neonatal nutrition. *Proc. Natl. Acad. Sci. USA* **74**, 3547–3549 (1977).

29. J. R. Duncan and L. S. Hurley, An interaction between zinc and vitamin A in pregnant and fetal rats. *J. Nutr.* **108**, 1431–1438 (1978).

30. G. W. Evans and P. E. Johnson, Purification and characterization of zinc-binding ligand in human milk (abstract). *Fed. Proc.* **38**, 2501 (1979).

31. G. W. Evans and P. E. Johnson, Characterization and quantification of a zinc-binding ligand in human milk. *Pediatr. Res.* **14**, 876–880 (1980).

32. K. M. Hambidge, P. A. Walravens, C. E. Casey, R. M. Brown, and C. Bender, Plasma zinc concentrations of breast-fed infants. *J. Pediatr.* **94**, 607–608 (1979).

33. E. J. Moynahan, Acrodermatitis enteropathica: a lethal inherited human zinc-deficiency disorder (letter to the editor). *Lancet* **2**, 399–400 (1974).

34. I. Lombeck, H. C. Schnippering, F. Ritzl, L. E. Feinendegen, and H. J. Bremer, Absorption of zinc in acrodermatitis enteropathica (letter to the editor). *Lancet* 1, 855 (1975).

35. C. E. Casey, K. M. Hambidge, P. A. Walravens, A. Silverman, and K. H. Neldner, Zinc binding in human duodenal secretions (letter to the editor). *Lancet* **2**, 423 (1978).

36. C. E. Casey, K. M. Hambidge, and P. A. Walravens, Zinc binding in human duodenal secretions. *J. Pediatr.* **95**, 1008–1010 (1979).

37. I. Krieger and G. W. Evans, Acrodermatitis enteropathica without hypozincemia: therapeutic effect of a pancreatic enzyme preparation due to a zinc-binding ligand. *J. Pediatr.* **96**, 32–35 (1980).
38. I. Krieger, Picolinic acid in the treatment of disorders requiring zinc supplementation. *Nutr. Rev.* **38**, 148–150 (1980).
39. K. T. Smith and R. J. Cousins, Quantitative aspects of zinc absorption by isolated vascularized perfused rat intestine. *J. Nutr.* **110**, 316–323 (1980).
40. R. J. Cousins, Regulation of zinc absorption: Role of intracellular ligands. *Am. J. Clin. Nutr.* **32**, 339–345 (1979).
41. R. J. Cousins, Regulatory aspects of zinc metabolism in liver and intestine. *Nutr. Rev.* **37**, 97–103 (1979).
42. J. Freeland-Graves, M. L. Ebangit, and P. J. Hendrikson, Alterations in zinc absorption and salivary sediment zinc after a lacto-ovo-vegetarian diet. *Am. J. Clin. Nutr.* **33**, 1757–1766 (1980).
43. B. C. Starcher, J. G. Glauber, and J. G. Madaras, Zinc absorption and its relationship to intestinal metallothionein. *J. Nutr.* **110**, 1391–1397 (1980).
44. D. L. Hamilton, J. E. C. Bellamy, J. D. Valberg, and L. S. Valberg, Zinc, cadmium and iron interactions during absorption in iron-deficient mice. *Can. J. Physiol. Pharmacol.* **56**, 384–389 (1978).
45. P. R. Flanagan, J. Haist, and L. S. Valberg, Comparative effects of iron deficiency induced by bleeding and a low-iron diet on the intestinal absorptive interactions of iron, cobalt, manganese, zinc, lead and cadmium. *J. Nutr.* **110**, 1754–1763 (1980).
46. N. W. Solomons and R. A. Jacob, Studies on the bioavailability of zinc in man. IV. Effect of heme and nonheme iron on the absorption of zinc. *Am. J. Clin. Nutr.* **34**, 475–481 (1981).
47. D. M. Burke, F. J. DeMicco, L. J. Taper, and S. J. Ritchey, Copper and zinc utilization in elderly adults. *J. Gerontol.* **36**, 558–563 (1980).
48. P. W. F. Fischer, A. Giroux, and M. L'Abbé, The effect of dietary zinc on intestinal copper absorption. Program, Western Hemisphere Nutrition Congress VI, Los Angeles, California (abstract), **84** (1980).
49. N. W. Solomons, R. A. Jacob, O. Pineda, and F. E. Viteri, Studies on the bioavailability of zinc in man. III. Effects of ascorbic acid on zinc absorption. *Am. J. Clin. Nutr.* **32**, 2495–2499 (1979).
50. J. T. McDonald and S. Margen, Wine versus ethanol in human nutrition. IV. Zinc balance. *Am. J. Clin. Nutr.* **33**, 1096–1102 (1981).

51. R. M. Welch, W. A. House, and D. Van Campen, Effects of oxalic acid on availability of zinc from spinach leaves and zinc sulfate in rats. *J. Nutr.* **107**, 929–933 (1978).

52. F. R. Keltz, C. Kies, and H. M. Fox, Urinary ascorbic acid excretion in the human as affected by dietary fiber and zinc. *Am. J. Clin. Nutr.* **31**, 1167–1171 (1978).

53. A. Huber and S. N. Gershoff, Effects of zinc deficiency on the oxidation of retinol and ethanol in rats. *J. Nutr.* **105**, 1480–1490 (1975).

54. J. C. Smith, J. A. Zeller, E. D. Brown, and S. C. Ong, Elevated plasma zinc: a heritable anomaly. *Science* **193**, 496–498 (1973).

55. J. R. Duncan and L. S. Hurley, An interaction between zinc and vitamin A in pregnant and fetal rats. *J. Nutr.* **108**, 1431–1438 (1978).

56. J. E. Smith, E. D. Brown, and J. C. Smith, Jr., The effect of zinc deficiency on the metabolism of retinol-binding protein in the rat. *J. Lab. Clin. Med.* **84**, 692–697 (1974).

57. W. J. Bettger, P. G. Reeves, E. A. Moscatelli, G. Reynolds, and B. L. O'Dell, Interaction of zinc and essential fatty acids in the rat. *J. Nutr.* **110**, 480–488 (1979).

58. W. J. Bettger, P. G. Reeves, E. A. Moscatelli, J. E. Savage, and B. L. O'Dell, Interaction of zinc and polyunsaturated fatty acids in the chick. *J. Nutr.* **110**, 50–58 (1980).

59. N. W. Solomons, Zinc and copper in human nutrition. In Z. A. Karcioglu and R. Sarper, eds., *Zinc and Copper in Medicine*, C. C. Thomas, Springfield, Ill., 1980, pp. 224–275.

60. N. W. Solomons, T. J. Layden, I. H. Rosenberg, K. Vo-Khactu, and H. H. Sandstead, Plasma trace metals during total parenteral alimentation. *Gastroenterology* **70**, 1022–1025 (1976).

61. C. R. Fleming, R. E. Hodges, and L. S. Hurley, A prospective study of serum copper and zinc levels in patients receiving total parenteral nutrition. *Am. J. Clin. Nutr.* **29**, 70–77 (1976).

62. S. L. Wolman, H. Anderson, E. B. Marliss, and K. N. Jeejeebhoy, Zinc in total parenteral nutrition: Requirements and metabolic effects. *Gastroenterology* **76**, 458–467 (1979).

63. American Medical Association. Department of Food and Nutrition. Guidelines for essential trace element preparations for parenteral use. *J. Am. Med. Assoc.* **241**, 2051–2054 (1979).

64. J. C. L. Shaw, Trace elements in the fetus and young infant. I. Zinc. *Am. J. Dis. Child.* **133**, 1260–1268 (1979).

65. K. M. Hambidge and C. E. Casey, Trace element requirements in premature infants. In E. Liebenthal, ed., *Gastrointestinal*

Development and Infant Nutrition, Raven Press, New York, 1980.
66. T. Arakawa, T. Tamura, Y. Igarashi, H. Suzuki, and H. H. Sandstead. Zinc deficiency in two infants during total parenteral alimentation for diarrhea. *Am. J. Clin. Nutr.* **29**, 197–204 (1976).
67. C. T. Strobel, W. J. Byrne, W. Abramovits, V. J. Newcomer, R. Bleich, and M. E. Ament, A zinc-deficiency dermatitis in patients on total parenteral nutrition. *Int. J. Dermatol.* **17**, 575–581 (1978).
68. L. P. Bos, W. A. van Vloten, A. F. Smit, and M. Nube, Zinc deficiency with skin lesions as seen in acrodermatitis enteropathica and intoxication with zinc during total parenteral nutrition. *Neth. J. Med.* **20**, 263–266 (1977).
69. J. Faintuch, J. J. Faintuch, M. Toledo, G. Nazario, M. C. Machado, and A. A. Raia, Hyperamylasemia associated with zinc overdose during parenteral nutrition. *J. Parent. Ent. Nutr.* **2**, 640–645 (1978).
70. N. W. Solomons, On the assessment of zinc and copper nutriture in man. *Am. J. Clin. Nutr.* **33**, 856–871 (1979).
71. B. E. Walker, I. Bone, B. H. Mascie-Taylor, and J. Kelleher, Is plasma zinc a useful investigation? *Int. J. Vitam. Nutr. Res.* **49**, 413–418 (1979).
72. R. W. Henry and M. E. Elmes, Plasma zinc in acute starvation. *Br. Med. J.* **4**, 625–626 (1975).
73. E. L. Giroux, P. J. Schechter, J. Schoun, and A. Sjoerdsma, Reduced binding of added zinc in serum of patients with decompensated hepatic cirrhosis. *Eur. J. Clin. Invest.* **7**, 71–73 (1977).
74. J. C. Smith, J. A. Zeller, E. D. Brown, and S. C. Ong, Elevated plasma zinc: A heritable anomaly. *Science* **193**, 496–498 (1976).
75. L. Soliman, S. El Safouri, G. M. Megahed, and G. El Maola, Copper and zinc levels in the blood, serum and urine of bilharzial hepatic fibrosis. *Experientia* **31**, 280–281 (1975).
76. R. I. Henkin and D. F. Bradley, Hypogeusia corrected by Ni^{++} and Zn^{++}. *Life Sci.* **9**, 701–709 (1970).
77. K. M. Hambidge, C. Hambidge, M. Jacob, and J. M. Baum, Low levels of zinc in hair, anorexia, poor growth and hypogeusia in children. *Pediatr. Res.* **6**, 868–874 (1972).
78. J. L. Greger and A. H. Geissler, Effect of zinc supplementation on taste acuity of the aged. *Am. J. Clin. Nutr.* **31**, 633–637 (1978).
79. E. Atkin-Thor, B. W. Goddard, J. O'Nion, R. L. Stephen, and W. J. Kolff, Hypogeusia and zinc depletion in chronic dialysis patients. *Am. J. Clin. Nutr.* **31**, 1948–1951 (1978).

80. K. Weissman, E. Christensen, and V. Dreyer, Zinc supplementation in alcoholic cirrhosis. *Acta Med. Scand.* **205**, 361–366 (1979).
81. D. Palin, B. A. Underwood, and C. R. Denning, The effect of oral zinc supplementation on plasma levels of vitamin A and retinol-binding protein in cystic fibrosis. *Am. J. Clin. Nutr.* **32**, 1253–1259 (1979).
82. N. W. Solomons, C. Rieger, R. Rothberg, R. A. Jacob, and H. H. Sandstead, Zinc nutriture and taste acuity in cystic fibrosis. *Nutr. Res.* **1**, 13–24 (1981).
83. L. M. Bartoshuk, The psychophysics of taste. *Am. J. Clin. Nutr.* **31**, 1068–1077 (1978).
84. S. A. Morrison, R. M. Russell, E. A. Carney, and E. V. Oaks, Zinc deficiency: A cause of abnormal dark adaptation in cirrhotics. *Am. J. Clin. Nutr.* **31**, 276–281 (1978).
85. C. J. McClain, D. H. Van Theil, S. Parker, L. K. Badzin, and H. Gilbert, Alteration in zinc, vitamin A and retinol-binding protein in chronic alcoholics: A possible mechanism for nightblindness and hypogonadism. *Alcoholism Clin. Exp. Res.* **3**, 135–141 (1979).
86. R. L. Gross, N. Osdin, L. Fong, and P. M. Newberne, Depressed immunological function in zinc-deprived rats as measured by mitogen response of spleen, thymus and peripheral blood. *Am. J. Clin. Nutr.* **32**, 1260–1265 (1979).
87. R. K. Chandra and B. Au, Single nutrient deficiency and cell-mediated immune response. I. Zinc. *Am. J. Clin. Nutr.* **33**, 736–738 (1980).
88. P. J. Fraker, S. M. Haas, and R. W. Luecke, Effect of zinc deficiency on the immune response of young adult A/J mouse. *J. Nutr.* **107**, 1889–1895 (1977).
89. R. S. Beach, M. E. Gershwin, R. K. Makishima, and L. S. Hurley, Impaired immunological ontogeny in postnatal zinc deprivation. *J. Nutr.* **110**, 805–815 (1980).
90. W. L. Weston, J. C. Huff, J. R. Humbert, K. H. Neldner, and P. A. Walravens, Zinc correction of defective chemotaxis in acrodermatitis enteropathica. *Arch. Dermatol.* **113**, 422–425 (1977).
91. B. Björksten, O. Back, K. H. Gustavson, S. G. Hallman, B. Hägglof, and A. Tarnik, Zinc and immune function in Down's syndrome. *Acta Paediatr. Scand.* **69**, 183–187 (1980).
92. J. M. Oleske, M. L. Westphal, S. Shore, D. Gorden, J. D. Bogden, and A. Nahmias, Zinc therapy of depressed cellular immunity in acrodermatitis enteropathica: Its correction. *Am. J. Dis. Child.* **133**,

915–918 (1978).

93. R. S. Pekarek, H. H. Sandstead, R. A. Jacon, and D. F. Barcome, Abnormal cellular immune response during acquired zinc deficiency. *Am. J. Clin. Nutr.* **32**, 1466–1471 (1979).

94. M. H. N. Golden, B. E. Golden, P. S. E. G. Harland, and A. A. Jackson, Zinc and immunocompetence in protein-energy malnutrition. *Lancet* **1**, 1226–1228 (1978).

95. P. Z. Sobicinski, W. J. Canterbury, Jr., E. C. Hauer, and F. A. Beall, Induction of hypozincemia and hepatic metallothionein synthesis in hypersensitivity reactions. *Proc. Soc. Exp. Biol. Med.* **160**, 175–179 (1979).

ADDITIONAL RECENT REFERENCES

W.J. Bettger and B. L. O'Dell, A critical physiological role of zinc in the structure and function of biomembranes. *Life Sci.* **28**, 1425–1438 (1981).

E. F. Gordon, R. C. Gordon, and D. B. Passal, Zinc metabolism: basic, clinical and behavioral aspects. *J. Pediatr.* **99**, 341–349 (1981).

M.H. Golden and B. E. Golden, Trace elements. Potential importance in human nutrition with particular reference to zinc and vanadium. *Br. Med. Bull.* **37**, 31–36 (1981).

A. S. Prasad, A. A. Abbasi, P. Rabbani, and E. DuMouchelle, Effect of zinc supplementation on serum testosterone level in adult male sickle cell anemia subjects. *Am. J. Hematol.* **10**, 119–127 (1981).

N. W. Solomons, Biological availability of zinc in humans. *Am. J. Clin. Nutr.* **35**, 1048–1075 (1982).

8

Recent Developments in Selenium Nutrition

ORVILLE A. LEVANDER, Ph.D.

U.S. Department of Agriculture
Beltsville Human Nutrition Research Center
Beltsville, Maryland

Address correspondence to Orville A. Levander, Ph.D., Research Chemist, Vitamin and Mineral Nutrition Laboratory, U.S. Department of Agriculture, Science and Education Administration, Beltsville Human Nutrition Research Center, Beltsville, Maryland 20705.

ABSTRACT

Beneficial nutritional responses to selenium in animals have been known for about 25 years, but only in the past few years has a nutritional role in humans been found for selenium. In 1979, selenium supplements were shown to alleviate muscular discomfort in a New Zealand patient receiving total parenteral nutrition and to prevent Keshan disease, a juvenile cardiomyopathy that occurs in certain low-selenium areas of China. In 1980, the U.S. National Research Council established for adults a safe and adequate range of selenium intake of 50–200 μg/day. Most North American diets provide quantities of selenium within that range. Some workers have noted inverse statistical associations between selenium status and the incidence of certain human diseases, especially cancer and heart disease, and are advocating selenium intakes of 250–300 μg/day as a preventive measure. The value of such elevated selenium intakes, however, has been questioned. Current research on selenium in human nutrition is directed at strengthening the scientific basis for present dietary recommendations. Any possible relationships between dietary selenium intakes and human diseases should also be examined further.

During the past few years, two major events occurred in the field of selenium nutrition. In 1979, the first reports of selenium deficiency in humans living in low-selenium areas appeared; and, in 1980, the U.S. National Research Council established a safe and adequate range of dietary selenium intake for humans. This review covers those recent developments in some detail, after providing a brief historical perspective of the selenium problem and giving a summary of progress in the understanding of the biochemical function of selenium. Human dietary selenium intakes and their possible relationship to human diseases are also discussed.

HISTORICAL PERSPECTIVE

During the 1930s, selenium toxicity was identified as the cause of alkali disease in livestock raised in certain areas of the Great Plains of the United States (1). In those regions, enough soil selenium is available for uptake by plants to cause chronic selenium poisoning in grazing animals. This discovery stimulated a great deal of research in the 1940s and early 1950s into the toxicologic properties of selenium and earned for selenium compounds a widespread reputation as poisons, with no beneficial biologic properties.

Then in 1957, Schwarz and Foltz (2) discovered that minute quantities of selenium in the diet protected against nutritional liver necrosis in vitamin E-deficient rats. This discovery led to a flurry of research in the late 1950s and 1960s as nutritionists attempted to link selenium with a wide variety of animal disorders associated with vitamin E deficiency. Several vitamin E-related animal diseases, such as white muscle disease in sheep and cattle and exudative diathesis in poultry, that have practical agricultural importance in low-selenium areas, were found to respond to selenium (3). In 1969, selenium was demonstrated to be an essential nutrient per se, since it protected against pancreatic atrophy in chicks fed selenium-deficient, but vitamin E-adequate, diets (4); selenium also prevented hair loss, cataract formation, and poor growth and reproduction in rats fed a selenium-deficient, vitamin E-adequate diet over two generations (5). In 1974, the U.S. Food and Drug Administration granted approval for the use of selenium as an additive to swine and poultry feeds to prevent nutritional deficiency diseases and has since approved addition to other animal feeds (6).

BIOCHEMICAL FUNCTION OF SELENIUM

In 1973, Rotruck et al. (7) reported that selenium was a component of glutathione peroxidase, an enzyme that destroys lipid peroxides. This finding clarified the metabolic relationship between selenium and vitamin E, since selenium, by virtue of its role in glutathione peroxidase, would remove any lipid peroxides that might be formed in vivo despite the antioxidant activity of vitamin E (8). The selenium at the active site of the enzyme is now thought to be in the form of selenocysteine, although the exact mechanism by which the selenoamino acid is incorporated into the protein molecule is still unresolved (9). Thus far, glutathione peroxidase appears to be the only well-characterized selenium protein in mammals. Numerous other selenoenzymes, however, have been reported in bacteria (10) and the search goes on for other possible roles for selenium in animal metabolism. Combs and coworkers, for example, have recently described a defect in the conversion of methionine to cysteine in the selenium-deficient chick (11), and Burk and associates have reported that selenium injection protected selenium-deficient rats against diquat toxicity by a mechanism that appeared to be independent of glutathione peroxidase activity (12).

Because of the vast amount of information generated in the 1960s showing that selenium is needed for the optimal nutrition of animals and because of the great progress made in the early 1970s characterizing the biochemical function of selenium, attention has recently focused on the implications of selenium for proper human nutrition.

HUMAN NEED FOR SELENIUM

Increasing evidence indicates that selenium is a required nutrient for humans. For example, addition of selenium compounds in vitro enhances the growth of human fibroblasts in culture (13), and selenium is a component of glutathione peroxidase purified from human red blood cells (14). Perhaps more significant, however, are the beneficial responses to selenium supplementation recently observed in certain persons living in low-selenium areas of New Zealand and the People's Republic of China.

The New Zealand case involved a patient who had been given total parenteral nutrition for 29 days because of complications after abdominal surgery (15). The patient suffered from severe bilateral muscular discomfort in the quadriceps and hamstring muscles. The muscle pain was aggravated by walking, and mobility was sharply restricted. The upper limb girdle was unaffected. The plasma selenium level of the patient at this time was only 9 ng/ml, one of the lowest levels ever recorded in humans. When 100 μg of selenium as selenomethionine was added daily to the intravenous feeding solution, all muscular symptoms disappeared within 7 days. The authors concluded that the favorable response to selenium treatment in this patient might represent the first clinical case documenting the essential role of selenium in human nutrition. Physicians are now gradually becoming more aware of the possible importance of selenium in patients receiving total parenteral nutrition.

The Chinese work implicating selenium in human nutrition concerns Keshan disease, an endemic cardiomyopathy that mainly affects children from 1 to 9 years old (16, 17). The disease occurs primarily in a region stretching from northeastern to southwestern China and is characterized by gallop rhythm, heart failure, cardiogenic shock, abnormal electrocardiograms, and heart enlargement. Selenium concentrations in the blood of residents often are below 10 ng/ml in the areas where Keshan disease occurs, but are seldom less than 40 ng/ml in other areas. Other indicators of poor selenium status in residents of the Keshan-disease areas included low hair selenium levels and depressed whole blood glutathione peroxidase activities. Analysis of several staple foods revealed that the selenium content was lower in Keshan-disease areas than in other areas.

The increasing evidence linking selenium deficiency with Keshan disease led the Chinese to carry out an intervention trial with sodium selenite in an affected area. In a trial in 1974, a group of 4510 children 1 to 9 years old was given the selenium supplement and 3985 children were given placebo controls (Table 1). Dosage was 0.5 mg sodium selenite/week for children of 1 to 5 years and 1.0 mg for those of 6 to 9 years. Morbidity due to Keshan disease was 2.2% (10/4510) and 13.5% (54/3985) in the selenium-supplemented and placebo groups, respectively. The effect of selenium was also positive in a 1975 trial, so the placebo group was eliminated in the 1976 and 1977 trials.

Table 1. Effect of Sodium Selenite Intervention on Incidence and Prognosis of Keshan Disease

Group	Year	Number of Subjects	Number of Cases		
			Alive	Dead	Total
Placebo	1974	3,985	27	27	54
	1975	5,445	26	26	52
Selenite	1974	4,510	10	0	10
	1975	6,767	6	1	7
	1976	12,579	2	2	4
	1977	12,749	0	0	0

Note: Data adapted from reference 16.

Selenium administration caused no detrimental side effects in those children. Isolated instances of nausea could be avoided by taking the supplement after meals. Physical examinations and liver function tests revealed no hepatic damage after continuous selenium dosing for 3 or 4 years.

Selenium deficiency accounted for most features of Keshan disease but did not easily explain seasonal variation. Therefore, other environmental factors might also play a role. The disease may involve a viral myocarditis that occurs in populations perhaps predisposed to infection by selenium deficiency (18). Recent studies have demonstrated that selenium deficiency increases the frequency and severity of myocardial necrosis in mice injected with a culture of Coxsackie B_4 virus (19).

SELENIUM IN THE HUMAN DIET

It is difficult to assign specific values for the selenium content of different foods because of the wide variations found, especially in plant materials. The most important factor affecting the selenium in foods of plant origin is the quantity of selenium available in the soil for translocation into the plant. Crop plants do not require selenium, so their selenium levels are directly proportional to the selenium available in the soil. An example of the extreme variation possible in the selenium content of plants was given by Schroeder et al. (20), who found that the selenium in wheat ranged from 0.04 to 21.4 $\mu g/g$. Such wide variations in the selenium content of cereals as consumed are uncommon in the U.S. food supply because of the blending and interregional shipment of grains. Some degree of variability is also possible in the selenium content of foods of animal origin, although animals exposed to extreme intakes are not likely to reach market. Other factors such as milling, cooking, processing, and so on may contribute to the variable selenium content of foods, but those effects are relatively minor compared to the effect of geographical origin (discussed in reference 21).

Although precise values for the selenium content of foods are difficult to assign, some generalizations are possible. Seafoods and organ meats are quantitatively the best dietary sources of selenium, followed, in decreasing order, by muscle meats, cereal products (depending on origin), dairy products, vegetables, and fruits (reviewed in reference 21). It must be emphasized that this ranking of food groups according to their selenium content is based upon generalizations, and exceptions can be expected. This uncertainty about the selenium content of foods greatly complicates estimation of the dietary intake of selenium. Samples representative of the foods actually eaten must be analyzed, either by analysis of foods typical of the particular region of interest or, preferably, by "duplicate plate" analyses (analysis of duplicate portions of diets collected as actually prepared and consumed) of foods from a specified area.

Little work has been done on the nutritional availability to humans of the selenium in foods. The bioavailability of selenium was recently estimated by comparison of the ability of various foods to induce glutathione peroxidase activity and to raise selenium levels in the livers of rats previously depleted of selenium (22). By the criterion of glutathione peroxidase induction, the selenium in freeze-dried, water-pack tuna was less readily available to rats than that in beef kidney or wheat from a high-selenium area. Thus, tuna, a good food source of selenium in the human diet, apparently has a low nutritional potency because of relatively poor bioavailability. Possibly the selenium in the tuna was not readily available because it complexed with mercury present in the fish. Complex formation might also partially explain the protection selenium provides against the toxic effects of mercury (23). A recent attempt to compare availability to humans of selenium from tuna and from wheat was frustrated by the relatively high mercury content of the fish (24).

HUMAN DIETARY SELENIUM INTAKES

Because of the great differences in the selenium content of soils in various countries, dietary selenium intakes vary widely among residents in different parts of the world (Table 2). The Keshan-disease areas of China, the south island of New Zealand, and certain regions of Finland have some of the lowest reported intakes, whereas Venezuela (due to a seleniferous agricultural region) and especially the endemic selenosis area of China have some of the highest. Intakes in Canada and the United States tend to fall somewhere between those extremes. A recent duplicate plate dietary survey of free-living Maryland residents consuming self-selected diets (29) showed that the mean selenium intake was 81 ± 41 μg/day. The results of this survey were remarkably similar to those of another Maryland survey that showed that the average intake among pregnant, lactating, and nonlactating women was 80 ± 37 μg/day (30). About 17–20% of all the daily diets in both surveys furnished less than 50 μg/day. Very few diets (3% or less) furnished more than 200 μg/day. Daily intakes in the second survey, estimated by analysis of separate 1-day dietary composites, ranged from 0.6–221 μg; intakes estimated by analysis of 3-day pooled composites ranged from 14–154 μg. Analysis of the diets in the first survey by food groups revealed that those diets that derived most protein and calories from seafoods were also highest in total selenium and were most selenium-dense; those diets that derived most protein and calories from dairy products and processed meats were lowest in total selenium and least selenium-dense.

**Table 2. Estimated Dietary Selenium Intakes in
Different Countries of the World**

Country	Dietary Selenium Intake (μg/day)	Reference
China (Keshan disease area)	11	G. Q. Yang, personal communication
New Zealand	28	(25)
Finland	30	(26)
USA ("market basket")	169	J. H. McLoughlin, personal communication
USA (South Dakota)	216	(27)
Venezuela (Caracas)	218	(28)
China (endemic selenosis area)	4990	G. Q. Yang, personal communication

HUMAN SELENIUM REQUIREMENTS

In 1980, the U.S. National Research Council set an estimated safe and adequate range of daily dietary intake of selenium for adults and children over 7 years old of 50–200 μg, with correspondingly lower levels for younger children and infants (Table 3). Most North American diets appear to furnish quantities of selenium within this safe and adequate range (see discussion above). The range was derived primarily by extrapolation from animal experiments, since few data from human studies were available. Several animal species apparently require selenium at a dietary level of 0.1 μg/g for optimal growth and reproduction. A person eating 500 g of a mixed diet daily (dry matter basis) containing that level of selenium would ingest 50 μg of selenium/day. To compensate for possible individual variations in selenium requirement or for the effects of other dietary factors in selenium metabolism, the range of safe and adequate intake was expanded to 200μg/day. The upper limit was established to protect against possible overdosing by abuse of nutritional supplements.

Table 3. Estimated Safe and Adequate Daily Dietary Intake of Selenium

Life Stage	Age (years)	Selenium Intake (μg/day)
Infants	0-0.5	10–40
	0.5-1	20–60
Children	1-3	20–80
	4-6	30–120
	7-11+	50–200
Adults		50–200

Note: Data adapted from reference 31.

There have been relatively few investigations of the human selenium requirement. Only 20 μg/day was needed to maintain balance in New Zealand women consuming low-selenium diets (32) and that level was suggested as a "minimum daily requirement." On the other hand, a balance trial conducted with young North American men during a selenium depletion/repletion study (24) indicated that about 70μg/day was needed to replace their urinary and fecal losses and maintain their body stores (unpublished results). The difference between selenium intakes needed to maintain balance in North Americans and New Zealanders is presumably due to differences in body pools of selenium between those two groups. The estimated whole body selenium content of North Americans is about 14.6 mg (20), whereas that of New Zealanders is only 6.1 mg (32). Some epidemiologic surveys have also helped to define human requirements. For example, the Chinese workers stated that Keshan disease was absent in those areas where the dietary selenium intake was at least 30 μg/day (17), and no known adverse human health effects have been observed in New Zealanders consuming 28–32 μg/day on a long-term basis (25).

SELENIUM AND HUMAN DISEASE

Some workers have made statistical associations suggesting that low selenium status might be related to a high incidence of certain major human diseases such as cancer or heart disease (33–35). However, those associations have been criticized by others as lacking strength and consistency (36, 37). The difficulties in assessing human selenium status by estimation of dietary selenium intake have been discussed above. Low blood selenium levels have been noted in cancer patients (38), but such levels could well be the consequence rather than the cause of the disease (39). Several experiments have shown that the incidence of virally or chemically induced cancers in rodents could be reduced by the feeding of selenium (40), but the levels of selenium fed were usually far in excess of nutritional requirements. A recent study, however, demonstrated that the incidence of chemically induced mammary tumors was increased in rats that were fed diets that were high in polyunsaturated fats and deficient in selenium (41).

Significant deleterious interactions of selenium with other nutrients have been observed in studies of experimental carcinogenesis. Pharmacologic doses of selenium combined with retinyl acetate had an additive effect in reducing the incidence of chemically induced mammary tumors in rats (42), but the combined treatment also caused changes in the estrous cycle of these animals and led to fibrotic changes in the ovary, oviduct, and uterus. In another study, supplements of high levels of either selenium or vitamin C alone decreased the incidence of chemically induced colon tumors in rats, but a combined supplement of selenium plus vitamin C increased the incidence of colon tumors (43).

Early studies indicated that selenium may have a carcinogenic rather than an anticarcinogenic effect in animals, but many of these studies were poorly designed and an elaborate later study showed no carcinogenic effect of sodium selenite or selenate in rats (see reference 44 for a review). On the other hand, the U.S. National Cancer Institute recently reported that selenium sulfide, an ingredient of some antidandruff shampoos, caused liver cancer in rats and lung cancer in female mice (45). This experiment has been criticized on the basis of inappropriate testing (i.e., very large doses that were administered by gavage), but the similarity of selenium sulfide to certain naturally occurring selenium/sulfur metabolic products suggests that further testing would be advisable.

The involvement of selenium with Keshan disease in China might seem to support the concept that selenium could be involved in those cardiovascular diseases that are rampant in Western societies, but the pathologies of the diseases differ markedly. No differences were observed in the selenium content of tissues from patients who died with or without myocardial infarctions (46, 47), and blood selenium levels of New Zealand hypertensives were similar to those of normotensives (48). However, a protective role of selenium against thrombosis was suggested on the basis of the high selenium content of human platelets (49). Rat platelet glutathione peroxidase activity is markedly depressed in selenium deficiency (50) and responds quickly and in a dose-dependent manner to shifts in dietary selenium intake (51, 52). Perhaps a role for selenium in platelet function could provide a rationale for linking low selenium intakes with high incidence of heart disease, but there is little evidence to suggest that selenium intakes greater than those commonly provided by the usual North American diet offer any additional protection against cardiovascular disease.

HUMAN SELENIUM SUPPLEMENTS

On the basis of studies showing a reduction in the incidence of experimental cancer in rodents fed selenium at levels in excess of their nutritional requirements, some workers (53) have promoted increased intakes of selenium by humans (250–300 μg/day), either by diet or by supplements, as a way to prevent cancer. Others, however, concluded that selenium supplements are not presently justified because of reasonable doubts that selenium has any practical value in preventing cancer (40). Before supplementation of the diet of humans with selenium can be advocated, its toxicity must be considered and proof obtained that it really acts against human cancer. The toxic dose of selenium for humans is not known precisely, but a tentative maximum acceptable daily intake of 500 μg was calculated (54). Moreover, the deleterious interactions of selenium with other nutrients, as discussed in the previous section, should be taken into account. One worker (55) recommended that humans take supplements of both vitamin C and selenium daily as "prudent precautions" against gastrointestinal cancer. But such dietary advice could be counterproductive if the results of rat studies indicating that the incidence of colon cancer was elevated in animals supplemented with both vitamin C and selenium (discussed above) should prove applicable to humans.

CONCLUSIONS

1. Long recognized as an essential trace element for animals, selenium is attracting more and more attention from those interested in human nutrition.
2. Two instances of beneficial responses in humans to selenium supplementation, one in a patient receiving total parenteral nutrition in a low-selenium area of New Zealand, the other in children living in a low-selenium area of China, have provided evidence for the essentiality of selenium for humans.
3. The U.S. National Research Council has established a safe and adequate range of selenium intake for adults of 50–200μg per day.
4. Most North American diets furnish levels of selenium within this range.
5. The richest dietary sources of selenium are organ meats and seafoods, followed, in decreasing order, by muscle meats, cereal products (depending on geographical origin), dairy products, vegetables, and fruits.

6. Statistical associations and animal experiments have led some workers to suggest that somewhat higher intakes of selenium (250–300 μg/day) might be of some benefit in the prevention of certain human diseases such as cancer or heart disease. Other workers, however, have disputed these claims.

7. Research planned or in progress should provide more complete information on actual human selenium requirements, but at present there appears to be little justification for North Americans to consume supplements to prevent selenium deficiency.

REFERENCES

1. I. Rosenfeld and O. A. Beath, *Selenium. Geobotany, Biochemistry, Toxicity, and Nutrition*, Academic Press, New York, 1964.
2. K. Schwarz and C. M. Foltz, Selenium as an integral part of Factor 3 against dietary necrotic liver degeneration. *J. Am. Chem. Soc.* **79**, 3292 (1957).
3. National Research Council, Agricultural Board, Committee on Animal Nutrition, Subcommittee on Selenium. *Selenium in Nutrition*, National Academy of Sciences, Washington, D.C., 1971.
4. J. N. Thompson and M. L. Scott, Role of selenium in the nutrition of the chick. *J. Nutr.* **97**, 335 (1969).
5. K. E. M. McCoy and P. H. Weswig, Some selenium responses in the rat not related to vitamin E. *J. Nutr.* **98**, 383 (1969).
6. D. E. Ullrey, Regulation of essential nutrient additions to animal diets (selenium—a model case). *J. Anim. Sci.* **51**, 645 (1980).
7. J. T. Rotruck, A. L. Pope, H. E. Ganther, A. B. Swanson, D. G. Hafeman, and W. G. Hoekstra, Selenium: Biochemical role as a component of glutathione peroxidase. *Science* **179**, 588 (1973).
8. W. G. Hoekstra, Biochemical function of selenium and its relation to vitamin E. *Fed. Proc.* **34**, 2083 (1975).
9. R. A. Sunde and W. G. Hoekstra, Structure, synthesis, and function of glutathione peroxidase. *Nutr. Rev.* **38**, 265 (1980).
10. T. C. Stadtman, Biological functions of selenium. *Trends Biochem. Sci.* **5**, 203 (1980).
11. M. J. Bunk, M. W. La Vorgna, and G. F. Combs, Jr., Evidence for an impairment in the conversion of methionine to cysteine in the selenium-deficient chick. *Fed. Proc.* **40**, 903 (1981).
12. R. F. Burk, R. A. Lawrence, and J. M. Lane, Liver necrosis and lipid peroxidation in the rat as the result of paraquat and diquat administration—effect of selenium deficiency. *J. Clin. Invest.* **65**, 1024 (1980).

13. W. L. McKeehan, W. G. Hamilton, and R. G. Ham, Selenium is an essential trace nutrient for growth of WI-38 diploid human fibroblasts. *Proc. Natl. Acad. Sci. USA*, **73**, 2023 (1976).
14. Y. C. Awasthi, E. Beutler, and S. K. Srivastava, Purification and properties of human erythrocyte glutathione peroxidase. *J. Biol. Chem.* **250**, 5144 (1975).
15. A. M. van Rij, C. D. Thomson, J. M. McKenzie, and M. F. Robinson, Selenium deficiency in total parenteral nutrition. *Am. J. Clin. Nutr.* **32**, 2076 (1979).
16. Keshan Disease Research Group. Observations on effect of sodium selenite in prevention of Keshan disease. *Chin. Med. J. (Engl. Ed.)* **92**, 471 (1979).
17. Keshan Disease Research Group. Epidemiologic studies on the etiologic relationship of selenium and Keshan disease. *Chin. Med. J. (Engl. Ed.)* **92**, 477 (1979).
18. He Guanqing. On the etiology of Keshan disease: two hypotheses. *Chin. Med. J. (Engl. Ed.)* **92**, 416 (1979).
19. B. Jin, The combined effect of selenium deficiency and viral infection on the myocardium of mice. *Acta Acad. Med. Sinicae* **2**, 29 (1980).
20. H. A. Schroeder, D. V. Frost, and J. J. Balassa, Essential trace metals in man: Selenium. *J. Chronic Dis.* **23**, 227 (1970).
21. O. A. Levander, Selenium in foods. In *Selenium—tellurium in the Environment*, Industrial Health Foundation, Pittsburgh, Pa., 1976, p. 26.
22. J. S. Douglass, V. C. Morris, J. H. Soares, Jr., and O. A. Levander, Nutritional bioavailability to rats of selenium (Se) in tuna, kidney, and wheat. *Fed. Proc.* **39**, 339 (1980).
23. H. E. Ganther, C. Goudie, M. L. Sunde, M. J. Kopecky, P. Wagner, S. H. Oh, and W. G. Hoekstra, Selenium: Relation to decreased toxicity of methylmercury added to diets containing tuna. *Science* **175**, 1122 (1972).
24. O. A. Levander, B. Sutherland, V. C. Morris, and J. C. King, Selenium metabolism in human nutrition. In J. E. Spallholz, J. L. Martin, and H. E. Ganther, eds., *Selenium in Biology and Medicine*, AVI Publishing, Westport, Conn., 1981, p. 256.
25. C. D. Thomson and M. F. Robinson, Selenium in human health and disease with emphasis on those aspects peculiar to New Zealand. *Am. J. Clin. Nutr.* **33**, 303 (1980).
26. P. Koivistoinen, Mineral element composition of Finnish foods: N, K, Ca, Mg, P, S, Fe, Cu, Mn, Zn, Mo, Co, Ni, Cr, F, Se, Si, Rb, Al, B, Br, Hg, As, Cd, Pb, and ash. *Acta Agric. Scand. Suppl.* **22**,

171 (1980).

27. O. E. Olson, I. S. Palmer, and H. Howe, Selenium in foods consumed by South Dakotans. *Proc. S. Dakota Acad. Sci.* **58**, 113 (1978).

28. M. C. Mondragon and W. G. Jaffe, Ingestion of selenium in Caracas, compared with some other cities. *Arch. Latinoam. Nutr.* **26**, 341 (1976).

29. S. O. Welsh, J. M. Holden, W. R. Wolf, and O. A. Levander, Selenium intake of Maryland residents consuming self-selected diets. *J. Am. Diet. Assoc.* **79**, 277 (1981).

30. O. A. Levander, V. C. Morris, and P. B. Moser, Dietary selenium (Se) intake and Se content of breast milk and plasma of lactating and non-lactating women. *Fed. Proc.* **40**, 890 (1981).

31. Food and Nutrition Board, *Recommended Dietary Allowances, 9th Revised Edition*, National Academy of Sciences, Washington, D.C., 1980.

32. R. D. H. Stewart, N. M. Griffiths, C. D. Thomson, and M. F. Robinson, Quantitative selenium metabolism in normal New Zealand women. *Br. J. Nutr.* **40**, 45 (1978).

33. R. J. Shamberger and D. V. Frost, Possible protective effect of selenium against human cancer. *Can. Med. Assoc. J.* **100**, 682 (1969).

34. G. N. Schrauzer, D. A. White, and C. J. Schneider, Cancer mortality correlation studies. III. Statistical associations with dietary selenium intakes. *Bioinorg. Chem.* **7**, 23 (1977).

35. R. J. Shamberger, C. E. Willis, and L. J. McCormak, Selenium and heart disease. III. Blood selenium and heart mortality in 19 states. In D. D. Hemphill, ed., *Trace Substances in Environmental Health-XII*, University of Missouri Press, Columbia, 1979, p. 59.

36. W. H. Allaway, An overview of distribution patterns of trace elements in soils and plants. *An. N.Y. Acad. Sci.* **199**, 17 (1972).

37. W. H. Allaway, Perspectives on trace elements in soil and human health. In D. D. Hemphill, ed., *Trace Substances in Environmental Health-XII*, University of Missouri Press, Columbia, 1979, p. 3.

38. R. J. Shamberger, E. Rukovena, A. K. Longfield, S. A. Tytko, S. Deodhar, and C. E. Willis, Antioxidants and cancer. I. Selenium in the blood of normals and cancer patients. *J. Natl. Cancer. Inst.* **50**, 863 (1973).

39. M. F. Robinson, P. J. Godfrey, C. D. Thomson, H. M. Rea, and A. M. van Rij, Blood selenium and glutathione peroxidase activity in normal subjects and in surgical patients with and without cancer in New Zealand. *Am. J. Clin. Nutr.* **32**, 1477 (1979).

40. A. C. Griffin, Role of selenium in the chemoprevention of cancer. *Adv. Cancer Res.* **29**, 419 (1979).
41. C. Ip and D. K. Sinha, Enhancement of mammary tumorogenesis by dietary selenium deficiency in rats with a high polyunsaturated fat intake. *Cancer Res.* **41**, 31 (1981).
42. H. J. Thompson, L. D. Meeker, and P. J. Becci, Effect of combined selenium and retinyl acetate treatment on mammary carcinogenesis. *Cancer Res.* **41**, 1413 (1981).
43. M. M. Jacobs and A. C. Griffin, Effects of selenium on chemical carcinogenesis. Comparative effects of antioxidants. *Biol. Trace Element Res.* **1**, 1 (1979).
44. National Research Council, Committee on Medical and Biologic Effects of Environmental Pollutants, Subcommittee on Selenium, *Selenium*, National Academy of Sciences, Washington, D.C., 1976.
45. National Cancer Institute, *Bioassay of Selenium Sulfide for Possible Carcinogenicity (Gavage Study)*, DHHS Publ. No. (NIH) 80-1750, National Institutes of Health, Bethesda, Md., 1980.
46. R. Masironi and R. Parr, Selenium and cardiovascular disease: preliminary results of the WHO/IAEA joint research programme. In *Selenium-tellurium in the Environment*, Industrial Health Foundation, Pittsburg, Pa., 1976, p. 316.
47. T. Westermarck, Selenium content of tissues in Finnish infants and adults with various diseases and studies on the effects of selenium supplementation in neuronal ceroid lipofuscinosis patients. *Acta Pharmacol. Toxicol.* **41**, 121 (1977).
48. C. D. Thompson, H. M. Rea, M. F. Robinson, and F. O. Simpson, Selenium concentrations and glutathione peroxidase activities in blood of hypertensive patients. *Proc. Univ. Otago Med. School* **56**, 1 (1978).
49. K. Kasperek, G. V. Iyengar, J. Kiem, H. Bobert, and L. E. Feinendegen, Elemental composition of platelets. Part III. Determination of Ag, Au, Cd, Co, Cr, Cs, Mo, Rb, Sb, and Se in normal human platelets by neutron activation analysis. *Clin. Chem.* **25**, 711 (1979).
50. R. W. Bryant and J. M. Bailey, Altered lipoxygenase metabolism and decreased glutathione peroxidase activity in platelets from selenium-deficient rats. *Biochem. Biophys. Res. Commun.* **92**, 268 (1980).
51. D. P. De Loach, V. C. Morris, P. B. Moser, and O. A. Levander, Platelet glutathione peroxidase activity in rats: An index of selenium status. *Fed. Proc.* **40**, 902 (1981).

52. V. C. Morris and O. A. Levander, Response of platelet glutathione peroxidase activity (GSH-Px) in rats fed selenite or high-selenium yeast (Se-Y). *Fed. Proc.* **40**, 902 (1981).
53. G. N. Schrauzer and D. A. White, Selenium in human nutrition: dietary intakes and effects of supplementation. *Bioinorg. Chem.* **8**, 303 (1978).
54. H. Sakurai and K. Tsuchiya, A tentative recommendation for the maximum daily intake of selenium. *Environ. Physiol. Biochem.* **5**, 107 (1975).
55. R. J. Shamberger, On your risk of stomach cancer from untreated beef. *Executive Health* **14**, (12), 4 (1978).

ADDITIONAL RECENT REFERENCES

J. S. Douglass, V. C. Morris, J. H. Soares, and O. A. Levander, Nutritional availability to rats of selenium in tuna, beef kidney and wheat. *J. Nutr.* **111**, 2180 (1981).

R. A. Johnson, S. A. Baker, J. T. Fallon, E. P. Maynard, J. N. Ruskin, Z. Wen, K. Ge, and H. J. Cohen, An Occidental case of cardiomyopathy and selenium deficiency. *N. Engl. J. Med.* **304**, 1210 (1981).

O. A. Levander, B. Sutherland, V. C. Morris, and J. C. King, Selenium balance in young men during selenium depletion and repletion. *Am. J. Clin. Nutr.* **34**, 2662 (1981).

O. A. Levander, Considerations in the design of selenium bioavailability studies. *Fed. Proc.*, in press.

C. D. Thomson, M. F. Robinson, D. R. Campbell, and H. M. Rea, Effect of prolonged supplementation with daily supplements of selenomethionine and sodium selenite on glutathione peroxidase activity in blood of New Zealand residents. *Am. J. Clin. Nutr.* **36**, 24 (1982).

9

Dietary Fiber in Human Nutrition

GENE A. SPILLER, Ph.D.
Mills College
Oakland, California

HUGH J. FREEMAN, M.D.
Faculty of Medicine
University of British Columbia
Vancouver, Canada

Address correspondence to Gene A. Spiller, Ph.D., Consultant in Nutrition Research, P.O. Box 123, Los Altos, California 94022.

ABSTRACT

Dietary fiber consists of a complex group of polymers found generally in the plant cell wall. With the exception of lignin, these polymers are all carbohydrates such as cellulose. Physiologically, dietary fiber can be defined as the sum of all plant carbohydrates and lignin that reach the colon undigested by gastrointestinal enzymes. In the early 1970s there was a resurgence of interest in dietary fiber, when certain chronic diseases common in Western countries—including colon cancer, diverticular disease of the colon, and diabetes—were found to be rare in societies consuming diets high in fiber. Extensive research in the 1970s with both humans and animals has shown that dietary fiber does have a protective effect. Of particular importance is the evidence from studies of animals of protection against chemically induced carcinogenesis and that from studies of humans of the value of diets high in unrefined carbohydrates in maturity-onset diabetes. In addition, some dietary fibers, especially gums, seem to lower blood cholesterol, but the correlation of this with the prevention of cardiovascular diseases is not yet clear. Undoubtedly, dietary fiber affects colon function, and low fiber diets almost inevitably lead to constipation. It appears that dietary fiber has an important role in nutrition.

Dietary fiber comprises a complex group of polymers (high-molecular-weight substances) found most frequently in the plant cell wall. With the exception of lignin, which is a high-molecular-weight derivative of different alcohols, such as coumaryl and coniferyl alcohols, all these polymers are carbohydrates with cellulose, hemicelluloses and pectin being the main components. Cellulose is truly the fibrous component of the cell wall and the most widely distributed. It typically constitutes about 3000 glucose units but sometimes many more. Hemicelluloses are less easy to define; they are complex mixtures of pentoses (five-carbon sugars) and hexoses (six-carbon sugars). They may contain such sugars as xylose, mannose, arabinose, galactose, glucose, and others as well as uronic acids. Pectins are usually present in smaller amounts, even though the white part of citrus peel (albedo) may

164

contain as much as 30% pectin on a dry basis. Pectins contain large amounts of galacturonic acid combined with other compounds (1).

Many other substances are associated with the plant cell wall, such as waxes and proteins. Other compounds, such as gums or mucilages, are considered part of dietary fiber, even though they are found inside the plant cell. These are often used as food additives because of their emulsifying properties.

Dietary fiber is the term that has become accepted by most researchers today. Because some of the components are not really fibrous, there have been many objections to this term and other terms, such as plantix (2), have been suggested. Nevertheless, the term dietary fiber is so widely accepted that we may be forced to use it in a manner similar to the way in which the term vitamins survived its original incorrect application (vital amines) and is today used for many substances that are not amines.

Dietary fiber can be physiologically defined as follows: dietary fiber is the sum of the plant carbohydrates and lignin that is not digested by human gastrointestinal enzymes and that, as a consequence, reaches the colon undigested (3). Once in the colon, the different polymers may, to various extents, be digested by the large number of microorganisms that make up the colonic flora. This digestion can be minimal or nil as in the case of lignin or total as in the case of pectin. Cellulose and hemicelluloses are usually partially digested by microorganisms in the colon. The degree of digestion depends on many factors, including the age of the plant.

HISTORY

Historically, it has been recognized that what we call today "unrefined carbohydrates," that is, plant foods high in plant cell wall material, prevented or relieved constipation in humans. To pick one example from the medical literature of the nineteenth century, the American physician Burne (4), in his treatise on constipation published in 1840, recommended "coarse brown bread" for the treatment of constipation. However, it was the American physiologist Cowgill who in the early 1930s did some experiments that proved that it was the fibrous part of wheat bran, rather than some other compound, that relieved constipation. After a flurry of studies in the early 1930s, fiber was set aside by nutritionists and physicians as having little benefit to humans beyond the treatment of constipation.

A tremendous revival in interest took place in the early 1970s. A British physician, Trowell, and a British surgeon, Burkitt, presented far-reaching hypotheses derived from their work in Uganda, where they had spent many years. They had noticed that certain diseases, so common in the United Kingdom and the Western world in general, were extremely rare in Uganda and Africa among people eating the local, more primitive diet high in fiber (1). Their work was supported by the careful studies of Walker (5) in South Africa who had accumulated similar evidence over many years but, not being as well-known to the medical world as Trowell and Burkitt, had not been able to find wide acceptance for his concepts. For similar reasons, the studies of Malothra in India had been largely overlooked by the scientific community (6). A careful review of the literature reveals that in the 1970s, following the Burkitt-Trowell hypotheses, the number of publications on "fiber" skyrocketed when compared to the previous 2 decades. Today, even though some of the hypotheses advanced in the early 1970s have not been totally proven, it appears that a higher intake of high-fiber carbohydrate foods could benefit many persons.

ANALYSIS

For many years, only the crude fiber values of plant foods were found in food composition tables. The crude fiber method of analysis dates back to the early nineteenth century and represents only a portion of the total fiber in feed and food. Analytical chemists agree that this is a very empirical method and that its application to human food is not desirable. In fact, it has been estimated that the recovery of fibrous polymers by the crude fiber methodology is approximately 50–80% of the cellulose, 20% of the hemicelluloses, and 10–50% of the lignin. All the pectins and gums are lost in the assay procedure.

Many methods have been developed to analyze for the total, true fiber in foods, but none of them have, as yet, been accepted as official methods in the United States. On the other hand, official food composition tables have been published in the United Kingdom that give total dietary fiber values (Table 1) (7).

Three basic approaches have been used to analyze for total dietary fiber: (1) methods based on special chemical detergents; (2) methods based on enzymes similar to those found in the human digestive system; and (3) methods based on the analysis of individual polymers or sugar components of these polymers.

Of the detergent methods, one of the most popular is the one perfected by Van Soest, referred to as the neutral detergent method. The values obtained are usually referred to as the neutral detergent fiber content of food (NDF) (8, 9). As water-soluble fractions such as pectins are lost in the analysis, NDF can be equated to the water-insoluble fraction of dietary fiber. This has physiologic and nutritional

Table 1. Dietary Fiber Content of Some Food as Analysed by Southgate

Food	Total Dietary Fiber (g/100 g)
Fruit	
Apples, raw (no peel)	2.0
Apple peel	3.7
Apricots, flesh and peel, no stone	2.1
Blackberries, raw	7.3
Cherries, raw	1.7
Currants, raw	8.7
Figs, green, raw	2.5
Figs, dried, raw	18.5
Grapes, white, raw	0.9
Lemons, whole with skin, no pips	5.2
Lemon juice, fresh	0.0
Melons, cantaloupe, raw	1.0
Oranges, no peel or pips	2.0
Pears, raw (cooking variety)	2.9
Pineapple, fresh, no skin	1.2
Prunes, dried	16.1
Strawberries, raw	2.2
Vegetables	
Beans, red kidney, raw	25.0
Cabbage, white, raw	2.7
Carrots, raw	2.9
Cauliflower, raw	2.1
Celery, raw	1.8
Lentils, boiled	3.7
Lettuce, raw	1.5
Onions, boiled	1.3
Peas, boiled	5.2
Potatoes, baked, flesh only	2.5
Sweet corn on-the-cob, kernels only	3.7
Tomatoes, raw, skin and seeds	1.5
Yam, boiled	3.9
Nuts	
Almonds	14.3
Peanut butter, smooth	7.6
Walnuts	5.2
Cereals	
Bran, wheat	44.0
Flour, wheat 100%	9.6
Flour, white (72%), breadmaking	3.0
Oatmeal, raw	7.0
Rice, polished, boiled	0.8
Bread, whole meal	8.5

Note: Data taken from reference 7.

meaning, as it is most often this fraction of the plant cell wall that increases fecal weight and alters colonic activity. The NDF methodology has undergone many improvements in the last few years to eliminate confounding effects of other components such as starch. In cereals, this was accomplished by using enzymes. As a method, NDF has the advantage of being fairly rapid and easy to use when a large number of analyses are needed, as in the cereal industry. Some commercial cereals list dietary fiber analyzed as NDF and, considering that cereals contain very little of the water-soluble fractions, these results are probably quite acceptable (8, 9) and equivalent to the total dietary fiber; the values would have poor correlation to total dietary fiber, however, should the food be high in pectins or gums.

The second analytical approach is the use of methods that would resemble the processes that take place in the human digestive system by use of enzymes at the proper acidity. This concept is very appealing to nutritionists as, if successful, it would give a good estimate of the undigested residue that reaches the colon in humans. None of the methods developed over the years has yet found wide application. Very recently, however, a great deal of progress has been made, and perhaps in a few years this approach may emerge as the best for total fiber analysis (8, 10).

The third analytical approach is the determination of individual polymers and/or of their component sugars. The Southgate method (8) has been used successfully in the past 10 years, but it is time-consuming and requires trained chemists to execute it properly. For research purposes, it is an excellent method but, like other related methods, is not yet applicable to daily, rapid analysis in industry or in the field.

As the term "plant fiber" is used very carelessly, even in the scientific literature, it is important for the reader of published research to know how the fiber was analyzed and possibly the percentage of individual polymers. Otherwise, results of nutritional studies can be very confusing, even to the experts in this field (8–10).

PHYSIOLOGIC, NUTRITIONAL, AND CLINICAL ASPECTS OF PLANT FIBERS

The effects of plant fibers on the human body can be conceptually divided into direct and indirect. Plant fiber exerts its major direct effect on the colon (large bowel); here, fiber acts as a regulatory factor preventing constipation and, even more important, possibly contributes to the prevention of some very common diseases such as diverticular disease and colon cancer. The other possible, but more controversial, direct effect is as a regulator of food intake. As such, the consumption of a high fiber diet could help prevent obesity, a major problem in affluent countries.

Plant fibers exert indirect effects on sugar and lipid metabolism, "indirect" because they are probably mediated through an effect on the absorption of these nutrients in the small intestine. All of these are beneficial effects. However, no nutrient is free of negative effects when taken in excess. When the diet is borderline in other important nutrients, excesses of plant fiber may cause poor absorption of some minerals. In the following sections, these various aspects of the function of fiber in humans will be discussed in detail.

Food Intake Regulation: Obesity

Energy intake may differ depending on the physical form of the diet ingested. In human volunteers, daily caloric intake was less on a fiber-rich diet than on a fiber-depleted diet (11). Total carbohydrate intake, especially in the form of refined sugar, correlated significantly with weight gain on the fiber-depleted diet. Dietary exclusion of refined carbohydrate resulted in an involuntary fall in total energy intake and weight, suggesting that weight loss was due mainly to removal of refined sugar rather than to increased fiber alone. Such information supports the fiber hypotheses in that avoidance of fiber-depleted foods will help to avert obesity and arrest its progress. Even though moderate weight loss may occur, evidence to date is insufficient to indicate that obesity will regress with inclusion of fiber-containing foods in the diet. For further weight loss, additional restrictions appear essential to reduce energy intake below requirements.

There are several physiologic factors resulting from fiber intake, however, that may play a role in the regulation of food intake. Depletion of fiber from food often results in the energy source becoming physically softer, more liquid and soluble. The satiating value of the energy source is reduced by fiber depletion, which is, in part, related to the reduced effort required for chewing. In addition, fiber-free plant food can be consumed more rapidly; for example, apple juice can be consumed more quickly than a whole apple of equal caloric value. Fiber-free carbohydrate also results in greater insulin secretion when ingested in the absence of plant fibers (12). Finally, many factors in food preparation cause fiber disruption, leading to more rapid absorption of carbohydrates in the intestine.

Lipid Metabolism: Atherosclerosis and Gallstones

Dietary fiber probably plays a role in the metabolism of lipids and in lipid-related disorders. Fiber may do this by absorbing and binding bile acids in the small intestine and carrying them to the feces, thus enhancing their elimination. To compensate for this, the liver will synthesize more bile acids, and, as cholesterol supplies the chemical (steroid) backbone for the synthesis of these bile acids, reduced serum and tissue cholesterol levels may result. In addition, fiber may displace food items containing fat and cholesterol and, thus, indirectly lower plasma lipid levels. Some types of fiber, such as guar gum and pectin, seem particularly effective in lowering total plasma cholesterol levels, whereas wheat bran has not proven effective. Guar gum has been valuable in the therapy of more severe lipid disorders such as type II hypercholesterolemia (13–15). A diet with 50% alfalfa meal fed to monkeys induced regression of preestablished atherosclerotic lesions in arteries, although the clinical value in humans and mechanism of action remain to be elucidated, and the effect might not be due to the fiber.

There seems to be an effect of some fiber on bile composition (the amount of individual bile acids in bile), which might be beneficial in a person with cholesterol gallstones, perhaps preventing their recurrence; but the therapeutic value of a high-fiber diet in this situation requires much more study (13).

Carbohydrate Metabolism: Diabetes Mellitus

Certain fiber-containing foods alter the metabolic response to meals containing glucose and other carbohydrates. The presence of water-soluble fibers such as guar gum alters the response to oral glucose solution administration. After a meal, there is a typical glucose rise in the plasma; this curve is flattened in the presence of guar gum, given the same amount of glucose intake. Furthermore, release of insulin and other hormones in response to a standard meal is diminished when the food is high in fiber. This altered response may be due to the sum of delayed gastric emptying, altered small intestine transit time, and delayed but not diminished absorption of sugars. Thus, it appears that the total sugar is absorbed but its rate and perhaps site of absorption in the intestine are changed.

High fiber diets appear to enhance sensitivity to insulin given to diabetic patients and permit significant reductions in insulin dosage in these patients. The effect of these changes on the reduction of clinical complications observed in diabetics after a certain length of time is unknown and needs long-term follow-up studies (11–14).

Effects of Dietary Fiber on Colonic Function and Fecal Weight

Fiber-containing food sources or specific fiber components exert profound effects on colonic function. In principle, any fiber that reaches the colon undigested will induce larger and softer feces. The exceptions are polymers, such as pectin, that are totally digested by intestinal bacteria. In common foods, it appears that the water-insoluble fraction of the plant cell wall is probably the most effective in inducing greater fecal weight.

This effect of fiber on the formation of feces is not just a simple physical effect of increased amounts of undigested matter being present. It is probably due to the sum of (1) residual fiber in the feces; (2) the water-holding capacity of the fiber particles; (3) production of various metabolites (e.g., volatile fatty acids such as acetic and butyric) by microorganisms that partially digest fiber, particularly in the cecum; (4) increased bacterial mass; and (5) increased colonic acidity.

One of the physiologically important results of increased fecal weight and soft, moist feces is the decrease of the cecum-to-anus transit time, which is the time taken by an undigested pellet to move from the cecum, the very first part of the colon after the small intestine, to the anus. This transit time varies greatly and in people who are constipated, with fecal weight of 20–40 g/day, may be as long as 5 to 7 days or more. When the fecal weight is sufficient (150–200 g/day or more), the transit time is usually 1 or 2 days (14–16).

Cancer of the Colon

The possibility that cancer of the colon might be prevented by high-fiber diets is extremely challenging. The hypotheses advanced by Malothra in India (6) and Burkitt in England (1) have stimulated intense animal research and human studies. The human studies on the precise role of fiber in colon cancer are inconclusive because such a complex disease is most likely due to many causes, some of which may be related to the food eaten—such as high fat, low fiber, perhaps low intake of antioxidants. In a study in Israel, there was a significant inverse correlation between colonic cancer and ingestion of fiber-containing foods. In other words, the more fiber ingested, the lower the incidence of cancer for that population. Similar observations have been reported in the black population of the San Francisco Bay area. In a more recent study, the diets of inhabitants of a low-incidence area of colon cancer (Kupopio, Finland) were compared to a high-incidence area (Copenhagen, Denmark). Significantly less fiber was found in the Danish diet. Even though we do not know whether it is the fiber itself or some other factor associated with high-fiber foods that is protective, the latter study points to the value of increasing the consumption of unrefined plant foods (17).

Because of the difficulty in long-term human studies, projects have been undertaken in rodents in which cancer was chemically induced. Although direct extrapolation to human disease is difficult, the use of animals has permitted examination of various isolated, purified fiber polymers. In these studies, purified cellulose, a typical water-insoluble fiber, appears protective, whereas pectin, a typical water-soluble fiber, has no protective effect. Moreover, certain forms of carrageenan, water-soluble algal gums, appear to enhance colon tumor development in animal models.

A variety of hypotheses have been advanced to explain the possible role of water-insoluble fiber in colon carcinogenesis. As the type of fiber that is protective also induces increased fecal bulk and weight and shorter transit times (17), it is possible that carcinogens are diluted in the bulkier, larger feces and their time of residence in the colon is much shorter. This is in agreement with the fact that the largest number of colonic tumors are found in the sigmoid colon and rectum, the last parts of the colon where the feces reside for a long time in constipated people. Dilution and faster elimination of cocarcinogens, that is, factors that may enhance the action of the carcinogen, would also be of value.

Other important factors are alteration of the composition and amount of the colonic microflora; changes in bacterial metabolites of various substances that reach the colon, such as bile acids; and binding of ammonia by fatty acids produced by bacteria from the fiber polymers (14, 15, 17).

Diverticular Disease of the Colon

A diverticulum is an outpouching of mucosa of the colon through the muscular, outside layer and is a common finding in older people in the Western world. Some studies have examined the effect of fiber, especially the fecal-bulking, water-insoluble fibers, on the development of diverticular disease as well as on the relief of its symptoms. This condition is very rare in certain parts of Africa where the diet is higher in fiber. In two excellent British studies, the presence of both symptomatic (painful) and asymptomatic (discovered by X-rays of the colon) diverticular disease was higher in groups consuming less dietary fiber (17). A controlled study using high-fiber or low-fiber crackers demonstrated lasting pain-relieving effects only for the high-fiber cracker. Similarly, comparison between wheat bran and a placebo in patients with symptomatic diverticular disease suggested greatest improvement in the bran group.

Observations on rodents tend to support these clinical studies, although differing colonic anatomy and possibly greater degradation of fiber in the large cecum of these rodents may limit their applicability to humans. In monkeys, the level of colonic pressure appears inversely related to the amount of fiber in the diet (14–17).

POSSIBLE ADVERSE EFFECTS: MINERAL METABOLISM AND VOLVULUS

Some evidence suggests that fiber-rich diets may reduce absorption of some essential minerals such as calcium, zinc, and iron. In spite of the large number of human and animal studies, a careful review of the literature does not provide the answer as to whether it is the fiber itself or some associated substance (e.g., phytates) that is responsible for this action. There is also evidence that the composition of the remainder of the diet may affect the degree of loss. From a practical point of view, it appears that a reasonable increase in high-fiber plant food in an otherwise balanced diet should have no deleterious effect. Undoubtedly, in extreme situations, such as that found in certain Middle Eastern diets where the majority of the calories are often derived from unleavened wheat breads, this could become a major problem. There is some evidence in favor of the hypothesis that it may not be the fiber polymers per se that cause increased loss of minerals. It appears that sprouted or yeast-leavened wheat breads cause less mineral loss than do unleavened wheat products. Similarly, in a recent monkey study, it has been shown that purified cellulose (a pure fiber polymer) did not cause any losses of calcium and iron, while wheat bran (in an unleavened biscuit) did increase these losses (18). The increased bacterial mass in the colon may also result in a slight increase in protein losses in the feces. Finally, in populations on extremely high-fiber intake, occasionally volvulus (a twisting) of the colon may take place.

Most fiber researchers agree that a balanced increase in fiber intake in the Western world should not lead to any of these problems. That an excess of an otherwise essential or beneficial substance may be harmful is true of almost any nutrient, including fiber (14, 15).

CONCLUSIONS

While some research on the effects of dietary fiber on human health has been going on for many years, it was only in the 1970s that scientists from various disciplines began an intensive study of the subject, and chemists, nutritionists, clinicians, and epidemiologists published extensively in this field. Certainly, a high intake of fiber prevents constipation in a healthy person. Even though more studies are needed to extend this effect in the colon to the prevention of such diseases as diverticular disease and colon cancer, the preliminary evidence seems to indicate that water-insoluble fibers have a beneficial effect in the prevention of these diseases and in the reduction of pain in diverticular disease.

   Diets high in unrefined, high-fiber carbohydrate food have been used
to treat adult-onset diabetes successfully in many centers, and high-
fiber diets may prevent overweight and adult-onset diabetes in many
people. The effect on the prevention of cardiovascular diseases is less
well defined, but it appears that certain gums lower serum cholesterol
and that a diet high in unrefined carbohydrates may indirectly lower
serum cholesterol because of the altered balance of fat-protein-
carbohydrate in this diet.

   There is still no agreement as to whether fiber should be called an
essential nutrient, but moderate increase in fiber intake appears
desirable for people on typical Western diets. The best way to achieve
this is by replacement of highly refined carbohydrate foods with whole
grains, legumes, vegetables, and fruits. Alternatively, fiber
concentrates such as wheat bran or guar gum may be used for specific
purposes such as the prevention of constipation (wheat bran) and
diabetes (guar gum). While a diet containing a variety of whole grains,
fresh vegetables, fruits, and beans is the optimal way to increase plant
fiber intake, this kind of change might be difficult for some people, and
the alternate method suggested (the use of a supplements) might be
the only choice. The 1980s should see additional, more conclusive
research on he effects of fiber on health and perhaps a better definition
of the desirable amount in the diet.

REFERENCES

  1. J. H. Cummings, What is fiber? In G. A. Spiller and R. J. Amen,
     eds., *Fiber in Human Nutrition*, Plenum Press, New York, 1976, p.
     1.
  2. G. A. Spiller, G. Fasset-Cornelius, and G. M. Briggs, A new term
     for plant fibers in nutrition, *Am. J. Clin. Nutr.* **29**, 934 (1976).
  3. H. Trowell, E. Godding, G. A. Spiller, and G. M. Briggs, Fiber
     bibliographies and terminology, *Am. J. Clin. Nutr.* **31**, 1489 (1978).
  4. J. Burne, *Treatise on the Causes and Consequences of Habitual
     Constipation*, Haswell, Barrington and Haswell, New Orleans, 1840.
  5. R. P. A. Walker, Gastrointestinal diseases and fiber intake with
     special reference to South African populations. In G. A. Spiller
     and R. J. Amen, eds., *Fiber in Human Nutrition*, Plenun Press, New
     York, 1976, p. 141.
  6. S. L. Malothra, Geographical distribution of gastrointestinal cancers
     with special reference to causation. *Gut* **8**, 361 (1967).
  7. A. A. Paul and D. A. T. Southgate, *McCance and Widdowson's The
     Composition of Foods*, Her Majesty's Stationery Office, London,
     1978.

8. D. A. T. Southgate, The analysis of dietary fiber. In G. A. Spiller and R. J. Amen, eds., *Fiber in Human Nutrition*, Plenum Press, New York, 1976, p. 73.

9. P. J. Van Soest and R. W. McQueen, The chemistry and estimation of fiber, *Proc. Nutr. Soc.* **32**, 123 (1973).

10. N. G. Asp, Critical evaluation of some suggested methods for assay of dietary fiber. In K. W. Heaton, ed., *Dietary Fiber: Current Developments of Importance to Health*, John Libbey Publisher, London, 1978, p. 21.

11. K. W. Heaton, Food intake regulation and fiber. In G. A. Spiller and R. McPherson Kay, eds., *Medical Aspects of Dietary Fiber*, Plenum Press, New York, 1980, p. 223.

12. D. J. A. Jenkins, Dietary fiber and carbohydrate metabolism. In G. A. Spiller and R. McPherson Kay, *Medical Aspects of Dietary Fiber*, Plenum Press, New York, 1980, p. 175.

13. J. W. Anderson, Effect of carbohydrate restriction and high carbohydrate diets on men with chemical diabetes, *Am. J. Clin. Nutr.* **30**, 402 (1977).

14. R. M. Kay and S. M. Strasberg, Origin, chemistry, physiological effects, and clinical importance of dietary fiber, *Clin. Invest. Med.* **1**, 9 (1978).

15. G. A. Spiller, E. A. Shipley, and J. A. Blake, Recent progress in dietary fiber (plantix) in human nutrition, *CRC Crit. Rev. Food Science and Nutrition* **7**, 31 (1978).

16. G. A. Spiller, M. C. Chernoff, R. A. Hill, J. E. Gates, J. J. Nassar, and E. A. Shipley, Effect of purified cellulose, pectin and a low residue diet on fecal volatile fatty acids, transit time and fecal weight in humans, *Am. J. Clin. Nutr.* **33**, 754 (1980).

17. G. A. Spiller and H. J. Freeman, Recent advances in dietary fiber and colorectal diseases. *Am. J. Clin. Nutr.* **34**, 1145 (1981).

18. G. A. Spiller, M. C. Chernoff, and J. E. Gates, Effect of increasing levels of four dietary fibers on fecal minerals in pig-tailed monkeys (*Macaca nemestrina*), *Nutr. Rep. Int.* **22**, 353 (1980).

ADDITIONAL RECENT REFERENCES

D. Kromhout, E. B. Bosschieter, and C. de Lezenne Coulander, Dietary fiber and 10-year mortality from coronary heart disease, cancer and all causes. *Lancet* **2**, 518 (1982).

D. J. A. Jenkins, T. M. S. Wolever, R. H. Taylor, C. Griffiths, K. Krzeminska, J. H. Lawrie, C. M. Bennett, D. V. Goff, and D. L. Sarson, Slow release dietary carbohydrate improves second meal tolerance. *Am. J. Clin. Nutr.* **35**, 1339 (1982).

D. A. Jenkins, Dietary fiber and other antinutrients: metabolic effects and therapeutic implications. In G. A. Spiller, ed., *Nutritional Pharmacology*, Alan R. Liss, Inc., New York, 1981, p. 117.

Nutrition in the Life Cycle

10
Nutrition and Developmental Disabilities

MARION TAYLOR BAER, Ph.D., R.D.
Childrens Hospital of Los Angeles
and
Clinical Associate and Lecturer
Department of Home Economics
California State University, Los Angeles

Address correspondence to Marion Taylor Baer, Ph.D., Director of Training in Nutrition, University Affiliated Training Program, Center for Child Development and Developmental Disorders, Childrens Hospital of Los Angeles, 4650 Sunset Boulevard, Los Angeles, California 90027.

ABSTRACT

This chapter presents a review of current knowledge regarding nutrition and the most common developmental disabilities. The introduction briefly refers to evidence for the role of nutrition in the etiology of some developmental disabilities through its relationship to low birth weight and birth defects, both of which place a child at risk of becoming handicapped. A discussion of the nutritional status of children with developmental disabilities follows, highlighting factors that are usually not considered in evaluating the normal child. These include abnormal growth patterns not related to nutrition that make growth per se difficult to use as a criterion of nutritional status.

Energy needs are discussed relative to children with Down's syndrome or neurologic handicaps, and alternative methods of determining these needs are suggested. The possibility of altered nutrient requirements based on research findings in children with Down's syndrome or with seizure disorders is presented. Finally, the importance of the interdisciplinary approach to the assessment and treatment of feeding problems is mentioned.

NUTRITION AND DEVELOPMENTAL DISABILITIES

A developmental disability has been defined by the federal government as a "severe, chronic disability which is attributable to a mental or physical impairment or combination of mental and physical impairments . . ." that is manifest before age 22 and is likely to continue indefinitely. It "results in substantial functional limitations in three or more of the following areas of major life activity: self-care, language, learning, mobility, self-direction, capacity for independent living and economic self-sufficiency . . ." and reflects the need for services of extended duration (1). The cause of the disability may be genetic transmission or may be a number of environmental factors, both physical and psychosocial, operative during pregnancy, delivery, infancy, or early childhood. Very often the origin of the problem cannot be clearly identified.

To date, the nutritional problems of children with developmental disabilities have received relatively little attention. Thus, much of the research to be presented here was published some time ago, although it still represents our current level of knowledge in many areas. Recently, through the impetus of state and federally funded programs, interest in the field has grown enormously, and publications have begun to appear that focus on or include information relative to nutrition and developmental disabilities (2–7). However, since it is still a subject with which most people are unfamiliar, the material covered by this chapter will be rather more inclusive than its title might suggest.

The purpose of the chapter is to present an overview of the relationship between nutrition and developmental disabilities. The majority of the discussion will focus on what is presently known about the nutritional status of children who have the most common developmental problems and how the nutritional needs of these children may differ from those of normal children. Metabolic disorders and other more rare disabilities will not be considered. Interested readers are referred to the book edited by Palmer and Ekvall (2) for current knowledge regarding these problems and for suggestions for dietary management.

Prior to this discussion, I would like to highlight the importance of nutrition in the prevention of developmental disabilities by referring briefly to some of the evidence that poor nutrition may be a cause, either direct or indirect, of certain handicapping conditions. For those interested in further information on the subject of "developmental nutrition," a term coined by Dr. Lucille Hurley, it is well reviewed in her text by the same name (8).

NUTRITION AND THE PREVENTION OF DEVELOPMENTAL DISABILITIES

The Surgeon General's 1979 report on health promotion and disease prevention states that ". . . the two achievements which would most significantly improve the health record of infants would be a reduction in the number of low birth weight infants and a reduction in the number born with birth defects" (9). Infants in both categories are at risk for developmental disabilities, and, in both cases, it is possible that improved nutrition could play a preventive role.

Low Birth Weight

Low birth weight has been termed "the greatest single hazard for infants" (9) because it is the leading cause of infant mortality. Table 1 indicates the magnitude of the problem. A relationship between low birth weight and poor maternal nutrition, as measured both by low prepregnancy weight and by low weight gain during pregnancy, has been observed repeatedly. It should be emphasized here that this relationship provides a potential indirect link between poor nutrition and developmental disabilities. In 1978, 236,342 infants were born in the United States who weighed 2500 g or less; this represents approximately 7% of the total number of births (3,333,279) in that year.[1] At the present time, infant deaths and birth weight are not linked at the National Center for Health Statistics. However, they are so indicated in California, so the death rate for 1977 in that state was used to estimate the number of survivors/birth weight category (see Table 1).

Table 1. Morbidity of Low-Birth-Weight (LBW) Survivors

Infant weight category (g)	<1000	1001−1500	1501−2000	2001−2500	Totals
Number of LBW infants in U.S., 1977 (National Center for Health Statistics)	17,708	21,044	45,428	152,162	236,342
Survival rate (%)[a]	23	73	92	98	
Estimated survivors in U.S., 1978	4,073	15,362	41,794	149,119	210,342
Estimated % survivors with moderate to severe handicaps	21[b]	14[c]	9[d]	6[e]	
Estimated numbers of affected children	885	2,151	3,761	8,947	15,714

[a] In California, 1977 (national rates unavailable).
[b] Average (10−13).
[c] Average (11, 13, 14).
[d] Average (11, 14).
[e] Estimate extrapolated from averages for other categories.

A certain number of low-birth-weight infants who survive develop moderate to severe handicaps. To arrive at this figure was difficult, as a developmental disability is not a reportable disease. However, recently published follow-up studies of the development of low-birth-weight infants permit an estimate of the numbers of children born that year who might have been expected ultimately to manifest a handicapping condition (10−14). The total, 15,714, or about 13% of low-birth-weight infants, may be a conservative estimate, as these figures refer only to moderate and severe disabilities. The number would undoubtedly be

[1] National Center for Health Statistics, personal communication.

higher if milder problems, such as learning disabilities, which are more difficult to detect and which may not become apparent before a child reaches school age, had been included. However, it is sufficient to demonstrate the importance of preventing low birth weight so that developmental disabilities may be prevented. This is not to say that adequate maternal nutrition would prevent all low birth weight; however, even a modest reduction in the number of these infants would mean a great savings, both in human and in economic terms.

Birth Defects

The mammalian fetus was long considered to be a parasite, taking whatever nutrients were needed from the mother, regardless of the maternal diet. We now know that this is not the case, but that the nutritional state of the mother may profoundly affect the development of her offspring.

Since the 1930s when Hale first showed that the birth defects seen in pigs born to vitamin A-deficient mothers were due to a lack of the vitamin rather than heredity (15), every species tested has proved to be vulnerable to deficiencies of vitamin A during pregnancy. Also, deficiencies of other nutrients such as riboflavin, folacin, manganese, and zinc have been associated with birth defects in animals (8).

The evidence for such a link in humans is very scanty, but it is accumulating. For example, in the Middle East where zinc deficiency is prevalent, the incidence of congenital malformations of the central nervous system is also high. In 1973, epidemiologists Sever and Emanuel suggested that the two might be associated, since abnormalities of the central nervous system are commonly seen in zinc-deficient animals (16). Recently it was reported that serum zinc levels of 10 Turkish mothers of anencephalic (without a brain) infants were significantly lower than those of 90 mothers of normal infants (17). Another recent study of infants with cystic spina bifida (a spinal column defect) and their mothers found significant differences in maternal hair zinc levels and in infant growth parameters that were suggestive of an abnormality in zinc availability or metabolism in the mothers of these infants (18).

Also, three out of seven documented pregnancies in women with acrodermatitis enteropathica, a genetic disorder of zinc metabolism, resulted in two newborns with major abnormalities (one anencephalic) and one spontaneous abortion (19). These suggestive reports are far from conclusive, and further investigation is needed. However, they strongly indicate that the importance of prenatal nutrition goes beyond prevention of the risks associated with low birth weight.

NUTRITIONAL STATUS OF CHILDREN WITH DEVELOPMENTAL DISABILITIES

Developmentally disabled children are susceptible to the same nutritional problems as are seen in the general population. But they also may be subject to additional nutritional risk factors due, either directly or indirectly, to their physical disabilities and/or cognitive delay, or to altered nutrient requirements caused by their medical diagnosis and/or the medications used to control the condition.

Physical Growth and Development

In children, the first clinical sign of poor nutrition is a deficit in weight for their height. If this condition is prolonged, the child's height is also affected. A slowing in growth rate or evidence of growth retardation is, therefore, an indication of poor nutritional status.

Children with developmental disabilities are often small in comparison to their normal peers (20). Many of the children have organic impairments which cause growth retardation; but, in the absence of those conditions, an explanation for the high incidence of reduced growth is not available. The question, then, is whether the small size is an indication of less-than-optimal nutritional status, as one might suspect among normal children, or whether it is simply another manifestation of the extradietary factor(s) that are responsible for the handicap, or both. Although the importance of considering nutrition in the evaluation of the growth patterns of developmentally disabled children was suggested as long ago as 1883 (21), no comprehensive study of the nutritional status of such children has been published. Therefore, the role of nutrition has not yet been elucidated.

Early studies of physical growth among mentally retarded subjects (21–23) tended to correlate size with intelligence quotient (I.Q.), and even some more recent investigators have suggested that the mechanism responsible for mental retardation also causes the growth failure (20, 24). Kugel and Mohr (24), for example, surveyed 811 retarded children between the ages of 2 days and 16 years. They reported that, with decreases in intellectual levels, greater proportions of the children fell below the 17th percentile of the Iowa scale in height and weight. They did not say this was a cause and effect relationship, but suggested that a "reasonable hypothesis" was that the brain defect was responsible. No apparent consideration was given to nutritional aspects, nor was any distinction made among the various causes of the mental retardation. Furthermore, the importance of such factors as heredity and socioeconomic status was seemingly ignored.

At the present time it is more generally recognized that impaired physical growth and mental retardation may be independent of each other and that it is necessary to consider all the possible reasons for small stature, including those that would apply to the mentally normal child. Such reasons could include any one or a combination of the following factors. In each case, growth retardation, with or without mental retardation, has been recognized as being a possible manifestation of the disorder.

1. *Defect of a Major System.* In cases of prenatal brain damage, associated congenital malformations are common. When these involve the cardiac, renal, or gastrointestinal system, there may be related growth retardation due to secondary malnutrition.

2. *Endocrine Disorders.* Disorders such as a thyroid abnormality or pituitary insufficiency may cause growth retardation.

3. *Chromosomal Defects.* A comprehensive list of conditions associated with growth retardation has been published by Langer (25). The most serious of these result from chromosomal aberrations. Children with Down's syndrome, for example, are known to have specific growth abnormalities (26, 27). They tend to be consistently below the normal range in standing height, which is typically due to failure of normal leg growth (sitting height approaches normal), so that infantile body proportions persist. Their heads are also small and grow very little after the age of 3 years so that many have abnormally small heads (28).

A recent longitudinal study of 90 children with Down's syndrome from birth to 3 years (29) has confirmed that these children are born small (mean birth weight was 0.61 SD below the normal mean), implying prenatal growth retardation. The growth rate continued to slow after birth until at 3 years it was over 2 SD below the control mean (Stuart data, see reference 29). Based on her data, Cronk (29) has published growth charts for the first 3 years which are perhaps more appropriate to use in assessing the growth of children with Down's syndrome. After this age, the measurements of a subsample, followed for 3 more years, indicated a normal growth rate; and data from an earlier longitudinal study (30) suggest that this normal rate is maintained, at about 2 SD below the mean, from ages 7 to 18. This would suggest that after age 3 normal growth charts may be used to monitor the child's growth rate.

4. *Certain Prenatal Infections.* Prenatal infections such as rubella, syphilis, cytomegalovirus, and toxoplasmosis are associated with growth retardation. One way in which viruses may cause stunted growth is through chromosomal damage. Boué and Boué (31) cultured embryonic cells with the rubella virus and found decreases in cell division and increases in chromosomal breaks which resulted in fewer viable cells. The combined result, a decrease in the absolute number of cells, would certainly affect the size of the fetus. One follow-up study of 50 persons with congenital rubella revealed that, as adults, 50% were below the 10th percentile for height and/or weight (32).

5. *Metabolic Disorders.* Following is a list of some major categories of metabolic disorders with selected examples of each. These will not be discussed further; their implications for growth are well recognized.

Amino acid: phenylketonuria, maple syrup urine disease, homocystinuria.
Organic acid: lactic acidosis.
Carbohydrate: galactosemia, glycogen storage disease.
Mucopolysaccharide: Hurler's syndrome, Hunter's syndrome.
Lipid: Niemann-Pick disease, Gaucher's disease, Tay-Sachs disease.
Protein: Marfan's syndrome, Ehlers-Danlos syndrome.
Mineral: Wilson's disease.
Vitamin: dependency syndromes such as vitamin B-6, vitamin D.

6. *Recognizable Syndromes.* Many, if not most, of the common syndromes causing or associated with mental retardation or growth retardation would be covered in the above categories. Some additional examples are listed below (33).
Syndromes associated with growths or skin lesions such as tuberous sclerosis.
Syndromes with facial defects or oral-facial-digital defects such as Treacher—Collins syndrome.
Syndromes with skeletal defects such as achondroplasia.
Others such as Menkes' syndrome and fetal alcohol syndrome.

7. *Specific Central Nervous System Lesions.* Knowledge of neurophysiologic growth-regulating mechanisms in the brain is as yet incomplete. Mosier and coworkers (26) summarized animal studies that have shown that lesions in various areas of the brain, including the hypothalamus, can affect growth patterns. Often this alteration in growth is due to nutritional and endocrine disturbances, such as reduced food intake, thyroid abnormalities, or pituitary insufficiency, which accompany the lesion. However, in other cases no metabolic abnormalities can be found that might be responsible for stunting (34).

Hypothalamic lesions in the human also may greatly retard growth (35, 36), but some mentally deficient children have no associated physical retardation (37). Apparently then, the theory of damage to a presumed growth center cannot explain all subnormal growth in this population.

8. *Neuromuscular Pathology.* Nutritional status has rarely been considered in a meaningful way in studies of the growth of handicapped children. Only in the case of children with neuromuscular damage has there been any real effort to look at this parameter, probably because the motor dysfunction of the oral-pharyngeal area often obviously affects food intake. Tobis and associates (38) found that growth depression in 86 children with cerebral palsy was associated, not with intelligence, but with the severity of the motor involvement as measured by the number of affected extremities. This was reflected in two specific areas. One was the inability to walk, which increased the probability of depressed growth. Normal muscle tone and motor activity are considered necessary for normal long bone growth. Also, immobilization produces negative nitrogen and calcium balances (39). The other area was dependence in feeding. Severity of motor involvement is also associated with decreased nutritive value of the diet (40) and poor food intake (41). Studies of the actual nutrient intakes of these children show that they are consistently and significantly below those of normal children on the basis of kcal/cm height or kcal/kg weight (42) and also below the Recommended Dietary Allowances (RDA) for calories (40, 41). These findings would tend to support the suggestion that nutritional deficits over the years could promote substandard growth. Delayed skeletal age is another finding in children with cerebral palsy and may, again, be due to inadequate nutrient intake (40, 42).

Children with cerebral palsy have also been reported to have increased extracellular water and a reduced body cell mass as compared to normal children (43). Inactivity and malnutrition were considered relevant causes. In another study carried out by these investigators, however, no increase in body cell mass and no growth spurt could be demonstrated following improvements in dietary intake or physical activity, although in the latter case oxygen utilization was improved (44).

9. *Use of Stimulant Drugs.* The chronic use of the stimulant drug methylphenidate hydrochloride (Ritalin) and dextroamphetamine sulfate (Dexedrine) to treat hyperkinesis in children has been reported to cause a significant depression in growth (45, 46), which does not always respond with a rebound when the treatment is stopped (47). It appears that the drugs cause appetite suppression; food intakes of

treated children are significantly reduced, especially in the case of dextroamphetamine sulfate (45, 48).

10. *Socioeconomic Status: Psychosocial Deprivation.* In over 50% of retarded children there is no recognizable brain lesion (49), and the terms functional retardation and cultural familial retardation have been applied to them. Reports concerning the incidence and severity of growth retardation among these children relative to others within the developmentally disabled population and to the general population have been inconsistent (20, 26, 28, 37, 50). In a study of 514 children, approximately 80% of whom were classified as moderately or severely retarded, Roberts and Clayton (20) observed that the children of "nonspecific subnormality" were not stunted greatly in their physical development, whereas the retarded children with associated organic dysfunctions were noticeably smaller. Others have reported similar differences in growth between the functionally retarded and the other segments of the developmentally disabled population (28, 35, 37). In contrast to these reports, however, Mosier and coworkers (26) found no difference in the degree of stunting among diagnostic categories, with the exception of "mongolism" (Down's syndrome). Although the stunted growth may be less prevalent among the functionally retarded than among other children with developmental disabilities, many of the causes of growth retardation in the other groups are not present in this one. Thus, the chances are greater that their stunted growth may be due to undernutrition. Certainly, however, the possible influence of other environmental factors cannot be ignored.

Within a population of 77 children with cultural–familial retardation but with no detectable organic damage, Bailit and Whelan (50) looked for factors besides I.Q. that might be associated with the smaller size of these children, including maternal age, parity, sibling size, birth weight, birth order, age at admission, and length of time in an institution. The last two factors were included because one explanation for growth retardation among institutionalized children has been the emotional as well as physical hardships of life there, as opposed to being reared at home. These workers found that I.Q. and size were not related within the sample, but that both were positively and significantly correlated with birth weight (although none was premature). In terms of five of the 11 physical measurements obtained, the children who had a lower birth weight were significantly smaller. The other six measurements approached significance. Leg length was especially affected, and it is interesting to recall that this is often the case in malnourished children, the reason being that the legs grow more from birth to adolescence than do other parts of the body and so are more affected. Other observations that have been made on the general population of retarded children, such as the fact that they have smaller head circumferences, grow at a slower rate for a longer period of time (26, 51), and experience delayed onset of puberty (52) are also reminiscent of undernourished children in developing countries.

Developmentally delayed children, particularly the functionally retarded, are found in greater numbers among the lower socioeconomic groups (38), and lower socioeconomic groups appear to be at greatest risk of nutritional deficiency (53—55). However, the nutritional status of functionally retarded children has not been studied in relation to their physical growth. In fact, all variables related to heredity and environment have received little attention in evaluations of growth retardation in the functionally retarded population. Normal populations, not controlled for socioeconomic status, race, parity, number of siblings, and so on, have been used as comparison groups (56). Thus, questions can be raised as to the true etiology of the apparently stunted growth. Undoubtedly, many factors are involved; yet, given the higher incidence of both functional retardation and malnutrition in lower socioeconomic groups and what is known relative to the effects of early malnutrition on the developing brain (57), it is interesting to speculate about the extent to which a connection may someday become apparent.

NUTRIENT REQUIREMENTS
Energy

Children with mental retardation who have no neuromuscular involvement have been reported to have the same energy requirements as normal children if stature, rather than age, is used as a criterion for estimating those requirements (58). In the case of children with Down's syndrome, for example, a study of well-nourished 5—12-year-olds (59) indicated that their energy consumption based on height was approximately that of the average normal child 4—10 years of age. The intake of the boys was 16.1 kcal/cm height and that of the girls was 14.3 kcal/cm height; the average, 15.2 kcal/cm height, is only slightly lower than the average of 16.2 kcal/cm height for normal children (as calculated from the recommendations of the National Research Council) (60).

Children with Prader—Willi syndrome, a disorder characterized by pathologic overeating and gross obesity, however, have greatly reduced energy needs. It has been reported that they may maintain their weight (during a weight control program) on as few as 8.4 kcal/cm height/day (61).

Children with cerebral palsy may also have altered energy needs. Swedish studies measuring oxygen uptake indicate a decreased energy requirement, or about 71% of that expected for normal children with the same body cell mass (43). No difference was seen between children with spasticity and those with athetosis, the two most common forms of cerebral palsy. Culley and Middleton (58) measured the dietary energy intake of children with cerebral palsy who were of normal weight for height (50th percentile ± 10%) in an attempt to determine their energy needs. The children were aged 5–12, institutionalized, and moderately to profoundly retarded. The results indicated that within this age group energy consumption/cm height was constant over a wide range of heights and, therefore, appeared to be a good criterion for estimation of need. The type of motor dysfunction also made no difference in this study. However, the child's ambulatory status did affect energy consumption, which increased from an average of 11.1 kcal/cm height for those who did not walk to an average of 13.9 kcal/cm height for those who were ambulatory with some motor dysfunction to an average of 14.7 kcal/cm height for those who walked normally. These averages are well below the average recommended energy intake of 16.2 kcal/cm height for normal children 4–10 years of age (60).

Individual Nutrients

To date there are very few indications that children with developmental disabilities have different nutrient requirements than do normal children due to their condition per se. An obvious exception is children with metabolic disorders. Children with other genetic, or chromosomal, disorders could also have potentially different nutrient needs because of the altered genetic material.

Down's Syndrome. The pathogenesis of many of the well-known symptoms of Down's syndrome is unknown. At least two of these, decreased muscle tone and decreased resistance to infections, have led to speculation about the possibility of an increased need for certain nutrients secondary to inefficient or altered metabolic pathways.

Pyridoxine (Vitamin B-6). Children with Down's syndrome have been reported to have abnormalities in pyridoxine and/or tryptophan metabolism as manifested, for example, by decreased urinary excretion of xanthurenic acid and indoleacetic acid following an oral tryptophan load and by lowered levels of pyridoxal phosphate in the white blood cells as compared to normal children. Furthermore, they have abnormally low levels of blood 5-hydroxytryptamine (serotonin), an important regulatory amine (62).

These observations have led some clinicians, concerned about the decreased muscle tone common to children with Down's syndrome, to attempt to treat this symptom with 5-hydroxytryptophan, the immediate precursor of serotonin, or pyridoxine, the cofactor necessary for the reaction. The results of such trials have been mixed, but have generally been negative (63–66). The studies did not adequately address the question of the vitamin B-6 status of these children; no dietary information is reported, for example. However, until such time as this research is done, it would appear that routine supplementation with this vitamin is not indicated.

Vitamin A. Certain clinical signs in children with Down's syndrome, such as a high incidence of upper respiratory infections, skin lesions, and inflammation of the eyelid, plus evidence of impaired dark adaptation and vitamin A absorption (62, 67), are suggestive of altered vitamin A absorption and/or metabolism. Serum vitamin A levels have usually, but not always (68), been reported to be decreased in comparison with both normal and mentally retarded controls. However, the actual values have generally been within the acceptable range, if the Interdepartmental Committee on Nutrition for National Defense (ICNND) criterion of 20 μg/dl is used as the lower limit of normal. There is apparently no defect in the mechanism of conversion of carotene to vitamin A (68).

In a recent intervention study, Palmer (67) paired children with Down's syndrome with their normal siblings and then supplemented half of the pairs with vitamin A (1000 I.U./kg/month) for 5 months. Significant findings at baseline were that the children with Down's syndrome had lower plasma vitamin A levels, decreased vitamin A absorption from an oily medium, and a higher incidence of infection and immunoglobulin levels (serum IgG and secretory IgA) than did the controls. At the end of the trial, the plasma vitamin A levels in the treated children with Down's syndrome had increased significantly and were no longer different from levels in the normal controls, although they were still significantly lower than those of the treated controls. A significant decrease in the incidence of infection, improvement in absorptive ability, and reduction of serum IgG were also reported in the treated children with Down's syndrome. In the control group, the children with Down's syndrome continued to show a higher frequency of infection than did their siblings, which led Palmer to hypothesize that abnormalities in vitamin A metabolism were linked to the increased susceptibility to infection.

Zinc. Low serum zinc levels have also been reported in children with Down's syndrome (69), and some of the clinical symptoms mentioned in conjunction with the hypothesized vitamin A deficiency above, such as the skin and eye lesions and decreased resistance to infection, are also common in zinc deficiency. Furthermore, zinc deficiency can result in lower serum vitamin A levels because zinc is essential for the mobilization of vitamin A from the liver. Also, a zinc-dependent enzyme mediates the conversion of retinol (vitamin A) to retinal (essential for dark adaptation) in the eye. Because of these interactions it is possible that some of the confusing data with respect to possible vitamin A deficiency in these children might be explained by a zinc deficiency. It is clear that further investigation of this subject is warranted; measurements of circulating vitamin A levels following the zinc supplementation might be especially interesting.

Recently, Swedish workers (70) reconfirmed the finding of lowered serum zinc concentration in children with Down's syndrome in conjunction with several signs of lowered immunity (depressed cell-mediated immunity and leucocyte chemotaxis), which were improved by the administration of zinc (135 mg/day) for 2 months. Again, no dietary information was given, so it is difficult to tell whether the apparent zinc deficiency was due to dietary inadequacy, to increased need due to poor absorption, or to utilization possibly related to the chromosomal abnormality.

Seizure Disorders. Children with seizures who are treated with anticonvulsant drugs may have an increased requirement for certain nutrients because of their medical treatment. To date, certain of these medications have been reported to affect the utilization of folacin, vitamin D, riboflavin, vitamin B-6, and vitamin E. The effects of many other commonly used drugs have not been tested; nor have the effects of drugs on all nutrients been evaluated (71).

Folacin. Treatment with phenytoin (Dilantin), phenobarbital, and primidone (Mysoline) has been associated with subnormal (5 ng/ml) serum folacin levels in 33−89% of tested nonanemic, drug-treated children (72−78). Macrocytosis (large red blood cells), when determined, was observed in fewer (19−25%) children (73, 74). Frank megaloblastic anemia is more infrequent, occurring in less than 1% of epileptic patients of all ages according to one estimate, although early megaloblastic changes in bone marrow have been reported to be more common than macrocytosis (79). Serum vitamin B-12 levels have generally been found to be within normal limits or transiently subnormal and correctable with folacin therapy (80).

The mechanism for the disturbance in folacin metabolism is still unknown; four hypotheses, proposed by workers in the field and summarized by Reynolds (79), are (1) folacin malabsorption, (2) drug-induced synthesis of folacin metabolizing enzymes, (3) competitive interaction between the structurally similar drugs and the folacin coenzymes, and (4) increased need for folacin as a coenzyme for hydroxylation of the drug metabolites or for other hepatic enzymes induced by the drugs (76–78).

Folacin supplementation causes a rapid rise in serum and whole blood folacin. The dosage given has usually been 15 mg/day (75, 77, 79). However, in one case, 5 mg/day was used (77) and, in another, the dosage was lowered to 5 mg/week after 4–6 weeks of therapy and was found to be sufficient to maintain normal serum levels (78).

Reynolds (80) reports an increase in the number of seizures experienced during long-term (up to 3 years) folacin supplementation of epileptic adults and has postulated that folacin and its derivatives have convulsant properties (79). However, other workers have found no such exacerbation of the condition in children for periods up to 18 months (73, 76–78).

Vitamin D. Bone development and the metabolism of vitamin D and calcium have also been shown to be affected by anticonvulsant drugs. Again, phenytoin, phenobarbital, and primidone have been implicated. Biochemical indications of vitamin D deficiency in treated children have included depressed serum calcium (81–85) and phosphorous (82–86) and significantly increased serum alkaline phosphatase (81–86).

Radiologic confirmation of osteomalacia was reported in three of 12 children found by Silver and coworkers (86) to have biochemical values suggestive of vitamin D deficiency. Other studies suggest that the incidence of rickets or osteomalacia among those treated with anticonvulsant drugs in the United States ranges from 8–56% (85, 87).

Where it has been determined, serum 25-hydroxycholecalciferol has been found to be significantly depressed in children treated with anticonvulsants as compared with controls (81, 83, 84). Winnacker and coworkers (82), however, found this to be true only of children receiving primidone. In their subjects, they also noted a slight, nonsignificant rise in immunoreactive parathyroid hormone, consistent with a mild degree of vitamin D deficiency; whereas Tolman and associates (85) found significant elevations.

The mechanism by which rickets develops in children with epilepsy is presumed to be induction by the anticonvulsant drugs of hepatic microsomal enzymes that convert cholecalciferol (vitamin D_3) to inactive metabolites rather than to 25-hydroxycholecalciferol. Hunter and coworkers (81) have shown that urinary D-glucaric acid excretion, a quantitative index of hepatic enzyme induction, was raised in 94% of the children on drugs whom they studied. The enzyme induction theory is also supported by the fact that although simple vitamin D therapy corrects the signs of osteomalacia (84, 86, 87), the use of 25-hydroxycholecalciferol is much more effective (88, 89).

It appears that factors other than drug dosage, duration of treatment, numbers of drugs, or serum levels of the drugs may be important in determining the susceptibility of the child (82). In some of the studies of vitamin D and calcium metabolism in children treated with anticonvulsant drugs (83, 84), the biochemical abnormalities have been impressive. In others (82), only a minimal degree of vitamin D deficiency was demonstrated. Also, the dosage of vitamin D required to normalize biochemical values may be as modest as 3000 I.U./week (86), whereas in other cases many times that amount may be necessary (90). A deficiency in the dietary intake of vitamin D is also not a consistent factor. In the studies by Lifshitz and Maclaren (83) and Hahn and associates (84), the children were consuming greater amounts of vitamin D but had more severe signs of vitamin D deficiency than did the subjects of Winnacker and coworkers (82) who had a lower vitamin D intake. However, the former studies, as well as that of Tolman and associates (85), were carried out on populations of institutionalized children who were more severely physically involved. It is possible that the associated reduction in physical activity and exposure to sunlight could explain the more abnormal serum chemistries in these children, since Winnacker's group carefully controlled for the amount of outdoor activity experienced by their subjects. Other investigators (91) have found a lower incidence of hypocalcemia in institutionalized adult epileptics who worked outdoors as compared with those working indoors. Another factor may be the individual variation in the degree to which liver enzymes can be induced, as evidenced by the wide range of urinary D-glucaric acid excretion seen in the investigation of Hunter and coworkers (81).

Riboflavin. One study of 24-hour urinary riboflavin excretion in children treated with a variety of anticonvulsants showed a significant decrease as compared with controls (92). This decrease occurred in spite of an adequate riboflavin intake which was not different from that of the normal children. The duration of drug treatment did not appear to be a factor; in fact, the younger children appeared to be the most affected.

Erythroid aplasia due to long-term treatment with phenytoin was prevented from recurring by the administration of 120 mg riboflavin/day (93). No mechanism of action was proposed.

Pyridoxine. A high percentage of children with seizures excrete abnormal amounts of tryptophan metabolites after a tryptophan load (94–97). A possibility exists that this may be due to a relative pyridoxine deficiency induced by anticonvulsant medication, although the data are not clear (98). Pyridoxine deficiency and dependency syndromes are characterized by seizures, and some authors have noted clinical improvement following pyridoxine therapy in several cases of seizures in children with adequate dietary B-6 (98).

Reinken and coworkers (99) measured erythrocyte glutamic oxalacetic transaminase (EGOT) activity and its response to in vitro saturation with pyridoxal-5-phosphate in 30 epileptic children (3 months to 12 years) treated with a variety of anticonvulsants, including phenobarbital, phenytoin, and primidone. The enzyme activity, both nonsaturated and saturated, was found to be significantly lower than that of a control group (25 normal children aged 2 months to 11 years). Relative increases, however, were significantly higher in the group with seizures. The authors concluded that there is a possibility that the changes in tryptophan metabolism seen in epilepsy may be due to drug-induced pyridoxine deficiency.

Vitamin E. A study was recently conducted (100) comparing the plasma α-tocopherol levels in 100 children (aged 2–12 years) receiving anticonvulsant drugs with those of 100 normal children of the same ages. The levels of the treated children as a group were significantly lower, although there were no differences in the values of the children in the lower age group (2–6). In the control group there was a significant positive relationship between plasma vitamin E and age; this rise was not seen in the treated children and accounted for the overall difference. No possible mechanisms were offered to explain this phenomenon, although it was established that the anticonvulsant drugs did not interfere with the analysis for α-tocopherol. The clinical significance is also unclear.

FEEDING PROBLEMS

All children are susceptible to the development of problems centered around feeding, a regularly occurring event that can easily become a focus of parent-child struggles. It has been estimated, in fact, that fully 25% of the children in the United States have some recognized feeding problem. It is probable that the incidence is actually higher, since published figures represent only those problems brought to professional attention (101).

Children with developmental disabilities are even more at risk for feeding problems than is the general pediatric population. An estimate of the incidence, again based on clinic attendance, has been placed at 33% (102). The greater prevalence in these children is due to the fact that, in addition to having the problems common to normal children, some developmentally delayed children are also susceptible to difficulties whose primary cause is neuromotor dysfunction and/or structural abnormalities and/or cognitive delays (2, 3, 7, 28, 39, 85).

In addition, many parents and professionals are not able to recognize cues indicating developmental readiness for the acquisition of feeding skills, and these must often be taught to a handicapped child. The failure to provide appropriate stimulation at critical times often leads to prolonged bottle feeding and delayed introduction of foods of increasing textures, and this compromises the child's nutritional status and dental health and results in his/her later refusal to accept new feeding techniques and foods of different textures.

Evaluation and treatment of complex feeding problems require the expertise of several disciplines — psychology, occupational therapy, physical therapy, speech pathology, and dentistry, as well as nutrition. There are several publications that address these areas in depth (101−104).

SUMMARY AND CONCLUSIONS

Although I have not stressed the importance of nutrition intervention in the case of children with developmental disabilities, the results in some cases of such intervention may be dramatic. It is well known, for example, that children with phenylketonuria, an inborn error of metabolism, can develop normally as a result of dietary treatment which regulates the level of phenylalanine in their blood. Untreated children become severely mentally retarded. It has also been recently reported that prevention of the gross obesity in children with Prader−Willi syndrome by strict caloric control and a behavior modification program can aid in preventing the decline in I.Q. with age which has been observed in these children (36).

In other cases, the results may be less dramatic, although the challenge to the clinician and the rewards for the parents and child just as great. Lowered energy requirements and possible increases in nutrient needs appear to be common in children with developmental disabilities. Therefore, the dietary goal for many of these children is that of meeting nutrient requirements while not exceeding energy needs. To this challenge is often added the need to evaluate the child's developmental level, particularly with regard to oral-motor and feeding skills, so that foods of an appropriate texture may be chosen.

The problems of children with developmental disabilities are just beginning to attract the attention of both clinicians and researchers in the field of nutrition. The establishment in the 1960s of federally funded university affiliated programs, whose mission is to provide service-oriented training and research in the area of mental retardation and handicapping conditions, has provided much of the impetus. One reason is the existence in these centers of the interdisciplinary expertise necessary to approach the complex nutritional problems of this population.

An example of this new activity is a major collaborative research project, undertaken by nutritionists from four university affiliated programs,[2] which is presently being concluded. This project represents the first attempt at a comprehensive assessment of the nutritional status of a large group of noninstitutionalized children with mental retardation of unknown etiology and will expand the basis for clinical guidelines for the provision of services to this population, as well as, it is hoped, provide a stimulus for further investigation.

ACKNOWLEDGMENTS

The author would like to acknowledge the contributions of several colleagues working in the field of mental retardation and developmental disabilities: Betty Whittle Kozlowski, Ph.D.; Martha L. Taylor, Ph.D., R.D.; Elaine M. Blyler, R.D., M.S.; and Cristine M. Trahms, R.D., M.S.

This work was funded, in part, by the Maternal and Child Health Training Grant MCT–000914–15–0.

REFERENCES

1. U.S. 95th Congress, Senate Report No. 95-890, Rehabilitation, comprehensive services and developmental disabilities act of 1978, 1978.
2. S. Palmer and S. Ekvall, eds., *Pediatric Nutrition in Developmental Disorders*, C. C. Thomas, Springfield, Ill., 1978.
3. P. Pipes, *Nutrition in Infancy and Childhood*, 2nd ed., C. V. Mosby, St. Louis, 1981. R. B. Howard, Nutritional support of the developmentally disabled child. In R. M. Suskind, ed., *Textbook of*

---

[2]Grant MCR 390400 to The Ohio State Research Foundation, Columbus, Ohio. Participating centers are The Nisonger Center, The Ohio State University; University Affiliated Program, Children's Hospital of Los Angeles; Child Development Center, Georgetown University, Washington, D.C.; Child Development and Mental Retardation Center, University of Washington, Seattle.

Pediatric Nutrition, Raven Press, New York, 1981.

5. M. T. Baer, Nutrition. In R. B. Johnston and P. R. Magrab, eds., *Developmental Disorders: Assessment, Treatment, Education*, University Park Press, Baltimore, Md., 1976.

6. B. Worthington, P. Pipes, and C. Trahms, The pediatric nutritionist. In E. Allen, V. Holm and R. L. Schiefelbusch, eds., *Early Intervention—A Team Approach*, University Park Press, Baltimore, 1978.

7. B. Worthington, P. Pipes, and C. Trahms, Infant and child nutrition: Concerns regarding the developmentally disabled, *J. Am. Diet. Assoc.* **78**, 443 (1981).

8. L. S. Hurley, *Developmental Nutrition*, Prentice-Hall, Englewood Cliffs, N.J., 1980.

9. U.S. Department of Health, Education, and Welfare. *Healthy People: The Surgeon General's Report on Health Promotion and Disease Prevention*, U.S. Government Printing Office, Washington, D.C., 1979.

10. R. Bhat, T. N. K. Raju, and D. Vidyasagar, Less than 1000-g infant, immediate and long-term outcome, *Pediatr. Res.* **11**, 560 (1977).

11. M. Hack, A. A. Fanaroff, and I. R. Merkatz, The low-birth-weight infant—evaluation of a changing outlook. *N. Engl. J. Med.* **301**, 1162 (1979).

12. J. J. Pomerance, C. T. Ukrainski, T. Ukra, D. J. Henderson, A. H. Nash, and J. L. Meredith, Cost of living for infants weighing 1000 grams or less at birth. *Pediatrics* **61**, 908 (1978).

13. R. A. K. Jones, M. Cummins, and P. A. Davies, Infants of very low birth weight: A 15 year analysis. *Lancet* **1**, 1332 (1979).

14. A. T. Shennan and J. E. Milligan, The growth and development of infants weighing 1000 to 2000 grams at birth and delivered in a perinatal unit. *Am. J. Obstet. Gynecol.* **136**, 273 (1980).

15. F. Hale, The relation of maternal vitamin A deficiency to micropthalmia in pigs. *Texas State J. Med.* **33**, 37 (1937).

16. L. E. Sever and I. Emanuel, Is there a connection between maternal zinc deficiency and congenital malformations of the central nervous system in man? *Teratology* **7**, 117 (1973).

17. A. O. Cavadar, A. Arcasoy, T. Baycu, and O. Himmetoglu, Zinc deficiency and anencephaly in Turkey. *Teratology* **22**, 141 (1980).

18. K. E. Bergmann, G. Makosch, and K. H. Tews, Abnormalities of hair zinc concentration in mothers of newborn infants with spina bifida. *Am. J. Clin. Nutr.* **33**, 2145 (1980).

19. K. M. Hambidge, K. H. Neldner, and P. A. Walravens, Zinc, acrodermatitis enteropathica and congenital malformations. *Lancet* **1**, 577 (1975).

20. G. E. Roberts and B. E. Clayton, Some findings arising out of a survey of mentally retarded children. Part II, physical growth and development. *Dev. Med. Child Neurol.* **11**, 584 (1969).

21. G. Tarbell, On the height, weight and relative rate of growth of normal and feeble-minded children. *Proc. Assoc. Med. Off. Am. Inst. Idiot. Persons* **1**, 188 (1883).

22. H. H. Goddertd, The height and weight of feeble-minded children in American institutions. *J. Nerv. Ment. Dis.* **39**, 217 (1912).

23. C. D. Mead, Height and weight of children in relation to general intelligence. *Pediatr. Sem.* **21**, 394 (1914).

24. R. B. Kugel and J. Mohr, Mental retardation and physical growth. *Am. J. Ment. Defic.* **68**, 41 (1963).

25. L. O. Langer, Jr., Short stature: Checklist of conditions associated with retarded longitudinal growth. *Clin. Pediatr.* **8**, 142 (1969).

26. H. D. Mosier, Jr., H. J. Grossman, and H. F. Dingman, physical growth in mental defectives. A study in an institutionalized population. *Pediatrics* **36**, 465 (1965).

27. H. B. Pryor and H. E. Thelander, Growth deviations in handicapped children: An anthropometric study. *Clin. Pediatr.* **6**, 501 (1967).

28. G. Dutton, The size of mental defective boys. *Arch. Dis. Child.* **34**, 331 (1959).

29. C. E. Cronk, Growth of children with Down's Syndrome: Birth to age 3 years. *Pediatrics* **61**, 564 (1978).

30. L. Rarick and V. Seefeldt, Observation from longitudinal data on growth in stature and sitting height of children with Down's Syndrome. *J. Ment. Defic. Res.* **18**, 63 (1974).

31. A. Boué and J. Boué, Effects of rubella virus infection on the division of human cells. *Am. J. Dis. Child.* **118**, 45 (1969).

32. M. A. Menser, D. C. Dorman, K. G. Kenrick, S. G. Purvis-Smith, R. F. Slinn, L. Dods, and J. D. Harley, Congenital rubella—long term follow-up. *Am. J. Dis. Child.* **118**, 32 (1969).

33. D. W. Smith, *Recognizable Patterns of Human Malformation*, 2nd ed., Saunders, Philadelphia, 1976.

34. D. L. Rimoin and W. A. Horton, Short stature Part II, *J. Pediat.* **92**, 697 (1978).

35. H. H. Van Gelderen, Studies in oligophrenia: Growth in mentally deficient children. *Acta Paediatr. Scand.* **51**, 643 (1962).

36. K. A. Crnic, S. Sulzbacher, J. Snow, and V. A. Holm, Preventing mental retardation associated with gross obesity in the Prader—Willi Syndrome. *Pediatrics* **66**, 787 (1980).
37. J. Pozsonyi and H. Lobb, Growth in mentally retarded children. *J. Pediatr.* **71**, 865 (1967).
38. J. S. Tobis, P. Saturen, G. Larios, and A. O. Posniak, Study of growth patterns in cerebral palsy. *Arch. Phys. Med. Rehabil.* **42**, 475–481 (1961).
39. H. M. Wallace, Nutrition and handicapped children. *J. Am. Diet. Assoc.* **61**, 127 (1972).
40. M. I. Hammond, M. N. Lewis, and E. W. Johnson, A nutritional study of cerebral palsied children. *J. Am. Diet. Assoc.* **49**, 196 (1966).
41. D. O. Ruby and W. D. Matheny, Comments on growth of cerebral palsied children. *J. Am. Diet. Assoc.* **40**, 525 (1962).
42. C. M. Leamy, A study of the food intake of a group of children with cerebral palsy in the Lakeville Sanatorium. *Am. J. Public Health* **43**, 1310 (1953).
43. K. Berg and B. Isaksson, Body composition and nutrition of school children with cerebral palsy. *Acta Paediatr. Scand. Suppl.* **204**, 41 (1970).
44. K. Berg, Effect of physical activation and ofimproved nutrition on the body composition of school children with cerebral palsy. *Acta Paediatr. Scand. Suppl.* **204**, 53 (1970).
45. D. Safer, R. Allen, and E. Barr, Depression of growth in hyperactive children on stimulant drugs. *N. Engl. J. Med.* **287**, 217 (1972).
46. D. Safer and R. Allen, Factors influencing the suppressant effects of 2 stimulant drugs on the growth of hyperactive children. *Pediatrics* **51**, 660 (1973).
47. D. Safer, R. Allen, and E. Barr, Growth rebound after termination of stimulant drugs. *J. Pediatr.* **86**, 113 (1975).
48. B. Lucas and C. Sells, Nutrient intake and stimulant drugs in hyperactive children. *J. Am. Diet. Assoc.* **70**, 373 (1977).
49. The President's Committee on Mental Retardation. Dept. Health, Education and Welfare. No. 0—413—182, U. S. Government Printing Office, Washington, D.C., 1971.
50. H. L. Bailit and M. A. Whelan, Some factors related to size and intelligence in an institutionalized mentally retarded population: An anthropometric study. *J. Pediatr.* **71**, 897 (1967).
51. C. D. Flory, The physical growth of mentally deficient boys. *Monogr. Soc. Res. Child Dev.* **1**, No. 6 (1936).

52. A. T. Rundle, Anthropometry: A ten-year survey of growth and sexual maturation. In B. W. Richards, ed., *Mental Subnormality: Modern Trends in Research*, Pitman Medical and Science Publishing, London, 1970.
53. Ten-State Nutrition Survey: Highlights. Dept. of Health, Education, and Welfare, No. (HSM) 72–8134, 1972.
54. G. M. Owen, K. M. Kram, P. J. Garry, J. E. Lowe, and A. H. Lubin, A study of nutritional status of preschool children in the United States, 1968–1970 (Part II). *Pediatrics* **53**, 597 (1974).
55. F. E. Johnston, B. Newman, J. Cravioto, E. Delicardie, and T. Scholl, A factor analysis of correlates of nutritional status in Mexican children, birth to 3 years. In L. S. Green and F. S. Johnston, eds., *Social and Biological Predictors of Nutritional Status, Physical Growth, and Neurological Development*, Academic Press, New York, 1980.
56. R. H. Bruininks, Physical and motor development of retarded persons. *Int. Rev. Res. Ment. Retard.* **7**, 209 (1974).
57. P. R. Dodge, A. L. Prensky, and R. D. Feigin, eds., *Nutrition and the Developing Nervous System*, C. V. Mosby, St. Louis, 1975.
58. W. J. Culley and T. O. Middleton, Calorie requirements of mentally retarded children with and without motor dysfunction. *J. Pediatr.* **75**, 380–384 (1969).
59. W. J. Culley, K. Goyal, D. H. Jolly, and E. T. Mertz, Calorie intake of children with Down's Syndrome (mongolism). *J. Pediatr.* **66**, 772 (1965).
60. Committee on Dietary Allowances, Food and Nutrition Board, National Research Council, *Recommended Dietary Allowances*, 9th ed., National Academy of Sciences, Washington, D.C., 1980.
61. V. Holm and P. Pipes, Food and children with Prader–Willi Syndrome. *Am. J. Dis. Child.* **130**, 1063 (1976).
62. S. Palmer, Down's syndrome. In S. Palmer and S. Ekvall, eds., *Pediatric Nutrition in Developmental Disorders*, C. C. Thomas, Springfield, Ill., 1978.
63. M. Baselon, R. S. Paine, V. A. Cowie, P. Hunt, J. C. Houck, and D. Mahanand, Reversal of hypotonia in infants with Down's syndrome by administration of 5-hydroxytryptophan. *Lancet* **1**, 1130 (1976).
64. P. Weise, R. Koch, K. N. F. Shaw, and M. J. Rosenfeld, The use of 5-HTP in the treatment of Down's syndrome. *Pediatrics* **54**, 165 (1974).
65. S. M. Pueschel, R. B. Reed, C. E. Cronk, and B. I. Goldstein, 5-hydroxytryptophan and pyridoxine: Their effects in young children with Down's syndrome. *Am. J. Dis. Child.* **134**, 838 (1980).

66. M. W. Partington, M. R. A. MacDonald, and J. B. Tu, 5-hydroxytryptophan in Down's syndrome. *Dev. Med. Child. Neurol.* **13**, 362 (1971).

67. S. Palmer, Influence of vitamin A nutriture on the immune response: findings in children with Down's Syndrome. *Int. J. Vit. Nutr. Res.* **48**, 189 (1978).

68. H. S. Barden, Vitamin A and carotene values of institutionalized mentally retarded subjects with and without Down's syndrome. *J. Ment. Defic. Res.* **21**, 63 (1977).

69. A. Milunsky, B. M. Hackley, and J. A. Halsted, Plasma, erythrocyte and leucocyte zinc levels in Down's syndrome. *J. Ment. Defic. Res.* **14**, 99 (1970).

70. B. Bjorksten, O. Back, K. H. Gustavson, G. Hallmans, B. Hagglof, and A. Tarnvik, Zinc and immune function in Down's Syndrome. *Acta Paediatr. Scand.* **69**, 183 (1980).

71. D. A. Roe, *Drug-induced Nutritional Deficiencies.* Avi Publishing, Westport, Conn., 1976.

72. M. B. Dahlke and E. Mertens-Roesler, Malabsorption of folic acid due to diphenylhydantoin, *Blood* **30**, 341 (1967).

73. N. Gordon, Folic acid deficiency from anticonvulsant therapy. *Dev. Med. Child Neurol.* **10**, 497 (1968).

74. D. R. Miller, Serum folate deficiency in children receiving anticonvulsant therapy. *Pediatrics* **41**, 630 (1968).

75. J. D. Maxwell, J. Hunter, D. A. Stewart, S. Ardeman, and R. Williams, Folate deficiency after anticonvulsant drugs; an effect of hepatic enzyme induction. *Br. Med. J.* **1**, 297 (1972).

76. J. C. Bowe, E. J. Cornish, and M. Dawson, Evaluation of folic acid supplements in children taking phenytoin. *Dev. Med. Child Neurol.* **13**, 343 (1971).

77. J. R. Moore and E. W. Ball, Folic acid replacement in folate deficient children on anticonvulsants. *Arch. Dis. Child.* **47**, 309 (1972).

78. C. Neubauer, Mental deterioration in epilepsy due to folate deficiency. *Br. Med. J.* **2**, 759 (1970).

79. E. H. Reynolds, Neurological aspects of folate and vitamin B_{12} metabolism. *Clin. Haematol.* **5**, 661 (1976).

80. E. H. Reynolds, Effects of folic acid on the mental state and fit frequency of drug-treated epileptic patients. *Lancet* **1**, 1086 (1967).

81. J. Hunter, J. D. Maxwell, D. A. Stewart, V. Parsons, and R. Williams, Altered calcium metabolism in epileptic children on anticonvulsant drugs. *Br. Med. J.* **4**, 202 (1971).

82. J. L. Winnacker, H. Yaeger, J. A. Saunders, B. Russell, and C. S.

Anast, Rickets in children receiving anticonvulsant drugs. *Am. J. Dis. Child.* **131**, 286 (1977).

83. F. Lifshitz and N. K. Maclaren, Vitamin D dependent rickets in institutionalized mentally retarded children receiving long-term anticonvulsant therapy: a survey of 288 patients. *J. Pediatr.* **83**, 612 (1973).

84. T. J. Hahn, B. A. Hendin, C. R. Scharp, V. C. Boisseau, and J. G. Haddad, Jr., Serum 25-hydroxycalciferol levels and bone mass in children on chronic anticonvulsant therapy. *N. Engl. J. Med.* **292**, 550 (1975).

85. K. G. Tolman, W. Jubiz, J. J. Sannella, J. A. Madsen, R. E. Belsey, and R. S. Goldsmith, Osteomalacia associated with anticonvulsant drug therapy in mentally retarded children. *Pediatrics* **56**, 45 (1975).

86. J. Silver, T. J. Davies, E. Kypersmitt, M. Orme, A. Petrie, and F. Vajda, Prevalence and treatment of vitamin D deficiency in children on anti-convulsant drugs. *Arch. Dis. Child.* **49**, 344 (1974).

87. C. J. Crosley, C. Chee, and P. H. Berman, Rickets associated with long-term anticonvulsant therapy in a pediatric outpatient population. *Pediatrics* **56**, 52 (1975).

88. N. Maclaren and F. Lifshitz, Vitamin D dependent rickets in institutionalized mentally retarded children on long-term anticonvulsant therapy II. Response to 25-hydroxy vitamin D_3 and vitamin D_2. *Pediatr. Res.* **7**, 914 (1973).

89. T. C. B. Stamp, J. M. Round, D. J. E. Rowe, and J. G. Haddad, Plasma levels and therapeutic effect of 25-hydroxycholecalciferol in epileptic patients taking anticonvulsant drugs. *Br. Med. J.* **4**, 9 (1972).

90. T. C. B. Stamp, Effects of long-term anticonvulsant therapy on calcium and vitamin D metabolism. *Proc. R. Soc. Med.* **67**, 64 (1974).

91. A. Richens and D. J. F. Rowe, Anticonvulsant osteomalacia. *Br. Med. J.* **4**, 684 (1971).

92. J. S. Lewis, M. T. Baer, and M. S. Laufer, Urinary riboflavin and creatinine of children treated with anticonvulsant drugs. *Am. J. Dis. Child.* **129**, 394 (1975).

93. A. A. Yunis, G. K. Arimura, C. L. Lutcher, J. Blasquez, and M. J. Halloran, Biochemical lesion in Dilantin induced erythroid aplasia. *J. Clin. Invest.* **44**, 1114 (1965).

94. B. D. Bower, Pyridoxine, tryptophan and epilepsy. *Dev. Med. Child Neurol.* **7**, 73 (1965).

95. B. Hagberg, A. Hamfelt, and O. Hansson, Tryptophan tolerance tests and vitamin B_6 (pyridoxine) metabolism in epileptic children. *Dev. Med. Child Neurol.* **7**, 50 (1965).
96. H. Ekelund, I. Gamstrop, and W. Von Studnitz, Apparent response to impaired mental development, minor motor epilepsy and ataxia to pyridoxine. *Acta Paediatr. Scand.* **58**, 572 (1969).
97. H. A. Peters, P. L. Eichman, J. M. Price, F. L. Kozelka, and H. H. Reese, Abnormal copper and tryptophan metabolism and chelation therapy in anticonvulsant drug intolerance. *Dis. Nerv. Syst.* **27**, 97 (1966).
98. O. Hansson, Tryptophan loading and pyridoxine treatment in children with epilepsy. *Ann. N.Y. Acad. Sci.* **166**, 306 (1969).
99. L. Reinken, L. Hohenauer, and E. E. Zeigler, Activity of red cell glutamic oxalacetic transaminase in epileptic children under antiepileptic treatment. *Clin. Chim. Acta* **36**, 270 (1972).
100. A. O. Ogunmekan, Relationship between age and vitamin E level in epileptic and normal children. *Am. J. Clin. Nutr.* **32**, 2269 (1979).
101. T. R. Linscheid, Disturbances of eating and feeding. In P. R. Magrab, ed., *Psychological Management of Pediatric Problems*, University Park Press, Baltimore, 1978, pp. 191–218.
102. S. Palmer and S. Horn, Feeding problems in children. In S. Palmer and S. Ekvall, eds., *Pediatric Nutrition in Developmental Disorders*, C. C. Thomas, Springfield, Ill., 1978, pp. 107–129.
103. H. L. Ogg, Oral-pharyngeal development and evaluation. *Phys. Ther.* **55**, 235–241 (1975).
104. M. A. Smith, ed., *Feeding the Handicapped Child*, University of Tennessee Child Development Center, Memphis, 1971.

ADDITIONAL RECENT REFERENCES

M. L. Taylor, B. W. Kozlowski, M. T. Baer, E. M. Blyler, and C. M. Trahms, Anticonvulsant therapy and differences in iron parameters among developmentally delayed children (abstract). *Fed. Proc.* **41**, 953 (1982).
B. W. Kozlowski, M. L. Taylor, M. T. Baer, E. M. Blyler, and C. M. Trahms, Anticonvulsant medication use and levels of retinol-binding protein and thyroxine in children (abstract). *Fed. Proc.* **41**, 943 (1982).
M. T. Baer, B. W. Kozlowski, E. M. Blyler, M. L. Taylor, and C. M. Trahms, Selected measures of vitamin D and calcium status in children with developmental delay (abstract). *Fed. Proc.* **41**, 950 (1982).

11
Dietary Risk Patterns During Pregnancy

JANET C. KING, Ph.D., R.D.
University of California, Berkeley

Address correspondence to Janet C. King, Ph.D., Associate Professor of Nutrition, Department of Nutritional Sciences, University of California, Berkeley, California 94720.

ABSTRACT

Nutritional risk in pregnant women is currently identified by 12 factors established by the American College of Obstetrics and Gynecology and the American Dietetic Association. Only one of the 12 factors refers specifically to dietary habits (adherence to a fad diet). Dietary histories carefully obtained from pregnant women could easily be used to identify their usual dietary pattern. At least three different dietary patterns could predispose women to the two most common nutritional problems in pregnancy, energy imbalance and iron deficiency anemia. These three dietary patterns are insufficient food intake, poor food selection, and poor food distribution throughout the day. After a discussion of the usual adjustments in nutrient utilization during pregnancy, the links between these three dietary patterns and clinical problems are explained. The paper concludes with general guidelines for nutrition education of pregnant women.

In 1978 the American College of Obstetricians and Gynecologists and the American Dietetic Association (1) established a set of factors to identify women who are at nutritional risk during pregnancy (Table 1). The first eight factors are aspects of the women's social, economic, and health environment that may be linked to altered or poor nutrition. The next three factors are standards for hemoglobin/hematocrit levels and weight gain that may have deviated from normal as a result of poor nutrition. These factors, then, are a consequence or a symptom of poor nutrition, not a predictor. Finally, the woman planning to breast feed is considered to be at risk because nutritional needs for lactation are so great.

These 12 factors, commonly used in prenatal clinics to identify women who need dietary counseling, do not use any information on dietary habits other than adherence to a fad diet. Dietary interviews can be used to determine habitual patterns of food intake that may put the woman at nutritional risk. Three dietary patterns which would not support optimal maternal and fetal nutritional needs are insufficient food intake, poor food selection, and poor food distribution throughout

Table 1. Nutrition Risk Factors during Pregnancy

Risk is very likely if at the onset of pregnancy:

She is an adolescent (15 years or less).

She has had three or more pregnancies in the last 2 years.

She has a history of poor obstetric or fetal performance.

She is economically deprived.

She is a food faddist.

She is a heavy smoker, drug addict, or alcoholic.

She requires a therapeutic diet for a chronic systemic disease.

She had a prepartum weight at her first prenatal visit of <85% or >120% of standard weight.

Risk is also very likely if during prenatal care:

She has a low or deficient hemoglobin/hematocrit (low is Hb < 11.0 g, HCT < 33; deficient is HB < 10.0 g, HCT < 30).

She has inadequate weight gain (any weight loss during pregnancy or gain < 2 pounds (1 kg) per month after the first trimester).

She has excessive weight gain [> 2 pounds (1 kg) per week].

She plans to breast feed her infant.

the day. If these patterns were added to the list of risk factors in Table 1, the criteria would be much more sensitive for nutritional risk. Women troubled by abnormalities in weight gain, iron depletion, and other nutritional problems during pregnancy may be following one of these three patterns. Thus, these patterns would be predictors of poor nutrition, which is a much more useful criterion for nutritional risk than is waiting for a clinical symptom of poor nutrition.

MATERNAL METABOLIC ADJUSTMENTS

Numerous adjustments occur in nutrient utilization during pregnancy. With good nutritional support, the adjustments are normal and are all geared toward protection of maternal health and support of fetal growth and development. However, poor nutrition resulting from an inadequate food supply, poor food choices, or poor food distribution can alter normal adjustments in nutrient utilization. Optimal conditions for maintenance of maternal health and support of fetal growth may then no longer exist. Before discussing the potential effects of these three dietary patterns on nutrient utilization, normal adjustments seen in healthy pregnant women will be reviewed.

Addition of Maternal Tissues and Stores

Overall, pregnancy is an active state of growth. The range of maternal weight change associated with this growth is wide, however, going from a loss to a gain of 50 lb or more (2). A net weight loss would mean that some loss of maternal tissue occurred while fetal tissue is gained. Birth weight is usually reduced in this condition, and, on the average, infants of mothers gaining no weight weigh 2/3 to 1 pound less than do the infants of mothers gaining 40 lb or more (3). The issue of how much to gain during pregnancy has been debated extensively and may never be resolved because there is very little information on what healthy women eating without restriction usually gain and because the amount gained seems to be individualized. In general, though, primigravidae (women pregnant for the first time) gain more than multigravidae (pregnant women who have been pregnant two or more times previously); the average total gain of healthy Western women is about 28 lb (12.5 kg), all but 2.5 lb (1.1 kg) is gained in the 2nd and 3rd trimester, and smaller women from developing countries usually gain less than Western women, about 17−20 lb (8−9 kg) (2). Two factors lead to the addition of new tissue: a change in maternal hormone milieu and an increase in appetite (4).

The fetus represents a small part, only about 30%, of the total average weight gain. Tissue supporting fetal growth (e.g., placenta, amniotic fluid, uterine muscle, mammmary gland, and blood) account for 40% of the weight. The remaining 30% is maternal stores, which are primarily fat (2).

Composition of Tissue Gained

Analysis of the total tissue gained in a pregnancy when the weight gain is about average shows that the largest component is water, 62%; next is fat, 31%; and protein is 7% (2). Small amounts of minerals would be gained along with the protein.

Water is not only the largest component of the tissue gained but it is also the most variable. The usual gain is about 8 kg (18 lb), but as much as 11 kg (24 lb) has been seen. Of the 8 kg of water normally gained, 5-1/2 kg (12 lb) is associated with the fetus and other tissues gained in pregnancy. The remaining 2-1/2 kg (6 lb) of fluid tends to accumulate in maternal interstitial tissue. Because of gravity, the fluid pools more in the lower extremities and leads to swelling of the ankles, which occurs quite often in pregnant women. When large amounts of fluid are retained, the amount associated with the fetus and other pregnancy tissues does not change appreciably. Instead more is deposited in maternal tissues.

No one knows why fluid retention is so variable among pregnant women, but it is probably related to differences in hormonal changes. It seems that connective tissue becomes more hygroscopic (moisture-retaining) during gestation due to some estrogen-induced changes in the ground substance (2). As a result, the connective tissue becomes softer and more mobile. This would facilitate delivery because the cervix and vagina are more readily distensible. Also, many pregnant women note edema of the gingiva which predisposes them to periodontal disease. Possibly, the changes occurring increase the diffusibility of solutes and facilitate the nutrition of the cells. At any rate, fluid retention during pregnancy seems to be a normal phenomenon and it has a positive effect on fetal growth. Women with edema tend to have bigger babies than do women without edema, and attempts to prevent edema by giving pregnant women diuretics result in a reduction in birth weight (2, 5).

Of the fluid gained during pregnancy, about 75% is extracellular. A little over 1 kg of fluid accumulates in the blood, increasing the plasma volume. The normal increase in plasma volume is about 1200 ml, or a rise of about 50% (2), but gains of as much as 1800 ml, or a 70% rise, have been seen. The number of red blood cells does increase during pregnancy, but not nearly as much as does the plasma volume. A gain of about 20% occurs in women not given iron supplements and 30% in those who do receive iron. Consequently, the percentage of the blood volume accounted for by red blood cells, that is, the hematocrit, normally drops during pregnancy. Also, the concentration of some of the solutes in the plasma will decrease if they do not increase as much as the plasma volume does. To account for these normal changes in blood composition during pregnancy, different standards must be established for use of blood measurements to evaluate health in pregnant women. Standards for some components are shown in Table 2. The effects of plasma volume expansion on the concentration of vitamins and minerals in the plasma are summarized in Table 2. The concentration of most of them is decreased, but some are increased due to other physiologic adjustments that occur during pregnancy.

Table 2. Normal Changes in Serum Levels of Vitamins and Minerals during Pregnancy (28)

Blood Components Increased	Variable Response[b]	Blood Components Decreased
Serum tocopherol	Serum folacin	Serum ascorbic acid
Serum vitamin A[a]	Serum	Serum vitamin B-12
Serum copper	25-hydroxycholecalciferol	Plasma pyridoxal phosphate
	Serum iron	Serum calcium
		Serum magnesium
		Serum inorganic phosphate
		Serum zinc
		Plasma inorganic iodine
		Serum selenium

[a] Data are conflicting.
[b] Responses vary with supplementation level or season of the year (25-hydroxycholecalciferol).

Rosso and Kava (6) recently showed that good nutrition is essential in pregnant rats for normal expansion of the plasma volume. Restriction of the food intake of a group of pregnant rats to 50% of that eaten by those allowed free access to food reduced blood volume expansion and decreased cardiac output and, therefore, placental blood flow. The decrease in placental blood flow resulted in a reduction in the transfer of nutrients to the fetus. The investigators showed this reduction by measuring glucose transfer across the placenta. A reduction in glucose transfer, the primary fetal energy source, in essence caused starvation of the developing offspring so that birth weight was reduced. This study is a good example of the important role of nutrition in facilitating the normal physiologic adjustments during pregnancy. Apparently, hormonal changes cannot bring about these changes if nutritional support is not also present. Or, good nutrition may be needed for even the hormonal changes to occur.

In women gaining about 12.5 kg during their pregnancy, approximately 3.8 kg of the gain is fat. Only about 0.5 kg of that fat is deposited in the fetus; the rest is accumulated by the mother primarily during the maternal phase or 2nd trimester of pregnancy (2). Women gaining more than 12.5 kg will presumably at some point begin gaining excessive fat stores. The point at which this occurs will vary with the individual, the size of the fetus, prepregnancy nutritional state, and differences in energy intake and expenditure.

The purpose of the maternal fat store is not known with certainty, but it is thought to be an energy reserve for the high cost of lactation, which is about 500 kcal/day. An association between maternal weight gain during the 1st and 2nd trimesters and the prematurity rate has been demonstrated. Women who had an average or greater gain in both trimesters had the lowest incidence of prematurity (7).

Considerable energy, about 9 kcal/g of fat, is required to store this fat during pregnancy. Since most of it is stored in the 2nd trimester, it boosts the daily energy needs in this period to about equal that in the 3rd trimester when energy is needed primarily for fetal growth and development. The additional energy need for pregnancy is constant at about 300 kcal/day throughout the 2nd and 3rd trimesters. This is about 13% of the woman's total need (8).

A little less than 1 kg of protein is gained by the average woman during pregnancy. About 75% of this gain is deposited in the fetus, placenta, and amniotic fluid; the rest is found in the gain of breast tissue and expanded blood volume (2). There is no evidence that protein is gained as lean tissue by the mother during the maternal phase for future support of fetal growth and development (9). Rats, however, who have a greater nutrient need/unit maternal body weight for development of multiple numbers of offspring, do appear to gain some lean tissue in the maternal phase which is catabolized later in the fetal phase (10). Nitrogen balance studies and measurements of potassium retention in adolescent pregnant girls with poor diet histories showed that they were gaining about twice as much protein in the last half of pregnancy as the estimated need for growth of the fetus and supportive pregnancy tissue (11). With improved dietary intakes while participating in the metabolic studies, these girls may have repleted their own protein reserves and/or grown some themselves.

Serum protein concentration tends to decrease during pregnancy from about 70 g/liter to about 62 g/liter at term (4). However, even though there is an overall decrease in serum protein concentration, there is a 30% increase in the beta-globulin fraction. Components of this protein fraction often function as carriers for nutrients in the blood, and an increase in concentration of the carrier in the serum usually leads to an increase in the concentration of the nutrient carried by the protein. For example, ceruloplasmin is a beta-globulin which is responsible for the transport of copper. The concentration of ceruloplasmin in the serum increases about twofold during pregnancy, even though the plasma volume expands by only about 50%. As a result of the increase in serum ceruloplasmin, serum copper also rises about the same amount. Transferrin, the transport protein for iron, also increases in the serum during pregnancy. But, without iron supplementation, comparable increases in serum iron are not seen, and the percent saturation of transferrin tends to fall. A decline to 20% saturation is considered normal. Albumin, which transports about 70% of the zinc in the serum, decreases from about 42 to 32 g/liter during gestation. Consequently, serum zinc levels normally decrease by about 20% during gestation.

Changes in Fat and Carbohydrate Metabolism

As stated above, most of the weight is gained during the 2nd and 3rd trimesters. These two trimesters are considered the maternal and fetal phase of pregnancy, respectively. This is because tissue accretion in the second trimester is primarily in the maternal compartment, presumably in preparation for future fetal demands. In the 3rd trimester, fetal growth is maximal, and there is essentially no deposition of tissue within the maternal compartment (4). In rats, maternal lean and fat tissues are catabolized during the fetal phase, which is the last week of gestation in this animal, to augment the dietary nutrient supply for fetal demands. In humans eating to appetite, however, there is no evidence that maternal tissue is normally catabolized in the last trimester to help meet fetal needs (5). Instead, an ingenious system is set up to conserve glucose, the preferred fetal energy source, for the fetus. Between meals, when blood glucose levels would fall since there is no incoming dietary supply, the mother alters her metabolism so that she makes greater use of fat as an energy fuel and "saves" glucose for the fetus. An increase in serum total lipid from about 6 g/liter to about 10 g/liter by term ensures that there is a readily accessible supply of fat for maternal energy. Increased mobilization of fatty acids from adipose tissue accounts for this rise in serum lipids. These fatty acids will not be used by a well-fed mother for energy, and hepatic triglyceride production will increase. The triglycerides would be stored in maternal adipose tissue so that there is no net loss of this tissue. In fact, there could be a gain if the dietary energy intake is above the need. Vitamins, such as vitamin E, which normally circulate with the lipid components of the blood, will also rise as a result of the higher levels of serum total lipids.

Besides making greater use of fatty acids for energy, maternal tissues also become insulin resistant and, therefore, resistant to the uptake of glucose. This is another way in which the mother "saves" as much glucose as possible for the fetus. The insulin resistance is thought to be due to the rise of several hormones, such as glucocorticoids, estrogen, progesterone, and human placental lactogen (4), during pregnancy.

Because of this insulin resistance, pregnant women normally have much larger outputs of insulin with food intake than do nonpregnant women (12). Women with marginally functioning pancreases are prone to develop gestational diabetes. In many cases, pancreatic function and glucose metabolism will return to normal following delivery.

Even though the mother tries to "save" glucose for the fetus by making greater use of fatty acids for energy and developing an insulin resistance in her tissues, plasma glucose levels still fall during gestation. The lowest level, approximately 68 mg/dl, is reached near term (4). This decline in plasma glucose is thought to be the effect of continuous glucose extraction by the fetus. Also, since maternal tissues become insulin resistant, there is not the usual gluconeogenic response that occurs with hypoglycemia. Absence of the gluconeogenic response conserves maternal skeletal muscle and protects the mother from severe lean tissue depletion if food is scarce during pregnancy. Instead, the fetus will suffer from a lack of energy and experience growth retardation or, if the lack is very severe, will die. It seems that nature has designed a system to protect the mother so that her tissues are spared during pregnancy in order to meet the even greater needs of lactation after the baby is born.

INSUFFICIENT FOOD

Although the food supply in the United States is sufficient to provide everyone with enough to eat, there are still individuals in this country who do not eat enough. This may be because of economic problems limiting food purchases or voluntary limitation of food intake in an effort to control body weight. Table 3 displays the usual dietary pattern of a 33-year-old strict vegetarian who was not eating enough food because she wanted to limit her weight gain. Although the case presented is that of a vegetarian, limiting food intake in pregnancy is common among women who are trying to conceal their pregnancy or who wish to prevent excessive weight gain. It is possible to meet the nutritional needs for pregnancy through the use of a vegetarian diet that includes dairy products and eggs.

The usual food intake pattern of this woman, determined in an interview, was only two meals at the beginning and end of each day with a light snack in the middle. Also, dairy products and eggs were not eaten on a daily basis, even though she was willing to include these foods in her vegetarian diet. Vitamin C-rich foods were also absent from her usual diet. The two meal/day pattern, absence of dairy products, eggs, and vitamin C-rich foods, and the very limited use of fat would suggest that the dietary energy content is less than

Table 3. Case Presentation of an Insufficient Food Intake Pattern by a 33-Year-Old Strict Vegetarian Pregnant Woman

	Usual Food Intake Pattern
Breakfast	1/2 cup hot cereal with 1 tbsp wheat germ, one apple, peanut butter sandwich on two slices whole wheat bread, water
Lunch	one piece of fresh fruit
Dinner	large spinach salad with apples, sesame seeds, radishes, green onions, mushrooms, and tomatoes; 1-1/2 cup baked beans; water

	Evaluation	
Food Groups	Servings Recommended (29)	Servings Eaten
Animal protein	0(for a vegetarian)	0
Vegetable protein	4	4
Milk and milk products	4	0
Breads and cereals	4	4
Vitamin C-rich fruits and vegetables	1	0
Dark green vegetables	1	2
Other fruits and vegetables	2	2

Nutrient Intake

Energy, kcal, 1322 (57% RDA)	Vitamins	Minerals, mg
Protein, g, 56.1 (76% RDA)	A, I.U., 3948	Calcium, 401[a]
Fat, % kcal, 40	D, I.U., 4[a]	Phosphorus, 1185
Carbohydrate, % kcal, 49	E, mg, 17	Sodium, 1166
	Ascorbic acid, mg, 43	Potassium, 2883
	Thiamin, mg, 1.2	Magnesium, 436
	Riboflavin, mg, 0.8[a]	Zinc, 12.5[a]
	Niacin, mg, 15	Copper, 2.2
	B-6, mg, 1.3[a]	Iron, 16.5
	Folacin, μg, 190[a]	
	B-12, μg, 0[a]	

[a] Less than two-thirds RDA (8)

recommended for pregnancy. A computer analysis of the diet confirms this conclusion. The energy intake is only about 60% of that recommended and her protein intake is about 75% of the standard. Seven of the other nutrients analyzed were below two-thirds of the pregnancy standard. These were vitamin D, riboflavin, and calcium, all normally contributed primarily by dairy products; folacin, which is high in vitamin C-rich foods; and vitamin B-6 and zinc, which are high in meats. Vitamin B-12 was also lacking due to the absence of animal products in the diet.

Health and Nutritional Consequences

If the woman had continued with this dietary pattern until term, fetal growth may have been limited and maternal prepregnancy reserves may have been mobilized. Analysis of data from both humans and rats fed insufficient food during gestation shows that maternal tissue is spared more than is fetal tissue under these conditions (4). Some of the pregnant women living in Holland during World War II gave birth to infants of normal birth weight whereas others had infants weighing about 300 g or more below the usual birth weight. It was found that those women who gave birth to normal birth weight infants weighed about the same postpartum as they did at conception, whereas those having the smaller infants lost about 1.5 kg during gestation. More detailed studies have been done in pregnant rats (4).

When the food intake of a group of pregnant rats was reduced to 50% of that of controls, there was a 25% reduction in birth weight of the offspring, but there was only a 10% decrease in maternal body weight. From a teleologic point of view, it is reasonable that the mother is more protected than is the developing fetus in times of food scarcity. It would be poor evolutionary adaptation if a mother became so severely depleted during gestation in order to deliver a full-grown infant that she was then unable to breast feed. The survival of the species would be much more likely if a growth-retarded infant is born to a moderately depleted mother who was then likely to recover and would be able to conceive again.

One of the reasons that fetal growth retardation occurs with reduced food intake is because protein in the diet must be used as a source of energy for maintenance of existing tissues rather than for synthesis of new tissue. Increased energy from a carbohydrate supplement given to a group of Guatemalan pregnant women was as effective in increasing birth weight as energy provided in a supplement of both carbohydrate and protein to another group of pregnant women (13). Apparently, the additional energy in the supplement of only carbohydrate spared the protein already in the women's diet so that it could be used for tissue synthesis. Also, the carbohydrate supplement was a good glucose supply, a primary fetal fuel, which may have been readily used for growth and development.

A classical study by Oldham and Sheft measured the relationship between energy intake and protein utilization during pregnancy (14). These investigators found that at least 36 kcal/kg pregnant body weight are required in the diet in order to support maximal utilization of protein for tissue synthesis.

Clinical Evidence

The clinical presentation of insufficient food intake during pregnancy will be a reduction in the rate of weight gain and possibly a decrease in accretion of maternal fat reserves. Pitkin (15) has defined an insufficient rate of weight gain as a gain of less than 1 kg/month during the 2nd and 3rd trimesters. Skinfold measurements could be used to

Table 4. Case Presentation of Poor Food Choices by a 31-Year-Old Housewife

Usual Food Intake Pattern

6:00 A.M.	two Twinkies, 12 oz milk
11:00 A.M.	tuna sandwich with two slices refined bread, 4 oz canned tuna, 3 tbsp mayonnaise, potato chips, one can diet soda
2:30 P.M.	ice cream cone (two scoops), one candy bar
6:00 P.M.	1/2 fried chicken, 1 cup french fries, 2 scoops chocolate ice cream, 1 Twinkie, 1 can diet soda

Evaluation

Food Groups	Servings Recommended (29)	Servings Eaten
Animal protein	2	4
Vegetable protein	2	0
Milk and milk protein	4	4
		(1-1/2 milk, 2-1/2 ice cream)
Breads and cereals	4	2
Vitamin C-rich fruits and vegetables	1	0
Dark green vegetables	1	0
Other fruits and vegetables	2	2
High fat or refined carbohydrate foods	---	8

Nutrient Intake

Energy, kcal, 3459 (150% RDA)
Protein, g, 127 (167% RDA)
Fat, % kcal, 50
Carbohydrate, % kcal, 36

Vitamins	Minerals, mg
A, I.U., 4086	Calcium, 1171
D. I.U., 383	Phosphorus, 1801
E, mg., 8	Sodium, 2700
Ascorbic acid, mg, 48	Potassium, 3695
Thiamin mg., 0.8[a]	Magnesium, 270[a]
Riboflavin, mg, 2.5	Zinc, 15.5
Niacin, mg, 35	Copper, 1.9
B-6, mg, 1.7[a]	Iron, 10.4[a]
B-12, μg, 5.0	
Folacin, μg, 99[a]	

[a] Less than two-thirds RDA (8).

assess maternal fat gain. In healthy, well-fed Western pregnant women, skinfold thicknesses increased at all of the usual sites measured up until 30 weeks of gestation; there was no further increase in the last 10 weeks. Change at the central sites, such as the thigh, suprailiac, and scapula, was greater than at the peripheral sites, biceps and triceps (16). Changes in skinfolds at central sites may provide a useful means of assessing maternal fat deposition during pregnancy. However, the weighing of women at each clinic visit and the plotting of their rate of weight gain on a graph would be as informative and much easier to carry out in a clinical situation.

POOR FOOD SELECTION

The second dietary pattern that would put a pregnant woman at nutritional risk is excessive use of foods with low nutrient density. This is usually due to the woman's making poor food choices. Diets falling into this category tend to be high in energy, but low in vitamins and minerals because the foods selected are not good nutrient sources.

An example of a diet of low nutrient density is shown in Table 4. The diet contains eight servings of foods which provide primarily fat or refined carbohydrate. Also, there are no servings of vitamin C-rich fruits and vegetables or dark green leafy vegetables. As expected from the number of foods high in fat or refined carbohydrate, the diet is high in energy, about 150% of the recommended intake. The protein content of this diet is also high because of the large servings of tuna fish and fried chicken. Five of the vitamins and minerals calculated are below two-thirds of the recommendation for pregnancy. Due to the limited use of cereal products, thiamin is low. This, along with the lack of dark green vegetables, contributes to the low intake of iron, magnesium, and folacin. Even though the servings of animal protein sources were more than sufficient and the protein intake was high, vitamin B-6 intake was still below two-thirds of the standard. This points out how difficult it is to obtain the 2.6 mg recommended intake from our food supply.

Health and Nutritional Consequences

If a pregnant woman followed this dietary pattern throughout gestation, her retention of maternal fat reserves would certainly be excessive. Pitkin's standard for an excessive rate of weight gain is greater than 3 kg/month at any time during gestation (15). The risk of obesity following pregnancy would be increased. A positive correlation between parity and body weight, as observed by McGanity, suggests that some women may be accumulating fat stores during gestation which are retained after delivery (W. J. McGanity, personal communication). In a reanalysis of the large collaborative Perinatal Project data, Naeye noted that a large weight gain in women who were above their standard body weight was associated with a significant reduction in birth weight (17). This intriguing observation needs to be verified by additional studies. However, it does suggest that large weight gains in overweight pregnant women may in some manner impair fetal growth.

Depletion of maternal nutrient stores may also occur with the use of a diet of low nutrient density during gestation. As discussed earlier, it seems that with lack of sufficient nutrients during pregnancy, maternal tissue is spared more than is fetal tissue. A possible exception to this is iron utilization. Both the fetus and placenta effectively parasitize iron from the mother, even if she is grossly deficient (18). Iron needs for the growing fetus and placenta and expansion of blood volume total about 1000 to 1100 mg. About 4 mg of iron would have to be absorbed from the diet daily throughout pregnancy to meet this need. Amenorrhea will partly offset the cost, and iron absorption does increase; but it is doubtful that these changes will ensure that the need can be met from dietary sources alone. The usual concentration of iron in the American diet is about 6 mg/1000 kcal. An intake of 2300 kcal by a pregnant woman would provide about 14 mg iron on the average. Iron absorption would need to average about 30% throughout pregnancy to provide 4 mg absorbed iron. Maximal iron absorption in pregnancy is only about 20%, and this peak is not reached until late in gestation (19).

A portion of the iron could be supplied by iron stores. In males, iron stores range from 500–1500 mg, but in females they tend to be much lower or even nonexistent (18). Since pregnant women are at risk of finishing their pregnancy in an iron-depleted state, the Food and Nutrition Board of the National Research Council recommends 30–60 mg of iron supplementation daily for pregnant women (8).

A recent paper by Rush, Stein, and Susser (20) has created some concern about high protein intakes, similar to the amount in this case (Table 4), and pregnancy outcome. These investigators studied three groups of women. Two groups received a liquid dietary supplement to be taken along with their usual diet; one group was given a high protein supplement (34% of the calories supplied as protein), the other group a low protein supplement (7% of the calories as protein). The third group, a control group, received only their usual prenatal vitamin/mineral supplements. Twenty-four-hour recalls were used to estimate the total protein intake of the groups. The high protein supplement group consumed about 102 g of protein/day, of which 28 g came from the liquid supplement and 74 g from their diet. The diets of the control group provided about 79 g of protein/day. Significant growth retardation of the fetus up to 37 weeks' gestation and increase in very early premature births which verged on being statistically significant were seen in the high protein supplementation group.

These differences between the high protein supplement group and the other groups were attributed to the differences in the protein content of the supplement. However, many other differences existed between the groups. The vitamin and mineral content of the high protein supplement and the low protein supplement differed; the amount of liquid supplement consumed differed between the two groups; there was no control of the quantity and quality of other food consumed; and weight gain prior to the intervention was not well randomized between the groups.

Because of these confounding variables, which were not controlled in this study, it is inappropriate to conclude that a 100-g protein intake impairs fetal growth. On the other hand, there is no evidence that protein intakes above the recommended 76 g/day for a woman of average pre-pregnancy weight (55 kg, 120 lbs) are beneficial. Highly controlled balance studies show that 76 g protein/day support a gain of about 1 g nitrogen (6.25 g protein) in the last trimester (12). It is estimated that this rate of protein gain will meet the needs for fetal growth and development at this stage of pregnancy (2).

Clinical Evidence

Usual clinical practices, such as measurement of body weights and hemoglobin concentrations, will detect any excessive weight gain or anemia resulting from a low nutrient-dense diet. The clinician can easily identify an excessive rate of gain by plotting the woman's weight at each visit on a graph or by determining the monthly gain and comparing it to the Pitkin standard, excessive gain being more than 3 kg/month (15).

Guidelines for assessing iron status of pregnant women are shown in Table 5. The first stage of iron depletion occurs when more iron is needed than is available from the diet, and storage iron must be mobilized. Serum ferritin is a good indicator of storage iron; 1 μg ferritin/liter of plasma is equivalent to 8 μg of storage iron (18). A fall in serum ferritin reflects a decrease in storage iron. A concentration of less than 10 ng ferritin/ml serum is associated with iron depletion erythropoiesis (18).

A rise in serum transferrin is a compensatory response to iron depletion. The result is an increase in the binding capacity of the blood and, without available iron, a decrease in the percent of transferrin saturated with iron. A saturation of less than 20% is indicative of iron deficiency in pregnancy (19).

With continued iron depletion, hemoglobin synthesis will decrease and, finally, the quantity of red blood cells produced will decline.

POOR FOOD DISTRIBUTION

Nutritionists commonly advise that food be eaten throughout the day, and that it be equally divided among meals at the beginning, middle,

Table 5.   Criteria for Evaluation of Iron Status in Pregnancy (19)

---

1. Decreased storage iron in bone marrow

    Serum ferritin, < 10 ng/ml

2. Reduced transport iron

    Serum iron, < 50 μg/dl

    Total iron binding capacity, < 350 μg/dl

    Percent saturation, $< 20\%$

3. Decreased erythrocyte iron

    Hematocrit, $< 30\%$

    Hemoglobin, < 9.5 g/dl

    Red blood cell count, $< 4 \times 10^6 / m^3$

---

and end of the day. However, a pattern like that of the case presented in Table 6 seems to be quite common. This pregnant woman regularly omitted breakfast, ate a light lunch, and had a large evening meal. Also, as is often seen, although the protein and energy content of the diet were appropriate, a number of vitamins and minerals were below two-thirds of the standard. Addition of vegetable protein sources, vitamin C-rich fruits and vegetables, and dark green vegetables, along with a reduction in the amount of bread, would have improved the quality of the diet. Use of whole grain breads instead of refined bread also would have increased the nutrient density. Consumption of seven cups of coffee/day during pregnancy may have been of concern as well.

Health and Nutritional Consequences

This woman was fasting about 16 hours out of each 24, from 7:30 P.M. when she had her evening meal until 11:30 A.M. the next day when she ate lunch. Even though the mother eats periodically during pregnancy,

Table 6. Case Presentation of Poor Food Distribution in a 21-Year-Old Pregnant Woman

	Usual Food Intake Pattern
6:00 A.M.	four cups coffee with cream and sugar
11:30 A.M.	bologna sandwich with two slices refined bread, two slices bologna, 1 tsp mayonnaise, 12 oz milk, 1 cup coffee
3:00 P.M.	one cup coffee with cream and sugar, four cookies
7:30 P.M.	fried pork (about 3 oz), 1 cup rice, 2 cups lettuce salad, two biscuits, 1/2 cup jello, one apple, 1 cup coffee

	Evaluation	
Food Groups	Servings Recommended (29)	Servings Eaten
Animal protein	2	2
Vegetable protein	2	0
Milk and milk products	4	2
		(1-1/2 milk, 1/2 cream)
Bread and cereals	4	6
Vitamin C-rich fruit and vegetables	1	0
Dark green vegetables	1	0
Other fruits and vegetables	2	3

Nutrient Intake

Energy, kcal, 2824 (123% RDA)	Vitamins	Minerals, mg
Protein, g, 94.5 (124% RDA)	A, I.U., 1995[a]	Calcium, 576[a]
Fat, % kcal, 45	D, I.U., 121[a]	Phosphorus, 1297
Carbohydrate, % kcal, 42	E, mg, 13	Sodium, 3906
	Ascorbic acid, mg, 24[a]	Potassium, 1914
	Thiamin, mg, 1.2[a]	Magnesium, 178[a]
	Riboflavin, mg, 1.5	Zinc, 12.4[a]
	Niacin, mg, 19	Copper, 1.4
	B-6, mg, 1.3[a]	Iron, 14.7
	B-12, μg, 6.8	
	Folacin, μg, 232[a]	

[a] Less than two-thirds RDA (8)

the fetus feeds continuously. As described earlier, to provide glucose to the fetus when the mother is going without food, the mother readily shifts to fat for her energy and spares glucose for the fetus. A pregnant woman is much more prone to ketosis, therefore, than is a nonpregnant woman. Coetzee et al. reported that, after a 12-hour fast, the blood beta-hydroxybutyrate and acetoacetate levels in pregnant women are twice that of nonpregnant women (21). These ketones cross the placenta and are used as fuel by some of the fetal tissues (9). There is one report in the literature of impaired central nervous system function in offspring of diabetic mothers who had acetoaciduria during pregnancy (22). However, this conclusion was based on single urinary ketone tests made by the nurses on the patient's day of delivery. Since many women do not ingest food during labor and delivery, it is not surprising that there would be some ketonuria during this energy-demanding process. No other reports of impaired central nervous system function have been reported in infants and children of diabetic pregnant women who are likely to have been ketotic periodically during gestation, and investigators and clinicians are beginning to doubt that some ketosis during pregnancy is harmful to the developing fetus. However, marked ketosis throughout pregnancy would reflect a lack of food intake and, therefore, a lack of optimal energy supply for growth and development of the fetus.

The woman in this case study regularly drank seven cups of coffee/day. After completing their own study of the teratogenic potential of fresh-brewed coffee and caffeine in rats (23), the Food and Drug Administration in 1980 urged pregnant women to limit their intake of caffeine-containing beverages (24). In animals, consumption of 80 mg caffeine/kg was associated with ectrodactyly (partial or complete absence of digits) (23). This defect is rare in humans, but three cases were recently reported in women who had consumed about 20—30 mg caffeine/kg daily during pregnancy (25). An "average" 150-ml cup of coffee contains 110 mg caffeine if the coffee is made by the percolator method. Therefore, our woman in the case study would have consumed 770 mg caffeine, or about 12 mg/kg. A safe level of caffeine consumption has not been established for pregnant women, but it does seem wise for them to limit their caffeine intake.

Half of the nutrients calculated in this woman's diet fell below two-thirds of the recommended intake. Vitamin A, ascorbic acid, and calcium intakes are likely to be below standard if the consumption of dairy products, vitamin C-rich fruits and vegetables, and dark green or yellow vegetables is limited. However, low intakes of thiamin, vitamin B-6, folacin, magnesium, and zinc are not as easily recognized because these nutrients are not associated with any one food group. It is not unusual to find that they are below standard (26), especially in diets lacking whole grain breads and cereals, legumes, and dark green vegetables.

Marginal intakes of vitamins and minerals can easily be corrected by the woman's ingesting a prenatal vitamin-mineral supplement. Prenatal supplements should only be given along with nutritional counseling. Most supplements contain only 12—17 nutrients, or about 35—40% of the total number of nutrients required daily from dietary sources. Without this information, the pregnant woman may have a false sense of security regarding her nutrient supply and may not carefully select the foods that the prenatal vitamin-mineral capsule is to supplement.

Use of a supplement with a poor quality diet could cause nutrient imbalances. Marked reduction in zinc absorption due to high rates of supplemental iron absorption is a potential nutrient imbalance. Solomons has reported that increased iron absorption from iron supplements in anemic patients decreased zinc absorption (27). Some anemic prenatal patients are given iron supplements containing 100 mg or more of iron without zinc supplements. It may be wise to give these patients zinc supplements providing about 20—40 mg daily to better balance the trace element dietary supply. Megadoses of vitamins and minerals, greater than 10 times the recommended intake, can certainly lead to nutrient imbalances and are not indicated for pregnant women.

Clinical Evidence

Long periods of food deprivation, greater than 12 hours, can be detected by tests for ketones in the urine (commonly done by dipping reagent strips in a urine sample). Although ketosis per se may not be harmful to the fetus, repeated positive tests for ketones, along with a pattern of insufficient weight gain, may be evidence of an inadequate food intake.

The clinician should also be aware that therapeutic iron supplementation of an anemic pregnant woman could compromise zinc status. Poor zinc status can be detected by measuring serum zinc concentration; a level below 50 μg/dl is considered marginal (19).

CONCLUSIONS

The two most common nutritional problems among pregnant women living in the United States are energy imbalance and iron deficiency anemia. The three food patterns described in this paper (insufficient food intake, poor food selection, and poor food distribution) all ultimately could lead to these two clinical problems. However, only a small percentage of the pregnant women following these dietary patterns will develop the clinical symptoms of these nutritional problems. Others may be in a subclinical nutritional state; a sudden change in their food intake may cause nutritional problems and/or they may finish pregnancy in a compromised nutritional state.

To assure that maternal nutritional status is not altered by pregnancy, all women who follow one of these three dietary patterns should receive nutritional counseling throughout their pregnancies. Potential problems associated with these dietary patterns should be explained, and information on how to improve their dietary habits should be given. At least four principles should be emphasized in the nutritional counseling session:

1. Add food to the diet that supplies the suggested additional energy (300 kcal) needed for pregnancy. A pint of lowfat milk, a cup of chili, or a peanut butter sandwich on whole grain bread each provide about 300 kcal.
2. Limit the use of low nutrient-dense foods for meeting energy needs. Although 10 french fried potatoes supply about 300 kcal, they only contribute two nutrients, niacin and ascorbic acid, above 10% of standard. One cup of chili contributes over 10% of standard for protein and all the minerals plus vitamins B-6, niacin, and riboflavin.
3. Select a wide variety of foods to give a good balance of nutrients. Substitution of legumes and nuts for some of the meat, and whole grain breads and cereals for refined products will improve diet quality. Dark green vegetables and vitamin C-rich fruits and vegetables are good sources of many nutrients.
4. Distribute food evenly throughout the day; limit the overnight fast to about 12 hours.

ACKNOWLEDGMENT

The author gratefully acknowledges the help of Mrs. Bitsy Kosovac in preparation of the manuscript.

REFERENCES

1. Task Force on Nutrition. Assessment of maternal nutrition, The American College of Obstetricians and Gynecologists and the American Dietetic Association, 1978.
2. F. E. Hytten, Weight gain in pregnancy. In F. Hytten and G. Chamberlain, eds., *Clinical Physiology in Obstetrics*, Blackwell Scientific Publications, Oxford, 1980.
3. F. E. Hytten and T. Lind, *Diagnostic Indices in Pregnancy*, CIBA–GEIGY, Basle, Switzerland, 1973.
4. P. Rosso and C. Cramoy, Nutrition and pregnancy. In M. Winick, ed., *Nutrition, Pre- and Postnatal Development*, Plenum Press, New York, 1979, p. 133.
5. D. M. Campbell and I. MacGillivray, The effect of a low calorie diet or a thiazide diuretic on the incidence of preeclampsia and on birth weight. *Br. J. Obstet. Gynaecol.* **82**, 572 (1975).
6. P. Rosso and R. Kava, Effect of food restriction on cardiac output and blood flow to the uterus and placenta in the pregnant rat. *J. Nutr.* **110**, 2350 (1980).
7. W. T. Tompkins, R. McN. Mitchell, and D. G. Wiehl, Maternal and newborn nutrition studies at Philadelphia Lying-In Hospital. In

Proceedings of the 1954 Annual Conference of the Milbank Memorial Fund, New York, 1955.

8. Committee on Dietary Allowances, Food and Nutrition Board, National Research Council, *Recommended Dietary Allowances*, 9th ed., National Academy of Sciences, Washington, D.C., 1980.

9. P. A. J. Adam and P. Felig, Carbohydrate, fat and amino acid metabolism in the pregnant woman and fetus. In F. Falkner and J. M. Tanner, eds., *Human Growth I. Principles and Prenatal Growth*, Plenum Press, New York, 1978, p. 461.

10. D. J. Naismith, Maternal nutrition and the outcome of pregnancy — a critical appraisal. *Proc. Nutr. Soc.* **39**, 1 (1980).

11. J. C. King, D. H. Calloway, and S. Margen, Nitrogen retention, total body 40K, and weight gain in teenage pregnant girls. *J. Nutr.* **103**, 772 (1973).

12. J. A. Appel, Protein and energy utilization in pregnant and nonpregnant women, Doctoral dissertation, University of California, Berkeley, 1980.

13. A. Lechtig, J.-P. Habicht, H. Delgado, R. E. Klein, C. Yarbrough, and R. Martorell, Effect of food supplementation during pregnancy on birthweight. *Pediatrics* **56**, 508 (1975).

14. H. Oldham and B. B. Sheft, Effect of caloric intake on nitrogen utilization during pregnancy, *J. Am. Diet. Assoc.* **27**, 847 (1951).

15. R. M. Pitkin, Obstetrics and gynecology. In H. A. Schneider, C. E. Anderson, and D. B. Coursin, eds., *Nutritional Support of Medical Practice*, Harper & Row, Hagerstown, Md., 1977, p. 407.

16. N. R. Taggart, R. M. Holliday, W. Z. Billewicz, F. E. Hytten, and A. M. Thomson, Changes in skinfolds during pregnancy. *Br. J. Nutr.* **21**, 439 (1967).

17. R. L. Naeye, Weight gain and the outcome of pregnancy. *Am. J. Obstet. Gynecol.* **135**, 3 (1979).

18. B. Luke, *Maternal Nutrition*, Little, Brown and Company, Boston, 1979, p. 59.

19. Committee on Nutrition of the Mother and Preschool Child, Food and Nutrition Board, *Laboratory Indices of Nutritional Status in Pregnancy*, National Academy of Sciences, Washington, D.C., 1978.

20. D. Rush, Z. Stein, and M. Susser, A randomized controlled trial of prenatal nutritional supplementation in New York City. *Pediatrics* **65**, 683 (1980).

21. E. J. Coetzee, P. U. Jackson, and P. A. Berman, Ketonuria in pregnancy — with special reference to calorie-restricted food intake in obese diabetics. *Diabetes* **29**, 177 (1980).

22. J. A. Churchill, H. W. Berendes, and J. Nemore,

Neuropsychological deficits in children of diabetic mothers. *Am. J. Obstet. Gynecol.* **105**, 257 (1969).

23. T. F. X. Collins, J. J. Welsh, T. N. Black, and E. V. Collins, A comprehensive study of the teratogenic potential of caffeine in rats when given by oral intubation. *J. Environ. Pathol. Toxicol.*, in press.

24. Editorial. FDA caffeine decision too early, some say. *Science* **209**, 1500 (1980).

25. M. F. Jacobson, A. S. Goldman, and R. H. Syme, Coffee and birth defects. *Lancet* **2**, 1415 (1981).

26. J. C. King and S. Charlet, Current concepts in nutrition—pregnant women and premature infants. *J. Nutr. Ed.* **10**, 158 (1978).

27. N. W. Solomons and R. A. Jacob, Studies on the bioavailability of zinc in humans: Effects of heme and nonheme iron on the absorption of zinc. *Am. J. Clin. Nutr.* **34**, 475 (1981).

28. V. A. Beal, *Nutrition in the Life Span*, Wiley, New York, 1980, p. 454.

29. Maternal and Child Health Unit, California Department of Health, *Nutrition during Pregnancy and Lactation*, California State Department of Public Health, Sacramento, 1975.

ADDITIONAL RECENT REFERENCE

Committee on Nutrition of the Mother and Preschool Child, Food and Nutrition Board, National Research Council. *Alternative Dietary Practices and Nutritional Abuses in Pregnancy*, National Academy of Sciences, Washington, D.C., 1982.

12

Recent Developments in Infant Feeding and Nutrition

CATHERINE BRIGGS, M.D., M.P.H.
Lafayette, California

Address correspondence to Catherine Briggs, M.D., Pediatric and Public Health Consultant, 3304 Berta Lane, Lafayette, California 94549.

ABSTRACT

Current advances in knowledge in the field of infant feeding and nutrition are reviewed in this chapter. Recent changes in recommendations for and practices in infant feeding in the United States show increases in breast-feeding as well as a trend toward later introduction of solid foods. Current recommendations for vitamin and mineral supplementation in infants' diets are also presented. Recent studies, which have shed further light on the many advantages, both nutritional and immunologic, of breast-feeding the infant are summarized. An update on the nutritional composition of breast milk with attention given to vitamins and minerals is also included. Also described are other components of human milk, such as prostaglandins, enzymes, and a newly described growth-promoting factor. The potential problems of drugs and pollutants in breast milk and published viewpoints regarding this topic are presented. Among other topics being studied in this important field and discussed in this chapter are relactation, problems with cow's milk for infants, and iron nutrition.

INFANT FEEDING PRACTICES AND RECOMMENDATIONS: RECENT TRENDS

Major changes in infant feeding practices and recommendations have occurred in the United States over the past decade. We have gone from a period when breast-feeding was chosen by only about one-fifth of all new mothers, and when solids were started as early as the first weeks of life, to the present era where over 50% of new mothers choose to start breast-feeding and where the introduction of solids is recommended at 4 to 6 months.

Forces behind the dramatic changes include research findings that point out health benefits of breast milk and of later introduction of solids, as well as support and information groups that communicate breast-feeding advantages and common sense feeding guidelines on a grass roots, mother-to-mother basis. The recent changes are not really new, many are a return to time-tested practices of previous generations. Now, however, substantial evidence supports the traditional practices.

228

Changes in Infant Feeding Practices

Martinez and Nalezienski (1, 2) have surveyed the progressive decline in breast-feeding from 1955 to 1971, followed by a resurgence of the practice through 1979. There are now more mothers breast-feeding as well as more who continue to do so for longer periods of time. There is a substantial increase in breast-feeding among lower-income, less-educated women and among women who attend public clinics, in addition to continuing increases among higher-income and better-educated women.

Rates of breast-feeding in hospitals ranged in 1979 from a low of 41% of new mothers in the southeastern states who started out breast-feeding their infants to a high of 71% in the western mountain states. The overall percentage of U.S. mothers breast-feeding their babies was 51% in 1979, up from 29% in 1955. This dramatic rate of increase amounts to nearly 10% a year. If this rate continues, 60% of the babies born in the United States during 1982 will be breast-fed.

In 1971, only 5.5% of 5- to 6-month-old infants were breast-fed. By 1979 this had risen to 23%. This means that nearly half of the mothers who began breast-feeding continued to do so for at least 5 or 6 months. During this same 1971–1979 period, the use of whole cow's milk or evaporated milk for 5- to 6-month-old infants dropped from 68% to 25%, and the use of prepared formula rose from 28% to 57%, with 40% being iron-fortified and 17% without iron. The use of iron-fortified prepared infant formula is the alternative to breast milk recommended by the American Academy of Pediatrics.

Need for Continuing Education

Andrews, Clancy, and Katz (3) looked at the infant feeding practices of one group of families in a large prepaid health plan in the Northeast. They demonstrated that there is much more to be done regarding both public and professional education about current infant feeding recommendations. Specifically there is need for education concerning breast-feeding, later introduction of solid foods, avoidance of skim milk under the age of 1 year, and recommendations regarding use of iron-fortified formula. Some selected findings of this report on infant feeding practices in New York include:

1. At 3 to 5 months of age, the use of whole cow's milk began to increase. Few infants over 6 months of age received prepared formulas or breast milk. Skim milk was given to about 10% of 5- to 11-month-olds. The diet of the children fed skim milk was low in calories and

total fat and, as a percentage of calories, protein was well above the recommended level. For half of the children fed skim milk, the dietary intake of linoleic acid was found to be less than the estimated dietary requirement for this essential fatty acid (1% of total calories).

2. The introduction of foods other than milk into the infants' diet was rapid. Beikost (foods other than milk) accounted for 4% of the mean caloric intake of infants in the 1st month, increased to 27% by 2 to 3 months, then linearly increased to 65% at 9 to 11 months. Two-thirds of all 1-month-olds had already been given some form of food other than milk or formula, and nearly all children were receiving solids by age 3 months. The authors point out that a large percentage of mothers introduced solids earlier than 3 months with the sanction of their pediatrician.

3. By 9 to 12 months, table foods contributed over 50% of the calories from solids. Prior to these ages, commercially prepared foods had made up most of the solid feedings.

4. A large proportion of infants were given unneeded supplements of thiamin, riboflavin, vitamin B-6, and vitamin C. The supplements were unnecessary because adequate amounts of these nutrients were supplied in the diet.

5. With the exception of vitamin D and iron, most infants received greater than the recommended intake of all nutrients examined. Use of iron-fortified cereal or formula was associated with greater iron intakes.

6. Average calorie intakes approached or were greater than the Recommended Dietary Allowances. Average sodium intakes were well above advisable intakes. (Since this study, most makers of commercial infant solid foods have discontinued the practice of adding salt to their preparations.)

7. Mothers sometimes added sugar to milk or formula, and a large proportion of children were given sweetened beverages, most given in a bottle. The authors point out that this is contrary to the recommendation that, in order to protect against dental caries, the feeding of sweetened beverages from the bottle be avoided once the first primary teeth have erupted.

Recommendations on the Introduction of Solid Foods

In 1980, the Committee on Nutrition of the Academy of Pediatrics published its latest statement on the introduction of solid foods in the infant's diet (4), the first on this topic since 1958. In this statement, the Committee makes the point that infant feeding should be considered in three overlapping stages: the nursing period, during which breast milk or an appropriate formula is the source of nutrients; a transitional period, during which specifically prepared foods are introduced in addition to milk; and a modified adult period, during which the majority of nutrients come from the foods available on the family table.

Progress through these stages is developmentally based, that is, determined by the rate of maturation of the infant's nervous system, intestinal tract, and kidneys. For example, during the nursing period, the intestinal tract has not yet developed the mechanisms for coping with foreign proteins, and the kidneys are not mature enough to handle large loads of protein and electrolytes.

The developmentally appropriate nursing stage lasts from 4 to 6 months; the transitional period from that age until about 1 year.

The Committee's statement also contains specific recommendations on the introduction of solid foods during the transitional period. For example, the first solids should be single-ingredient foods, which are started one at a time at weekly intervals. This system of introduction allows for easy identification of possible food intolerances. Infant iron-fortified cereals —rice, for example —are an excellent choice for the first solid food. Other foods —vegetables, meats and fruits, commercial or prepared at home —can then be introduced, one by one.

After the introduction of solids, the load on the kidney tends to increase and the infant may need additional water. Water should be routinely offered as a part of feeding, so that the infant may meet its fluid needs without obligatory intake of extra calories.

The Committee also pointed out that potential food allergies offer fairly strong arguments for exclusive breast-feeding during the nursing period, and that only hypoallergenic foods be used during the transitional period. These recommendations are especially emphasized for those infants with a family history of allergy.

In regard to obesity and the early introduction of solids, the Committee felt that additional studies are required before specific recommendations can be made, since some investigations have found no relationship between the age at the introduction of supplemental foods and the later development of obesity. The report does cite some studies which have documented that bottle-fed infants develop and gain weight more rapidly than do breast-fed infants, and that solid foods when started early appear to constitute an additive supply of calories rather than replacement calories from the infant's milk intake.

The major compelling developmental reasons given by the Committee for their revised guidelines on supplemental food introduction include:

1. Neuromuscular mechanisms that allow proper chewing and swallowing of nonliquid foods are not in place in the first months of life.

2. Intestinal maturation that would allow digestion and absorption of a variety of foods is not fully developed in the early months.

3. Immunologic protection against foreign proteins as well as full renal competence to handle extraosmolar loads, such as those found in supplements, develop only after the first 4—6 months of life.

Another pertinent objection to the introduction of solids before 4—6 months of age is based on the possibility that this practice may interfere with the establishment of sound eating habits and may contribute to overfeeding (5); that is, until about the middle of the 1st year, the infant is not fully capable of expressing desire for or disinterest in the food offered, and, thus, there is the possibility of feeding beyond the point of satiety.

Recommendations on Breast-feeding

In a recent publication (6), Barness states the following position regarding the method of early infant feeding: "The dietary goals of the United States might well include breastfeeding for all infants who can nurse. . . ." He also recommends that supplemental foods need not and should not be introduced to the breast-fed infant before 6 months; however, in cases of formula feeding, it is judicious to add solids at 4 months, since multiple foods would decrease the chances of any possible not-yet-described nutrient deficiencies.

A joint WHO/UNICEF statement (7) provides an international position in agreement with the above: "A healthy well-nourished mother who is fully breastfeeding her infant should not need to introduce any complements during the first four to six months of life, according to the needs of the infant."

UPDATE ON LATEST RECOMMENDATIONS FOR SUPPLEMENTS FOR INFANTS

Solid Food Supplementation

Ahn and MacLean (8) showed that most infants breast-fed by healthy mothers do not need solid food supplements during the first half of the 1st year of life in order to grow normally. The study demonstrated that the weight and length curves of the infants studied during the period of exclusive breast-feeding remained above the 50th percentile of the National Center of Health Statistics' growth charts throughout at least the 6th month. It should be emphasized that this study's subjects were otherwise healthy infants and that the mothers were themselves well nourished.

Water Supplementation for Breast-Fed Infants

In a recent report on the water requirements of breast-fed infants in hot climates (9), Almroth concluded that healthy, exclusively breast-fed infants, even in hot and humid weather, managed well without additional water. However, this would not necessarily apply to any infants being fed according to fixed and rigid schedules, nor would it apply to ill infants. The study was carried out in Jamaica.

Vitamin and Mineral Supplement Needs

In 1980, the American Academy of Pediatrics published a statement regarding usual vitamin and mineral supplement needs for infants and children living in the United States (10). As a background for their recommendations, they pointed out that essential vitamins and minerals have been incorporated into processed formulas with the aim of providing an essentially complete food for infants, and that specific nutrients likely to be lacking in the diet of older infants and children have been used to fortify certain food products, such as infant cereal. The overuse of vitamin and mineral supplements by the general public and the possible reasons for this misuse are discussed. Food and Drug Administration regulations relating to supplements for infants and children, as well as common types of commercially available vitamin and mineral supplements, are reviewed.

The Academy has published a summary of guidelines for the use of supplements in healthy infants and children (Table 1).

To meet the needs of breast-fed term infants, vitamin D should be given if the infant has little exposure to sunlight. A supplemental source of iron, such as iron-fortified cereal, is needed after 6 months. For term infants fed commercial formulas, no vitamin supplements are required, and, after 4 months, an iron-fortified formula or cereal should be routinely used as an iron source. In general, there is little basis for routine vitamin and mineral supplementation in normal children, especially after infancy as the growth rate decreases. The one exception, fluoride, is discussed below.

The Academy concluded that the normal breast-fed infant of a well-nourished mother has not been shown conclusively to need any specific vitamin and mineral supplement; similarly, that there is no evidence for any necessary supplementation for the full-term, formula-fed infant and for the properly nourished child. In general, in the United States, the level of use of supplements for infants far exceeds demonstrated need.

Table 1. Guidelines for the Use of Supplements in Healthy Infants and Children (10)

		Vitamins			Minerals
Child	Multivitamin/ Multimineral	D	E	Folacin	Iron
Term infants					
Breast-fed	0	±	0	0	±[a]
Formula-fed	0	0	0	0	0[b]
Normal infants					
after 6 months	0	0	0	0	±[a]
Normal children	0	0	0	0	0

Note: symbols indicate: 0, that a supplement is not usually needed; ± that it is possibly or sometimes needed. Vitamin K for newborn infants and fluoride in areas where there is insufficient fluoride in the water supply are not shown.

[a] Iron-fortified formula and/or infant cereal is a more convenient and reliable source of iron than is a supplement.
[b] Iron supplements are not usually necessary if iron-fortified formulas are used, or iron-fortified cereals are started by about 4 months.

Table 2. Supplemental Fluoride Dosage Schedule (mg/day)[a] (11)

	Amount of Fluoride to Be Added to Diet (mg/day) When Fluoride in Drinking Water is		
Age	<0.3 ppm	0.3–0.7 ppm	>0.7 ppm
2 weeks–2 years	0.25	0	0
2–3 years	0.50	0.25	0
3–16 years	1.00	0.50	0

[a] 2.2 mg sodium fluoride contains 1 mg fluoride.

Fluoride

The most recent statement on fluoride supplementation by the Committee on Nutrition of the Academy of Pediatrics presents some revisions of previous recommendations (11). The revised dosage schedule takes into consideration the concentrations of fluoride in local drinking water, and it assumes that prepared formulas are not manufactured with fluoridated water.[1] The Academy's recommended fluoride supplements are presented in Table 2. In this table, there is no differentiation between breast-fed and bottle-fed infants. The Committee favors the initiation of fluoride supplementation shortly after birth in breast-fed infants (0.25 mg/day); and recommends that fluoride be supplemented according to the fluoride content of the drinking water in formula-fed infants. These recommendations are made in the expectation that early supplementation would have a beneficial effect during a period of active mineralization of bone and teeth. It was also felt that the starting of a regimen in early infancy might influence long-term compliance. The supplementation is recommended for infants who are exclusively breast-fed, whether or not they live in optimally fluoridated communities, since such infants frequently receive little or no water, and breast milk, like cow's milk, contains very little fluoride, irrespective of the local water supply.

Ranges of intake of fluoride from 0.1–1.0 mg/day during the 1st year of life and 0.5–1.5 mg during the next 2 years are considered adequate and safe (12). Amounts over 2.5 mg/day may result in mottling of the teeth.

Vitamin E Update

In a recent review (13) on the role of vitamin E in the nutrition of premature infants, Bell and Filer critically examine this vitamin's reported benefits. They point out that published studies of vitamin E supplementation for premature infants do not agree on the magnitude or even the existence of a protective effect of this vitamin in the anemia that often occurs 4 to 6 weeks after premature birth. Vitamin E has frequently been recommended to prevent this hemolytic anemia, which has been reported to exist in proportion to the depression of serum tocopherol, and to resolve the condition once it has appeared. Based on the authors' analysis of a dozen studies on this subject over the past 18 years, they state that, given current feeding practices and

---

[1]There is, however, at least one report of certain infant formulas containing as much fluoride as 1 mg/liter [E. Wiatrowski, L. Kramer, D. Osis, and H. Spencer, Dietary fluoride intake of infants. *Pediatrics* **55**, 517 (1975)].

formula compositions, vitamin E deficiency anemia is a rare problem, appearing perhaps in the presence of unusual oxidant stresses (for example, diets high in polyunsaturated fatty acids and supplemented with the oxidant iron). They conclude that vitamin E supplementation is not necessary for the prevention of the hemolytic anemia of premature infants.

Further, vitamin E has been reported to have specific pharmacologic effects that include protection against two common diseases of prematurity which are thought to be at least partially due to the toxic effects of oxygen: retrolental fibroplasia (RLF) and bronchopulmonary dysplasia (BPD). The authors' analysis of these reported protective effects concludes that final determination of the efficacy of the vitamin will have to await the results of additional large controlled trials. Specifically, regarding bronchopulmonary dysplasia, the most recent reports have failed to demonstrate that vitamin E affords protection.

BREAST-FEEDING: UPDATE ON THE ADVANTAGES

The many recognized advantages of breast milk and breast-feeding to the infant have been well reviewed (14, 15). In addition to advantageous biochemical, nutritional, antibacterial, and immunologic factors, breast-feeding may provide enhanced psychosocial interaction between mother and infant, with possible long-term benefits for mental and emotional health. More recent studies, described below, have continued to identify potential benefits as well as areas for further research.

Marmot and coworkers (16) reported that women in their early thirties who had been breast-fed as infants had significantly lower mean plasma cholesterol levels than did women who had been bottle-fed. The apparent difference in cholesterol between the groups of men with different infant feeding histories was not significant.

Another study, which dealt with endocrine responses in bottle-fed and breast-fed infants, demonstrated that there are differences in pancreatic and intestinal hormone release according to the type of feeding (17). The authors point out that these hormones may play a key role in postnatal adaptation. Specifically, in their study of 77 6-day-old healthy term infants, those who were bottle-fed had significant changes in plasma concentrations of the hormones insulin, motilin, enteroglucagon, neurotensin, and pancreatic polypeptide after feeding, whereas in breast-fed infants these changes were reduced or absent. Basal levels of gastric inhibitory peptide, motilin, neurotensin, and vasoactive intestinal peptide were also higher in the bottle-fed than in the breast-fed. It was concluded that these findings may partly explain the differences in the deposition of subcutaneous fat as well as stool frequency between breast-fed and bottle-fed neonates.

One major benefit of breast-feeding is the protection this mode of feeding gives against infection. This subject was reviewed in a 1980 article (18), which also discusses in detail the role of lipids as host-resistant factors in human milk. The author proposes that the antiviral property in human milk, reported since 1950, can now be defined in terms of the specific molecular structures of fatty acids and/or monoglycerides. The data, the author asserts, point to a strong relationship between the lipase activity in human milk and the antimicrobial activity, that is, the formation of fatty acids and monoglycerides. Cow's milk and commercially-prepared milk, having high levels of triglycerides and low levels of monoglycerides, lack this lipid-mediated antiviral activity. Based on his description of the role of lipids in protecting the infant against infection, the author calls for improved formula lipid composition by stating that commercially prepared infant formulas should be fortified with monoglycerides rather than with unsaturated vegetable oils. This particular article also includes a list of 80 references, many of which review the various other important host defense factors that are present in human milk.

In an important study (19), Fallot et al. compared rates of hospitalization for infections in infants according to their method of feeding. Exclusive breast-feeding during the first 3 months was significantly associated with a reduced rate of infections that required hospital admissions. Among the hospitalized group, only 11% were exclusively breast-fed, although the community breast-feeding rate was 25%. The authors feel that their data suggest that breast-feeding in the early months of life offers definite protection against infections severe enough to require hospitalization. They do point out that the occasional occurrence of acute infection in breast-fed infants indicates that the protection should not be considered total.

The authors cite evidence suggesting that breast-feeding must be exclusive to achieve full benefits in terms of the protective effects on the microflora and the immune system. Their data support this statement. There were no bacterial illnesses in the exclusively breast-fed infants, whereas 25% of the partially breast-fed and the bottle-fed infants did have documented bacterial infections. Criticism of this study involves the fact that it was retrospective in design and that the conclusions may be applicable only to private patients.

In another study on this topic (20), Cunningham presents data that show that breast-feeding is associated with improved morbidity, independent of the factors of lower educational level, lower maternal age, low birth weight, parental smoking, and the presence of older siblings and day care exposure. This study has also been reviewed and commented upon elsewhere (21).

France et al. (22) have studied the effect of breast-feeding in protecting the infant against the bacterial disease, caused by salmonella, that can produce severe gastroenteritis as well as a more generalized and systemic illness, including meningitis. They found that even partial breast-feeding seemed to provide protection that was equally as effective as full breast-feeding against salmonella infection. The authors stress that the protection lasted only as long as breast-feeding was actually in progress; 12 infants who were nursed for a period of time subsequently became infected when breast-feeding was discontinued.

When diarrheal illness supervenes in a breast-fed infant, is it necessary to discontinue the breast-feeding as part of the treatment of oral fluid restriction? This question is especially important in the developing world where the benefits of continued breast-feeding are great, and interruptions such as those caused by medically imposed proscriptions against breast milk can result in a mother unable to reinitiate successful lactation. This problem was studied recently in infants hospitalized with gastroenteritis in Bangladesh. In report of the study, Hoyle et al. (23) note that breast-feeding can be easily maintained during the infant's diarrheal episodes, even when anorexia (lack of appetite) is present. The authors' data show that continued breast-feeding during acute episodes of gastroenteritis clearly protects a child against overall reduction of caloric and protein consumption during the illness. They state that "the promotion of continued breastfeeding during diarrhea should be the most emphasized nutritional component of a diarrhea treatment program."

The above studies have dealt with recent clinical and epidemiologic observations on how infant feeding choices can influence the health of children. For complete reviews of the microbiologic and immunologic data on host defense mechanisms of human milk, see the references of Welsh and May (24) and Chandra (25).

In addition to protection against infections, breast-feeding may also help protect against the development of allergies. A Finnish study reported in *Lancet* (26) presented data that indicate that prolonged breast-feeding can act as a prophylactic measure against allergic disease. In the study, three groups of newborns were followed for 3 years. In one group, breast-feeding was discontinued before 2 months of age; in another, infants were exclusively breast-fed for 2 to 6 months; and in a third, infants were fed breast milk as their sole source of milk for over 6 months. All infants had the same pattern of solid food intake under the age of 1 year.

The results showed that, compared with formula feeding, prolonged breast-feeding resulted in a lower incidence of severe or obvious allergic disease, particularly in babies with a family history of allergies. Specifically, prolonged breast-feeding decreased the incidence of allergic dermatitis (eczema) in babies, with and without a family history of allergy, up to 1 year of age; it also decreased the incidence of food allergies in babies with a positive family history. There was no increased protection found in commercially prepared infant formulas as compared with regular cow's milk.

The authors' data indicate that prolonged breast-feeding is prophylactic for allergic disease in infants at hereditary risk; the longer that breast-feeding continued, the fewer atopic symptoms were subsequently documented. In babies who were solely breast-fed for at least 6 months, food allergy was suppressed for up to 1 year of age, and eczema up to 3 years. This study does not make any claims for prophylactic effects longer than those mentioned; other articles which question the prophylactic effect of breast-feeding against allergies simply state that long-term prevention of allergies has not been proven. Fewer allergies in early infancy and young childhood alone can be beneficial to the infant and the family.

The report suggests that the benefits of prolonged breast-feeding derive not only from the elimination of cow's milk protein from the diet, but also from some kind of local protection by human milk in the gastrointestinal tract. This protection could result from the coating of the mucosa with secretory IgA and consequent blockage of the entrance of antigens through the mucosa, which would have led to the setting up of the allergic reaction. The clinical observations documented in the study accord with the higher concentration of serum total IgE (an immunoglobulin associated with the allergic state) found in formula-fed babies as compared with those who are breast-fed (27).

The data indicated that the hereditary risk of early allergies seemed to be significantly decreased by 6 months of exclusive breast-feeding. They conclude that infants from allergic families should be breast-fed for at least 6 months, longer when possible, to lessen the risk and severity of atopic disease. In addition, the most potent or most common allergic foods — fish, citrus, chocolate, eggs, and tomatoes in this study — should be avoided during the 1st year of life. They stress that they do not claim that breast-feeding will totally prevent any occurrence of allergies; however, they believe that for most infants, breast-feeding seems to offer, in addition to the many nutritional, anti-infective, and psychologic benefits, a natural and safe means of giving some extra protection against allergic disease.

In another informative recent article (28) on the subject of allergy and breast-feeding, Gerrard points out that there are chances of the susceptible infant developing allergic symptoms to certain ingredients in breast milk. There have been cases when breast-feeding has been discontinued due to the problem of allergy to the mother's milk, but the author calls instead for a modification of the mother's own diet if the infant develops symptoms suggestive of allergy. Thus, rather than discontinuing breast-feeding and placing the infant on a cow's milk or soy formula, both of which have their own allergenic potentials, the mother can continue breast-feeding once the offending allergen has been identified and removed from *her* diet. Gerrard also advises that if allergies, food allergies in particular, are present on either or both sides of the family, the mother should vary her diet so that a large intake of any one specific food, particularly cow's milk and egg products, is avoided.

BREAST MILK: COMPOSITION

Update on Nutritional Composition

More specific information on the nutritional composition of human milk has been reported in the last few years. See references 29 and 30 for excellent summaries of the total picture of the nutrient make-up of breast milk and reference 31 for a summary of factors affecting its composition.

Vitamins

The vitamin content of human milk has been reviewed recently by the Committee on Nutrition of the American Academy of Pediatrics (30).

The objective of a series of recent studies (32–34) regarding the vitamin composition of breast milk was to determine if vitamin supplementation during lactation is beneficial to healthy, well-nourished women. No vitamin level in the milk was less than the published norm for that vitamin. However, some vitamins were consumed at levels below 100% of the RDAs, and vitamin B-12 was found in significantly lower concentrations in the unsupplemented group than it was in the supplemented mothers during the 2nd postpartum month. A follow-up study done 6 months postpartum, which included data on all the above vitamins as well as folacin, showed that there were no differences in milk vitamin concentrations between the supplemented and nonsupplemented groups. All vitamins, in fact, were within normal limits for milk concentrations.

The conclusion of these studies was to reconfirm that for healthy, well-nourished, lactating women, vitamins C, B-6, B-12, thiamin, and riboflavin concentrations in milk can be maintained by normal diets alone, and that vitamin supplementation up to 6 months postpartum did not affect the breast milk concentrations of these vitamins.

It should be emphasized that all the above studies had well-nourished mothers as subjects, and results cannot necessarily be applied to those with less optimal nutrition intake. There have been occasional reports, for example, of infants of mothers who are strict vegetarians who developed symptoms of vitamin B-12 deficiency (35). In addition, Sneed et al. (36) have recently reported that milk vitamin levels increased with vitamin supplements in lower socioeconomic lactating women.

There has been some discussion and debate in the recent literature on the vitamin D content of breast milk and the consequent need for vitamin D supplementation of the breast-fed infant. The latest pediatric commentaries (37, 38) on this topic conclude that since there has been no confirmation of water-soluble vitamin D activity in human milk, it is judicious to continue 400 I.U. vitamin D supplementation daily for breast-fed infants, pending further information. Occasional cases of rickets, as reported in the United States, may be associated with long-term unsupplemented breast-feeding as well as with other factors (39).

Salt Content of Breast Milk

An interesting study of the sodium and potassium concentrations in breast milk during the 1st month postpartum was reported in 1979 in the Scandinavian literature (40). The concentration of sodium in colostrum of mothers delivered at term was found to be highest—61mM/liter on the 1st day of life. It then fell to 20mM/liter in from 2—11 days, then dropped further after 11 days to approximately 3—4mM/liter. The potassium concentration of breast milk was found to be fairly constant after delivery. According to the authors, the results suggest that infants who are not breast-fed may benefit from the temporary and judicious use of salt supplements. They state that this is probably more important for preterm infants, since they have greater urinary salt losses than do the full-term infants and may easily develop hyponatremia (low blood sodium). In addition, sodium and chloride have been found to be higher in preterm milk, and a sodium supplement has been reported to induce accelerated growth in preterm infants (41).

It should be pointed out that the call for salt supplementation of all non-breast-fed infants for the first few weeks has not appeared in the recent U.S. pediatric literature. There has been a recent statement by the Committee on Nutrition of the American Academy of Pediatrics regarding the sodium intake of U.S. infants (42) that emphasizes the infant's capability to tolerate a range of sodium intakes and calls for an end to efforts to further decrease sodium intake for infants.

The occurrence of hypernatremia (too much salt in the blood) has also received some attention in the recent literature. A case of hypernatremia was reported in an infant whose mother's breast-milk sodium concentration varied between 28–31 meq/liter (milliequivalents per liter) when the infant was 18–23 days old (43). There were no external signs of breast infection. The infant's hypernatremia apparently resulted from decreased fluid intake and elevation of the sodium level in the breast milk.

Based on this report, the suggestion has been made that, since a breast-fed infant who is gaining weight poorly may be ingesting breast milk with a high sodium content or possibly a low chloride content (44), an analysis of the sodium content of the mother's milk as well as of the infant's electrolytes might be considered (45). One possible cause of elevated sodium levels in breast milk is breast infection (46). If this is the case, the mother is usually able to continue nursing after proper treatment has been obtained.

Minerals

Atkinson and coworkers (47) studied the sodium, chloride, potassium, magnesium, calcium, and phosphorus content of milk from preterm mothers and compared it with milk of term mothers. They found that the mineral composition of milk from mothers of full-term and preterm infants was similar during the 1st month of lactation. They estimated infants' intakes of the breast milk of mothers of preterms as measured against mineral requirements and concluded that the quantities provided of sodium, chloride, potassium, and magnesium, but not of calcium and phosphorus, would be adequate to meet the requirements of premature infants during the early weeks of life.

Also regarding mineral content, a longitudinal study was reported by Vaughan et al. (48) which looked at the effect of length of lactation time on the mineral composition of breast milk and the changes that occur with the duration of lactation. The authors pointed out that studies prior to and during the early 1970s have shown that there is considerable variation in the composition of human milk, and that the variation is found among women as well as in individuals over time and even within feedings. But long-term studies for determination of variation in human milk content have been limited. Most trace mineral levels in milk decreased over the months of the study. Zinc and calcium decreased appreciably, copper and iron moderately, and magnesium and manganese showed little change. No significant correlations were found between milk mineral levels and (1) maternal hair levels of the minerals, (2) maternal serum levels, or (3) maternal dietary intake.

A recent study in India was done with the objective of determining the influence of maternal diet and nutritional status on the trace element content of breast milk (49). The investigators sought to learn if there were differences in the trace element profiles of subjects from differing socioeconomic groups. The groups studied included urban low- and high-income women as well as rural low-income women. The results showed:

1. Copper and zinc levels in milk fell by 7 to 12 months of lactation.

2. Concentrations of copper and zinc in serum did not correlate with their concentrations in breast milk.

3. There were no significant variations secondary to timing of the sampling of the breast milk. (Thus, the authors felt that analysis of one sample did give satisfactory information.)

4. There were no differences in amounts of copper, zinc, and magnesium in breast milk between rural and urban low-income women.

5. High-income (urban) mothers had significantly higher levels of copper and zinc in their milk than did low-income women in the first to third months of lactation only. Beyond this time, the milks were similar with regard to the minerals studies, despite dietary variations which were present in the intake of these elements between groups.

The authors concluded that the mean values for copper and zinc in the groups studied are essentially similar to those of women in the United States. Also, the finding that there was no correlation between the copper and zinc levels in serum and milk led to their suggestion that there is active transfer from plasma to milk for these minerals. In addition, they noted that, although both urban and rural poor women had low concentrations of copper and zinc in their milk samples, the growth and clinical condition of the infants being fed with this breast milk was satisfactory.

Another study regarding the concentration of copper and zinc in human milk was reported earlier in the Scandinavian literature. Vuori and Kuitunen (50) took samples of breast milk during the course of lactation. They found that concentrations of copper and zinc were dependent on the stage of lactation. The median copper and zinc concentrations decreased during the course of lactation from approximately 0.60 mg/liter and 4.0 mg/liter to 0.25 mg/liter and 0.5 mg/liter, respectively. The importance of a consideration of the stage of lactation in the evaluation of the nutritional value of trace elements in breast milk needs emphasizing, according to these authors.

Another study by Vuori et al. (51) reported that maternal intake of copper, iron, and zinc did not seem to affect the corresponding trace element levels in human milk.

Iron and Zinc

The concentration of iron in breast milk was evaluated in a longitudinal study, said by the authors to be the first of this type published (52). Lactating Finnish women were followed up to 9 months postpartum. The median value for iron declined during the course of lactation from 0.6 mg/liter early to 0.3 mg/liter after 5 months, with a wide range of values. The results indicated either that the concentration of iron is lower than usually stated or that it is unusually low in Finnish mothers. There was also a great variation in individual samples, from 0.11 mg/liter to 1.14 mg/liter.

The authors feel that as a consequence of the demonstrated low values of iron in their study, some infants may require iron supplementation during prolonged breast-feeding, even though the high bioavailability of iron in breast milk helps to prevent the development of iron deficiency.

There is evidence to support the view that trace minerals in human milk are utilized with greater efficiency than those present in cow's milk. Studies made during the past few years have established that iron is more efficiently absorbed from human milk than from cow's milk.

Zinc bioavailability has been receiving attention as well. Lönnerdal et al. (53) have isolated in human milk a low-molecular-weight compound that binds zinc. It has been hypothesized that this zinc-binding compound may enhance zinc transport in the neonatal period, before the development of an intestinal mechanism for zinc absorption.

More recently, Casey et al. (54) have studied the uptake of zinc in human subjects, with results that support the concept of increased bioavailability of zinc from human milk compared with cow's milk or infant formulas.

Lipids

For a review of the lipid composition of human milk as well as of infant formula, see the 1978 review by Jensen et al. (55). Many aspects of lipid composition, including the fatty acid composition of milk, and details of lipid content are discussed. For example, it is recognized that 98% of the lipid content of breast milk is in the form of triacylglycerol (normal triglycerides). At least 167 fatty acids have been identified in breast milk, and the fatty acid composition can be changed by diet, whereas diet has no effect on the total lipid content level. A mother can increase the polyunsaturated-to-saturated ratio of the fatty acids of breast milk by ingesting a diet rich in polyunsaturates, and the infant's polyunsaturated fatty acid levels will rise accordingly.

Recent articles have appeared on the usefulness of a simple and practical technique which is used to determine the creamatocrit, the relative lipid content of a sample of breast milk. The procedure involves filling a capillary tube with milk and centrifuging it, measuring the cream layer and calculating the percentage of total volume (56).

Nutrient Composition of Breast Milk in Poorly Nourished Communities

Studies on the volume and nutrient composition of breast milk in poorly nourished communities were reviewed in 1978 (57). Most investigators who compared the composition of breast milk between developing and Western countries have found the quality to be generally equivalent (58).

Further, it has been shown that the duration of lactation over 1 year does not appreciably affect breast milk composition and that by having the benefit of breast feeding into the 2nd year of life, children in developing countries will generally receive about one-third of their total protein requirement via breast milk (59).

Nutrient Composition of Breast Milk from Women using Oral Contraceptives

Nitrogen and protein composition were determined in milk from women using oral contraception during lactation (60). Total nitrogen and nonprotein nitrogen as well as lactose and the milk proteins lactoferrin, alpha lactalbumin, and serum albumin were analyzed before the introduction of oral contraceptives (four different types) and thereafter during the lactation period. Significant changes in protein content were observed between groups and controls for all parameters studied. The changes, however, resulted in values that were still within the normal broad range of values for well-nourished subjects. No differences were found in lactose content, and minerals and vitamins were not studied.

Other Recently Described Components of Human Milk

Besides macro- and micronutrients, breast milk contains other important cellular and molecular elements. For example, the presence of the following components has already been described in the literature over the past years: a growth enhancer of lactobacilli, an antistaphlococcal agent, immunoglobulins, certain complement components, lysozyme, lactoperoxidase, lactoferrin, and macrophages and lymphocytes (15, 61, 62).

In addition to the nutrients essential for the rapid growth and maturation of the infant, other components of breast milk have recently been discovered. The subject of hormones in human milk has been reviewed by Koldovsky (63). Hormonal components include: prolactin, thyroid-stimulating hormone, thyroid hormones, and corticosteroids (63, 64). The exact metabolic significance for the infant of the presence of these hormones is still being investigated.

Reid et al. (65) measured the levels of prostaglandins E_2 and F_2 by radioimmunoassay in milk aliquots from six term mothers. The two prostaglandins were detected in all fresh human milk samples, but not in formulas that used cow's milk as a base. Prostaglandins E_2 and F_2 are derivatives of the fatty acids linoleic and arachidonic acid. The prostaglandins affect a variety of physiologic functions including gastric acid and mucus secretion, smooth muscle contraction, local circulation, water, glucose and ion transport, zinc absorption, and protection of the gastrointestinal epithelium.

Prostaglandins in human milk could be derived from local synthesis in the mammary gland, from the cellular elements of human milk, or from the maternal circulation; the exact source is not yet clear. It is possible that prostaglandins from human milk could have a cytoprotective effect on the gastrointestinal tract of the neonate. Their specific physiologic role in the infant awaits further clarification.

Nucleotides

One recent study (66) reports the presence of the cyclic nucleotides AMP (adenosine monophosphate) and GMP (guanosine monophosphate) in breast milk. These nucleotides are known to participate in the regulation of the processes of cellular proliferation and differentiation, processes important to maturation of the neonate. Although these nucleotides are distinct components of the complex network of hormone-regulated physiologic regulations, exact delineation of their role in breast milk, if any, must await further studies.

Enzymes

The possible physiologic significance of enzymes found in human milk has been recently discussed by Shahani et al. (67). They stress that human milk is a highly complex fluid that contains numerous active enzymes. However, the significance, if any, of each enzyme in human milk, its possible origin, and its nutritive value to the infant are not clear.

A Newly Described Growth-Promoting Factor in Human Milk

Recently, researchers have reported a substance with growth-promoting activity in breast milk (68). It has been further determined to be a polypeptide termed epidermal growth factor (EGF) (69), which had previously been identified as a growth factor present in human plasma, saliva, urine, and amniotic fluid. This growth factor has been shown to produce significant biologic effects in the mammal, particularly in the fetus and newborn. It has also been shown to stimulate DNA synthesis and induce division in cells grown in culture. Effects on the fetus and neonate include the following:

1. Enhanced proliferation and differentiation of the epidermis.
2. Increased growth and maturation of the fetal pulmonary epithelium.
3. Stimulation of DNA synthesis in the digestive tract. These researchers concluded that the demonstrated ability of breast milk to stimulate DNA synthesis and cell multiplication is probably due to the presence of this epidermal growth factor. In fact, breast milk was more potent than purified EGF in this activity; it has been speculated that milk may contain molecules that enhance the activity of EGF.

There is no reported similar growth-promoting activity found in commercially available infant formulas. Epidermal growth factor is a small polypeptide with a molecular weight of about 6000 and is found in many mammalian species. It is acid stable and, thus, able to survive passage through the stomach with its acid pH, possibly enabling it to act directly on the tissues of the digestive tract and perhaps to be absorbed into the circulation where it may affect proliferation of other tissues as well.

Colostrum has the highest activity of this growth-promoting factor, where it is about 15 times as active as 3rd day milk which, in turn, is 10 times as active as 57th day milk. The activity, although decreased, could still be identified at 6 months (68).

It has been speculated that this growth-promoting factor may be involved in the growth and development of mucosal cells of the neonate, in preventing and aiding recovery from enterocolitis and peptic ulceration in the newborn, as well as affecting growth of cells in the ductal system of the mother's breast.

DRUGS AND POLLUTANTS IN BREAST MILK

Drugs

It is axiomatic that any drug that can enter the maternal bloodstream can also enter breast milk. Piatzker et al. (70) have listed drugs and toxins that can be transmitted to the infant by the lactating mother's milk. The reviewers list more than 200 drugs and drug categories for which published studies exist, give evidence for drug secretion or nonsecretion in milk, and evaluate whether a nursing mother's ingestion of the drug is compatible with breast-feeding. The authors point out that decisions as to the use of incompatible drugs, with at least temporary discontinuation of breast-feeding, versus the use of alternate, compatible drugs, need to be made in individual situations with the mother's and infant's physicians. When a mother requires treatment, the clinician can consider altering doses, changing the schedule of doses, or substituting an alternate drug, while closely monitoring the infant for adverse effects. The decision is made after weighing the risks and benefits of the drug alternatives to the mother and infant, as well as the factor of the benefits of breast milk to the infant. Hence, no arbitrary generalized recommendations can be given.

Pollutants

Polychlorinated biphenyl (PCB) contamination of human tissues is a matter of great current interest. The Committee on Environmental Hazards of the Academy of Pediatrics, in its most recent statement on PCBs in breast milk (71), concludes "unless women have a history of exposure to PCB's, they should be encouraged to breastfeed their infants as usual." If there is a known history of PCB exposure (for example, those who have worked with PCBs, have been in contaminated areas, or who are known to have ingested large amounts of sports fish from PCB-contaminated waters), it is suggested that the mother's PCB level be measured and advice sought from state health departments if high levels are found.

A study of breast milk from lactating mothers in Michigan, where there was contamination of dairy milk products with polyhalogenated biphenyls (a family of toxic compounds that includes PCBs) after an industrial accident in the 1970s, was recently published (72, 73). All 1000+ samples of breast milk collected throughout the state contained PCB residues ranging from trace to significant levels. The median level was only slightly less than the FDA's present tolerance limit of 1.50 ppm for PCBs in cow's milk and dairy products.

The authors of this study also point out in a 1981 report (74) that, although there have been no case reports of illnesses due to transmission of PCBs through breast milk, the lasting effects of this chemical contamination are unclear. They do not recommend any major changes in current breast-feeding practices, but they do echo recommendations for breast milk testing if there is a question of high PCB exposure. If PCB level is high (the levels are discussed in the article), a shorter duration of breast-feeding may be advised.

Pollutants in general in breast milk are reviewed in another recent article (75). The toxicity, intake, and "safe" levels of DDT, PCBs, and other compounds are discussed. The authors' conclusion, similar to that in the above study, is that "a clinical assessment of risk is difficult because, although virtually all studies of the value of breastmilk have shown definite benefits, the role of milk contaminants in the production of disease in children is virtually unstudied." Recommendations on this subject included the avoidance of excessive weight reduction in pregnant and lactating women, as this might mobilize the chemicals from fat stores.

There is general agreement that continued efforts to decrease the levels of contaminants and, thus, the potential of harm are needed, as is further research on the precise impact of environmental pollution on the health of the fetus and newborn.

RELACTATION AND INDUCED LACTATION

There have been a number of articles in the recent literature which describe and study aspects of relactation and induced lactation, including the nutritional composition of the breast milk produced in these processes. Relactation is defined as the resumption of breast-feeding following cessation of, or significant decrease in, milk production. Induced lactation is breast-feeding without a previous recent pregnancy.

Relactation

The major message in these articles is that relactation is frequently possible and successful, both in fulfilling or contributing to the complete nutritional requirements of an infant and in promoting enhancement of the mother-infant relationship.

In one of the recent studies (76), 75% of 336 women who had relactated evaluated their experience positively, even when there was a need for supplemental fluids in addition to the breast milk produced. Preparation and techniques of relactation are discussed.

In another report (77), six mothers initiated the relactation process from 10 to 150 days postpartum, and three were eventually able to completely nourish their infants by the breast. Two others provided at least 50% of the infants' nutritional needs, and one failed to provide significant quantities of milk, although some milk was produced. It took from 8 to 58 days to reach maximal milk production, and both the likelihood of successful relactation and the rapidity of onset of lactation correlated with shorter postpartum interval and the degree of postpartum breast involution. All the mothers expressed positive feelings about the process whether or not the relactation was complete. Relactation, the authors point out, may offer the mother who desires to breast-feed an alternative if she does not maintain lactation in the immediate postpartum period.

Induced Lactation

A review of the experiences of 240 women who attempted to induce lactation after adopting an infant has recently appeared (78). Preparation included breast and nipple stimulation, supplementation of the maternal diet, and occasional use of hormones.

It was found that a history of previous lactation was related to an increased likelihood of milk production. The increased willingness of the under-8-week-old infant to suck as compared with the older infant was also felt to be a factor.

Nearly all women in the study reported supplementing their own milk supply. Sixteen percent were able to discontinue the supplements before 1 month had elapsed, and 54% continued throughout the time they chose to nurse. The most frequent method of supplementation was the nursing trainer, which utilizes a small flexible tube attached to a small bag containing the supplemental milk supply, positioned so that it is sucked along with the mother's nipple at the time of feeding.

As in the studies of relactation, the majority of the mothers reported that the mother-infant relationship was a more important issue to them than reaching a certain level of success with milk production, and most (76%) evaluated the experience positively. No infants were reported to have required hospitalization as a result of inadequate weight gain or dehydration in this study.

Kleinman et al. (79) recently studied the protein content of milk produced by induced lactation and found that, during the first 5 days of lactation, total protein concentrations were similar in amount to values obtained from milk from biological mothers. This induced milk is lower in IgA (an immunologically active protein) and total protein and is higher in alpha-lactalbumin than is colostrum. Thus, sucking alone, without pregnancy and delivery, does not seem to be a sufficient stimulus for the production of colostrum, although sucking can and does produce milk essentially indistinguishable from mature milk of biologic nursing mothers.

Other investigators reporting on the milk composition of lactating women who had not experienced a recent pregnancy (80) agreed with the above in their conclusions that: (1) the average concentrations of the induced milk constituents were in close agreement with those obtained from women during established lactation after normal pregancy; and (2) with proper preparation, it is possible to induce lactation successfully in nonpostpartum women.

POTENTIAL PROBLEMS WITH COW'S MILK IN INFANTS

Potential problems and adverse effects of cow's milk and cow's milk formulas on the infant's gastrointestinal tract are reviewed and summarized in a 1979 article (81).

Since that time, Fomon and colleagues have studied the problem of occult blood loss from the gastrointestinal tract in older infants (3 to 6 months old) receiving pasteurized bovine milk (82). The study groups were fed either whole cow's milk (pasteurized, homogenized), a commercial formula, or heat-treated cow's milk (time and temperature treatments were identical to those used in the commercial formula). All groups were receiving recommended intakes of iron. The stools were checked for blood loss by the guaiac test; and hemoglobin, serum iron concentration, and transferrin saturation were analyzed.

The researchers showed that the number of infants with guaiac-positive (showing blood loss) stools in the age interval 112–140 days was significantly greater in the groups fed whole cow's milk than for those fed the formula or heat-treated cow's milk. A total of about 10% of 294 stools of infants fed whole cow's milk were guaiac-positive, whereas about 3% of 244 stools of infants fed a commercially prepared formula were guaiac-positive. The iron nutritional status comparisons between groups showed no statistically significant differences. Since these hematologic values remained satisfactory, the authors felt it was likely that daily supplementation of 12 mg iron from ferrous sulfate permitted sufficient absorption of iron to compensate for the documented gastrointestinal blood losses.

Because of their finding of significantly more blood loss occurring at ages under 140 days in the group fed pasteurized whole cow's milk, the authors conclude that pasteurized cow's milk should not be fed to infants before 140 days of age.

Other workers (83) have pointed out a nutritional problem emanating from the process of boiling pasteurized cow's milk for infants and young children. They showed that infants who are fed boiled pasteurized cow's milk may rapidly develop low serum and whole blood folacin levels indicative of folacin deficiency. The authors demonstrated that the folacin concentrations in the boiled milk samples were considerably lower than they were the preboiling levels, but that the addition of sodium ascorbate, 1 mg/ml, before the heating procedure, would prevent this loss.

Naveh and colleagues have recently reported (84) a case of copper deficiency in a 6-month-old infant fed an unmodified cow's milk formula. The child presented with anemia and neutropenia, which was reversed only with the administration of copper sulfate. It is thought to be the first such reported case.

A new immunologic assay for cow's milk allergy has recently been described by Ashkenazi and colleagues (85). A hypersensitivity reaction to cow's milk in infants and children occurs in approximately one infant out of 100. Signs and symptoms can include vomiting, diarrhea, respiratory problems, skin rashes, fever, gastrointestinal blood loss, and failure to thrive. A new test has been described which consists of identifying a lymphokine (LIF, or leukocyte inhibitory factor) produced by peripheral blood lymphocytes. This substance is produced in response to an in vitro challenge with bovine betalactoglobulin, which is the most common sensitizing antigen in cow's milk. The study demonstrates that this cell-mediated immunologic assay is a reliable test for the diagnosis of sensitivity to milk protein in infants and children and can be used to determine the need for dietary treatment and to ascertain when this treatment may be safely discontinued.

Also of interest was the finding by the same authors that when the infant is placed on a diet free of cow's milk, the above test returns to normal in most cases within several months to a year; cow's milk can then be reintroduced cautiously after the LIF has become negative (less than 16%). This finding agreed with clinical observations that most children with an allergy to cow's milk lose their hypersensitivity with time, which may be explained by the development of tolerance to milk antigens. The authors feel this tolerance may possibly be due to the action of a subpopulation of suppressor cells.

Butler et al. (86) studied depressed neutrophil function in infants with cow's milk and/or soy protein intolerance. They found in their study infants that both cow's milk and soy protein were capable of inducing mucosal injury, along with local inflammatory cell response in the small intestine and colon. By 2 years of age, most affected infants were once again able to tolerate these proteins. The authors feel that neutrophil function may be involved in formula protein intolerance. The neutrophil may play a role in protecting the gut against foreign proteins in normal situations, and there may be some loss of this role in formula intolerance.

UPDATE ON IRON: NUTRITIONAL CONSIDERATIONS FOR INFANTS

Recent developments concerning the subject of diet and iron absorption in infants in the first 12 months were highlighted in a review in 1979 (87). The exceptionally high bioavailability of iron in human milk is stressed. For example, the reviewers reported a study in which breast-fed infants absorbed up to 49% of a trace dose of extrinsic iron administered during a breast-feeding, whereas an approximate 10% to 20% level of iron absorption has been reported with feedings with cow's milk. In a 1979 study, Saarinen and Siimes (88) demonstrated that other ingredients in infants' diets, as well as in the diets of children and adults, can have an inhibitory effect on this high iron absorption rate. The high bioavailability of iron in breast milk rapidly dropped in the study group of infants after solid foods were introduced at 4 months of age.

A 1980 study on this topic was recently reviewed by Dallman (89). It confirmed and refined the above results, indicating that timing as well as choice of solid foods for infants appear to have a greater influence on iron nutrition than was previously recognized. For example, orange juice with a meal has been shown to more than double the iron absorbed from the entire meal. Meat, poultry, or fish in a meal resulted in the absorption of about four times as much iron from a meal compared with cheese, milk, or eggs in equivalent amounts. It now appears fairly well recognized that the iron in the "old favorites," spinach and eggs, is in a form that is not well absorbed.

Specifically, examples of common substances that decrease the absorption of non-heme iron are phytate, calcium, phosphorus, and fiber. It is now recognized that the most important factor in iron nutrition is not the iron content in the food or milk but how efficiently that iron is absorbed.

Owen and colleagues have recently reported on a prospective study of iron nutriture in infants (90) in which 6-month-old infants fed mainly breast milk appeared to be iron sufficient at age 2. If, however, iron supplements were routinely given to breast-fed infants, those infants had greater iron stores at age 6 months than did nonsupplemented breast-fed infants.

From what is presently known regarding different iron absorption levels from individual foods and mixtures of foods, we can advise certain infant feeding guidelines.

1. If breast-feeding, one should follow recommendations to defer solid food introduction for the term infant until around the middle of the first year (4—6 months). When this is done, breast-feeding alone has been found to be sufficient to meet iron needs during the first 6 months for the term infant.

2. A good choice for initial solid food is iron-fortified dry infant cereal. The canned baby cereal preparations have much less iron than the dry preparations.

3. After about 6 months of age, the infant could receive one meal a day with orange juice instead of milk. The meal should contain iron-fortified cereal or an iron-rich food such as meat. Then the milk feed (for example, breast milk if breast-feeding) could be given later as a snack, in place of juice. Also, combinations of animal and vegetable foods should be encouraged at each meal, or iron-rich vegetables alone with a vitamin C-containing juice.

4. If the infant is being fed by formula, the mother should choose one that is fortified with iron. This will give the infant an ample supply of iron and will offer less dependency on solid food sources of iron, as is the case when nonfortified formulas are used.

It should be added that a recent double blind randomized study (91) found no difference in the bowel habits of infants fed either iron-fortified or nonfortified formulas in the first weeks of life. Mild gastrointestinal symptoms were noted equally in each of these formula-fed groups.

PROTEIN—CALORIE MALNUTRITION IN CHILDREN

Although one usually thinks of protein—calorie malnutrition (PCM) as a problem of the developing world, there are occasional reports of severe malnutrition here in the United States. In a recent paper (92), four children in one medical center were reported to have developed kwashiorkor 6 weeks to 6 months after a low-protein, nondairy creamer (commonly sold along with dairy products in supermarkets throughout the country), was introduced into their diets as a milk substitute. This substitution was initiated in an attempt to control suspected milk protein sensitivity (however, only one of the four patients was subsequently proven to have this entity). In these children, each of whom demonstrated hypoproteinemia, edema, and hepatic abnormalities during the course of their illness, the nondairy milk substitute had become their major or only source of nutrients. The infants apparently became rapidly satiated with the high-calorie, high-fat product and refused to eat solid foods. All recovered after reinstitution of a nutritionally adequate diet. The nondairy creamer, in addition to having a very low protein content, had inadequate amounts of vitamins A and C, thiamin, riboflavin, niacin, calcium, and iron.

These cases serve as a reminder to all of the importance of following suspected allergic infants' and children's diets very closely, with careful attention being paid to nutritional adequacy. Furthermore, a careful diagnosis of the suspected allergic condition should be carried out before an elimination diet or food substitution regimen is instituted. In addition, parents need to be educated that commercial "milk substitutes," such as the one mentioned above, are not meant to replace infant formulas.

CONCLUSIONS

There have been many changes and new findings in the realm of infant feeding and nutrition within the past few years. The nutritional status and overall health of infants and children, both in the United States and abroad, should benefit from these developments and new knowledge. It is hoped that further research, as well as the active application of research findings, will continue to flourish in the coming years.

REFERENCES

1. G. A. Martinez and J. P. Nalezienski, The recent trend in breast-feeding. *Pediatrics* **64**, 686 (1979).
2. G. A. Martinez and J. P. Nalezienski, 1980 Update: The recent trend in breast-feeding. *Pediatrics* **67**, 260 (1981).
3. E. M. Andrews, K. L. Clancy, and M. G. Katz, Infant feeding practices of families belonging to a prepaid group practice health care plan. *Pediatrics* **65**, 678 (1980).
4. Committee on Nutrition, Academy of Pediatrics. On the feeding of supplemental foods to infants. *Pediatrics* **65**, 1178 (1980).
5. S. A. Fomon, L. J. Filer, Jr., T. A. Anderson, and E. E. Zeigler, Recommendations for feeding normal infants. *Pediatrics* **63**, 52 (1979).

6. L. Barness, Formula manufacture and infant feeding [editorial]. *J. Am. Med. Assoc.* **243**, 1075 (1980).
7. WHO/UNICEF Statement on infant and young child feeding. *WHO Chron.* **33**, 435 (1979).
8. C. H. Ahn and W. C. MacLean, Jr., Growth of the exclusively breast-fed infant. *Am. J. Clin. Nutr.* **33**, 183 (1980).
9. S. G. Almroth, Water requirements of breast-fed infants in a hot climate. *Am. J. Clin. Nutr.* **31**, 1154 (1978).
10. Committee on Nutrition, American Academy of Pediatrics. Vitamin and mineral supplement needs in normal children in the United States. *Pediatrics* **66**, 1015 (1980).
11. Committee on Nutrition, American Academy of Pediatrics. Fluoride supplementation: revised dosage schedule. *Pediatrics* **63**, 150 (1979).
12. Committee on Dietary Allowances, Food and Nutrition Board, National Research Council. *Recommended Dietary Allowances*, 9th ed., National Academy of Sciences, Washington, D.C., 1980.
13. E. F. Bell and L. J. Filer, The role of vitamin E in the nutrition of premature infants. *Am. J. Clin. Nutr.* **34**, 414 (1981).
14. Committee on Nutrition, American Academy of Pediatrics. Breastfeeding. *Pediatrics* **62**, 591 (1978).
15. D. B. Jelliffe and E. F. P. Jelliffe, *Human Milk in the Modern World*, Oxford University Press, London, 1978.
16. M. G. Marmot, C. M. Page, E. Atkins, and J. W. B. Douglas, Effects of breastfeeding on plasma cholesterol and weight in young adults. *J. Epidemiol. and Commun. Health* **34**, 164 (1980).
17. A. Lucas, L. A. Blackburn, A. Aynsley-Green, D. L. Sarson, T. E. Adrian, and S. R. Bloom, Breast vs. bottle: Endocrine responses are different with formula feeding. *Lancet* **1**, 1267 (1980).
18. J. J. Kabara, Lipids as host-resistance factors of human milk. *Nutr. Rev.* **38**, 65 (1980).
19. M. E. Fallot, J. L. Boyd III, and F. A. Oski, Breast-feeding reduces incidence of hospital admissions for infection in infants. *Pediatrics* **65**, 1121 (1980).
20. A. S. Cunningham, Morbidity in breast-fed and artificially fed infants. II. *J. Pediatr.* **95**, 685 (1979).
21. Anonymous, Morbidity in breast fed and artificially fed infants. *Nutr. Rev.* **38**, 114 (1980).
22. G. L. France, D. J. Marmer, and R. W. Steele, Breast-feeding and *Salmonella* infection. *Am. J. Dis. Child.* **134**, 147 (1980).
23. B. Hoyle, M. Yunus, and L. C. Chen, Breast-feeding and food intake among children with acute diarrheal disease. *Am. J. Clin.*

Nutr. **33**, 2365 (1980).

24. J. K. Welsh and J. T. May, Anti-infective properties of breast milk. *J. Pediatr.* **94**, 1 (1979).

25. R. K. Chandra, Immunological aspects of human milk. *Nutr. Rev.* **36**, 265 (1978).

26. U. M. Saarinen, M. Kajosaari, A. Backman, and M. A. Siimes, Prolonged breast-feeding as prophylaxis for atopic disease. *Lancet* **2**, 163 (1979).

27. U. M. Saarinen, F. Bjorksten, P. Knekt, and M. A. Siimes, Serum IgE of infants and influence of type of feeding. *Clin. Allergy* **10**, 593 (1980).

28. J. W. Gerrard, Allergy in breast fed babies to ingredients in breast milk. *Ann. Allergy* **42**, 69 (1979).

29. B. Blanc, Biochemical aspects of human milk: Comparisons with bovine milk. *World Rev. Nutr. Diet* **36**, 1 (1981).

30. Committee on Nutrition, American Academy of Pediatrics. Nutrition and lactation. *Pediatrics* **68**, 435 (1981).

31 S. A. Atkinson, Factors affecting human milk composition. *J. Can. Diet. Assoc.* **40**, 213 (1979).

32. M. R. Thomas, J. Kawamato, S. M. Sneed, and R. Eakin, The effects of vitamin C, vitamin B_6 and B_{12} supplementation on the breast milk and maternal status of well-nourished women. *Am. J. Clin. Nutr.* **32**, 1679 (1979).

33. P. N. Nail, M. R. Thomas, and R. Eakin, The effect of thiamin and riboflavin supplementation on the level of that vitamin in human breast milk and urine. *Am. J. Clin. Nutr.* **33**, 198 (1980).

34. M. R. Thomas, S. M. Sneed, C. Wei, P. A. Nail, M. Wilson, and E. E. Sprinkle III, The effects of vitamin C vitamin B_6, vitamin B_{12}, folic acid, riboflavin, and thiamin on the breast milk and maternal status of well-nourished women at 6 months postpartum. *Am. J. Clin. Nutr.* **33**, 2151 (1980).

35. M. C. Higginbottom, L. Sweetman, and W. O. Nyhan, A syndrome of methylmalonic aciduria, homocystinuria, megaloblastic anemia and neurologic abnormalities in a vitamin-B_{12} deficient breast fed infant of a strict vegetarian. *N. Engl. J. Med.* **229**, 317 (1978).

36. S. M. Sneed, C. Zane, and M. R. Thomas, The effects of ascorbic acid, vitamin B_6, vitamin B_{12}, and folic acid supplementation on the breast milk and maternal nutritional status of low socioeconomic lactating women. *Am. J. Clin. Nutr.* **34**, 1338 (1981).

37. L. Finberg, Human milk feeding and vitamin D supplementation: 1981 [editorial]. *J. Pediatr.* **99**, 228 (1981).

38. L. E. Reeve, H. F. DeLuca, and H. K. Schnoes, Synthesis and biological activity of vitamin D_3-sulfate. *J. Biol. Chem.* **256**, 823 (1981).
39. D. Edidin, L. Levitsky, W. Schey, N. Dumbovic, and A. Campos, Resurgence of nutritional rickets associated with breastfeeding and special dietary practices. *Pediatrics* **65**, 232 (1980).
40. A. Aperia, O. Broberger, P. Herin, and R. Zetterström, Salt content in human breast milk during the three first weeks after delivery. *Acta Paediatr. Scand.* **68**, 441 (1979).
41. G. W. Chance, I. C. Raddle, D. M. Willis, and E. Park, Postnatal growth of infants of less than 1.3 kg birthweight: Effects of metabolic acidosis, of caloric intake, and of calcium, sodium, and phosphate supplementation. *J. Pediatr.* **91**, 787 (1977).
42. Committee on Nutrition, Academy of Pediatrics. Sodium intake of infants in the United States. *Pediatrics* **68**, 444 (1981).
43. S. K. Anand, C. Sanborg, R. G. Robinson, and E. Lieberman, Neonatal hypernatremia associated with elevated sodium of breast milk. *J. Pediatr.* **96**, 66 (1980).
44. R. S. Asnes, D. H. Wisotsky, P. F. Migel, R. L. Siegle, and J. Levy, The dietary chloride deficiency syndrome occurring in a breast-fed infant. *J. Pediatr.* **100**, 923 (1982).
45. J. M. Arboit and E. Gildingers, Breast feeding and hypernatremia (letter). *J. Pediatr.* **97**, 335 (1980).
46. A. E. Conner, Elevated levels of sodium and chloride in milk from mastitic breast. *Pediatrics* **63**, 910 (1979).
47. S. A. Atkinson, I. C. Raddle, G. W. Chance, M. H. Bryan, and G. H. Anderson, Macromineral content of milk obtained during early lactation from mothers of premature infants. *Early Human Development* **4**, 5 (1980).
48. L. A. Vaughan, C. W. Weber, and S. R. Kemberling, Longitudinal changes in the mineral content of human milk. *Am. J. Clin. Nutr.* **32**, 2301 (1979).
49. K. Rajalakshmi and S. G. Srikantia, Copper, zinc and magnesium content of breast milk of Indian women. *Am. J. Clin. Nutr.* **33**, 664 (1980).
50. E. Vuori, and P. Kuitunen, The concentrations of copper and zinc in human milk: A longitudinal study. *Acta Paediatr. Scand.* **68**, 33 (1979).
51. E. Vuori, S. M. Makinen, R. Kara, and R. Juitunen, The effects of dietary intakes of copper, iron, manganese, and zinc on trace element content of human milk. *Am. J. Clin. Nutr.* **33**, 227 (1980).
52. M. A. Siimes, E. Vuori, and P. Kuitunen, Breast milk iron — A declining concentration during the course of lactation. *Acta.*

Paediatr. Scand. **68**, 29 (1979).

53. B. Lönnerdal, A. G. Stanislowski, and L. S. Hurley, Isolation of a low molecular weight zinc-binding ligand from human milk. *J. Inorg. Biochem.* **12**, 71 (1980).

54. C. E. Casey, P. A. Walravens, and K. M. Hambidge, Availability of zinc: Loading tests with human milk, cow's milk, and infant formulas. *Pediatrics* **68**, 394 (1981).

55. R. G. Jensen, M. M. Hagerty, and K. E. McMahon, Lipids of human milk and infant formulas: A review. *Am. J. Clin. Nutr.* **31**, 990 (1978).

56. J. A. Lemons, R. L. Schreiner, and E. L. Gresham, Simple method for determining the caloric and fat content of human milk. *Pediatrics* **66**, 626 (1980).

57. D. Jelliffe and E. F. P. Jelliffe, The volume and composition of human milk in poorly nourished communities: A review. *Am. J. Clin. Nutr.* **31**, 492 (1978).

58. E. Lauber and M. Reinhardt, Studies on the quality of breast milk during 23 months of lactation in a rural community of the Ivory Coast. *Am. J. Clin. Nutr.* **32**, 1159 (1979).

59. D. Boediman, D. Ismail, S. Iman, I. Goen, and S. Ismadi, Composition of breast milk beyond one year. *J. Trop. Pediatr. and Environ. Child Health* **25**, 107 (1979).

60. B. Lonnerdal, E. Forsum, and L. Hanbraeus, Effect of oral contraceptives on the composition and volume of breast milk. *Am. J. Clin. Nutr.* **33**, 816 (1980).

61. A. S. Goldman and C. W. Smith, Host resistance factors in human milk. *J. Pediatr.* **82**, 1082 (1973).

62. L. A. Hanson, S. Ahlstedt, and B. Carlsson, New knowledge in human milk immunoglobulins. *Acta Pediatr. Scand.* **67**, 577 (1978).

63. O. Koldovsky, Hormones in milk. *Life Sci.* **26**, 1833 (1980).

64. Thyroid hormones in human milk. *Nutr. Rev.* **37**, 140 (1979).

65. B. Reid, H. Smith, and Z. Friedman, Prostaglandins in human milk. *Pediatrics* **66**, 870 (1980).

66. J. P. Skala, O. Koldovsky, and P. Hahn, Cyclic nucleotides in breast milk. *Am. J. Clin. Nutr.* **34**, 343 (1981).

67. J. M. Shahani, A. J. Kwan, and B. A. Friend, Role and significance of enzymes in human milk. *Am. J. Clin. Nutr.* **33**, 1861 (1980).

68. D. Tapper, M. Klagsbrun, and J. Neumann, The identification and clinical implications of human breast milk mitogen. *J. Pediatr. Surg.* **14**, 803 (1979).

69. G. Carpenter, Epidermal growth factor as a major growth-promoting agent in human milk. *Science* **210**, 198 (1980).

70. A. C. Piatzker, C. C. Lew, and D. Stewart, Drug "administration" via breast milk. *Hosp. Pract.* **15**, 1114 (1980).
71. Committee on Environmental Hazards, American Academy of Pediatrics. PCBs in breast milk. *Pediatrics* **62**, 407 (1978).
72. T. Wickizer, L. Brilliant, R. Copeland, and R. Tilden, Polychlorinated biphenyl contamination of nursing mothers' milk in Michigan. *Am. J. Public Health* **71, 132 (1981)**.
73. M. Barr, Environmental contamination of human breast milk [editorial]. *Am. J. Public Health* **71**, 124 (1981).
74. T. M. Wickizer and L. B. Brilliant, Testing for polychlorinated biphenyls in human milk. *Pediatrics* **68**, 411 (1981).
75. W. J. Rogan, M. Bagniewska, and T. Damstra, Pollutants in breast milk. *N. Engl. J. Med.* **302**, 1450 (1980).
76. K. G. Auerbach and J. L. Avery, Relactation: A study of 366 cases. *Pediatrics* **65**, 236 (1980).
77. C. L. Bose, J. D'Ercole, A. G. Lester, R. S. Hunter, and J. R. Barrett, Relactation by mothers of sick and premature infants. *Pediatrics* **67**, 565 (1981).
78. K. G. Auerbach and J. L. Avery, Induced lactation. *Am. J. Dis. Child.* **135**, 340 (1981).
79. R. Kleinman, L. Jacobson, E. Hormann, and W. A. Walker, Protein values of milk samples from mothers without biologic pregnancies. *J. Pediatr.* **97**, 612 (1980).
80. J. K. Kulski, P. E. Hartmann, W. J. Saint, P. F. Giles, and D. H. Gutteridge, Changes in the milk composition of nonpuerperal women. *Am. J. Obstet. Gynecol.* **139**, 597 (1981).
81. E. J. Eastham and W. A. Walker, Adverse effects of milk formula ingestion on the gastrointestinal tract, an update. *Gastroenterology* **76**, 365 (1979).
82. S. J. Fomon, E. E. Ziegler, S. E. Nelson, and B. B. Edwards, Cow milk feeding in infancy: Gastrointestinal blood loss and iron nutritional status. *J. Pediatr.* **98**, 540 (1981).
83. J. Ek and E. Magnus, Plasma and red cell folacin in cow's milk-fed infants and children during the first 2 years of life: The significance of boiling pasteurized cow's milk. *Am. J. Clin. Nutr.* **33**, 1220 (1980).
84. Y. Naveh, A. Hazani, and M. Berant, Copper deficiency with cow's milk diet. *Pediatrics* **68**, 397 (1981).
85. A. Ashkenazi, S. Levin, D. Idar, A. Or, I. Rosenberg, and Z. T. Handzel, In vitro cell-mediated immunologic assay for cow's milk allergy. *Pediatrics* **66**, 399 (1980).

86. H. L. Butler, W. J. Byrne, D. J. Marmer, A. R. Euler, and R. W. Steele, Depressed neutrophil chemotaxis in infants with cow's milk and/or soy protein intolerance. *Pediatrics* **67**, 264 (1981).
87. Diet and iron absorption in the first year of life. *Nutr. Rev.* **37**, 195 (1979).
88. U. M. Saarinen and M. A. Siimes, Iron absorption from breast milk, cow's milk, and iron-supplemented formula: An opportunistic use of changes in total body iron determined by hemoglobin, ferritin, and body weight in 132 infants. *Pediatr. Res.* **13**, 143 (1979).
89. P. R. Dallman, Inhibition of iron absorption by certain foods. *Am. J. Dis. Child.* **134**, 453 (1980).
90. G. M. Owen, P. J. Garry, E. M. Hooper, B. A. Gilbert, and D. Pathak, Iron nutriture of infants exclusively breast-fed for the first five months. *J. Pediatr.* **99**, 237 (1981).
91. F. A. Oski, Iron-fortified formulas and gastrointestinal symptoms in infants: A controlled study. *Pediatrics* **66**, 168 (1980).
92. F. R. Sinatra and R. J. Merrit, Iatrogenic kwashiorkor in infants. *Am. J. Dis. Child.* **135**, 21 (1981).

ADDITIONAL RECENT REFERENCES

Policy Statement, American Academy of Pediatrics, The promotion of breast-feeding. *Pediatrics* **69**, 654 (1982).

D. L. Yeung, M. D. Pennell, J. Hall, and M. Leung, Food and nutrient intake of infants during the first 18 months of life. *Nutr. Res.* **2**, 3 (1982).

B. A. Underwood and Y. Hofvander, Appropriate timing for complementary feeding of the breast fed infant: a review. *Acta Paediatr. Scand.*, Supplement 294 (1982).

A. Ashworth, International differences in child mortality and the impact of malnutrition. *Human Nutr.: Clin. Nutr.* **36**, 279 (1982).

A. S. Goldman, C. Garza, B. L. Nichols, and R. M. Goldblum, Immunologic factors in human milk during the first year of lactation. *J. Pediatr.* **100**, 563 (1982).

G. G. Graham, B. Adrianzen, J. Rabold, and E. D. Mellits, Later growth of malnourished infants and children. *Am. J. Dis. Child.* **136**, 348 (1982).

A. W. Myres (and authors of four other papers), Special issue on Pediatrics, *J. Can. Diet. Assoc.* **43**, 284 (1982).

13

The Role of Nutrition in the Onset and Treatment of Metabolic Bone Disease

LINDSAY H. ALLEN, Ph.D., R.D.
University of Connecticut, Storrs

Address correspondence to Lindsay H. Allen, Ph.D., Associate Professor of Nutritional Sciences, University of Connecticut, Storrs, Connecticut 06268.

ABSTRACT

Loss of bone, or metabolic bone disease, occurs in all of us as we grow older. It causes an increased risk of bone fractures, pain, and disability. Osteoporosis is the most common bone disease. It is most prevalent in women after menopause, probably as a result of the hormonal changes that occur at this time of life. The symptoms include an increase in bone breakdown, a decrease in the intestinal absorption of calcium, and a greater loss of calcium in urine. While estrogen therapy temporarily improves these symptoms, dietary calcium supplements may be a more useful long-term remedy. It is now recognized that inadequate calcium intakes, even in earlier years, may cause loss of bone. A dietary calcium deficiency is even more harmful in the elderly, who cannot absorb calcium as efficiently as younger persons. Osteomalacia is a bone disease resulting from vitamin D deficiency. Most cases arise secondarily to diseases in which vitamin D absorption or metabolism is impaired. Low exposure to sunlight and a reduced capacity of the elderly to synthesize vitamin D in their skin may also be risk factors. From a nutritional perspective, the risk of bone disease may be reduced by consumption of diets adequate in calcium and vitamin D and by avoidance of excessive intakes of fiber, protein, and alcohol.

INTRODUCTION

The term metabolic bone disease is used here as a general term describing bone loss. Bone loss occurs in all of us as we grow older, but it is especially severe in women. This loss is associated with an increased number of fractures, pain, disfigurement, and disability. Six million spontaneous fractures occur annually in the United States in persons over 45 years of age. In spite of the tremendous costs of this phenomenon, in terms of both health care and personal discomfort, we have been relatively slow to understand why it occurs and what

Scientific contribution number 935, Agricultural Experiment Station, University of Connecticut, Storrs, Connecticut 06268.

treatment to use. Part of the difficulty lies in the fact that the disease is usually gradual in its onset and is difficult to detect in its earlier stages.

The most common bone disease is osteoporosis, which is a term used to cover a number of conditions in which there is a reduced bone mass. This disease is most prevalent in postmenopausal women, probably because of the hormonal changes that occur at this time. It has been estimated that one-third of all women have osteoporosis after menopause, and one-fourth of them have clinical symptoms after the age of 60 years. Osteoporosis does occur in men but usually at a later age than in women and at a slower rate.

Another factor that increases the individual's risk of developing the symptoms of bone loss is a low amount of bone at the onset of menopause or old age. This may explain the more frequent occurrence of osteoporosis in Caucasians as compared to Blacks, since Blacks have heavier bones. Although osteoporosis is not usually caused exclusively by dietary calcium deficiency, there is evidence to suggest that dietary calcium intakes play a role in the etiology of osteoporosis, and that calcium supplements can be an effective therapy for the disease.

Osteomalacia is also a bone disease that occurs more frequently in the elderly. Associated with vitamin D deficiency, it will generally respond to some degree to treatment with this vitamin.

DIAGNOSIS AND SYMPTOMS

Osteoporosis is characterized by a decrease in the amount of bone mineral (calcium and phosphorus) as well as in the amount of matrix in which these minerals are deposited. The bone becomes more porous, although that which remains has relatively normal amounts of minerals. Ordinary chemical analyses are poor at detecting any abnormalities in the blood or urine of individual patients with osteoporosis. Although osteoporotics as a group may have a slightly increased urinary excretion of calcium and hydroxyproline (an amino acid present in bone and connective tissue), there is still considerable overlap between these values in osteoporotics and age-matched controls.

Histologically, osteomalacia is characterized by the occurrence of large amounts of uncalcified bone matrix (osteoid), so that the mineral is lost but the matrix remains. Chemically, there is usually a low serum calcium and phosphorus, secondary hyperparathyroidism, and elevated serum alkaline phosphatase. Conventional X-ray techniques cannot detect these problems until about 25–40% of the skeletal mineral has been lost or fractures have occurred, although X-rays of the bones of the hand are considerably more sensitive. More advanced techniques, which have recently become available for following the progress of a patient on treatment, can provide a means of evaluating the effectiveness of the various therapies that will be discussed later in this chapter. These techniques include photon absorptiometry (1), computed tomography (2), neutron activation (3), and the use of nonradioactive calcium isotopes (4). However, none of these methods is very effective for diagnosing the disease in an individual patient because the amount of bone mass in healthy persons varies widely. Patients with pain and fractures caused by bone loss may have more or less bone than persons without these symptoms.

The most common places for osteoporotic bone loss to occur are in the vertebrae, where the trabecular bone has a relatively high rate of formation and resorption (turnover); and in the endosteal bone, which is adjacent to the bone marrow in the radius and ulna of the arm, the neck of the femur, and the ribs. In addition, osteoporosis occurs in the trabecular bone of the jaw, which can result in loosening of teeth. This may lead to an increased risk of periodontal disease, which involves infections and shrinkage of the gums.

The clinical symptoms that signal the presence of osteoporosis are usually back pain caused by compression or fractures in the lower vertebrae, "dowager's hump," and loss of height. Since osteoporotic bone is more fragile, the incidence of fractures resulting from trauma is greatly increased, especially in the forearm, hip, and femur. By far the majority of hip and leg fractures in the elderly are due to osteoporosis.

The symptoms of osteomalacia also include bone pain, although this may be more diffuse and felt more frequently in the limbs and ribs. The vertebrae become more biconcave and have fewer fractures than in osteoporosis.

PATHOGENESIS OF OSTEOPOROSIS

The reason why osteoporosis develops is not yet known, although much progress has been made in recent years in our understanding of this disease.

In the healthy person, bone is continually being remodelled, by "coupled" formation and resorption (breakdown). Bone formation in the adult skeleton occurs mostly in bone remodelling units, at the sites where bone has previously been resorbed (5). Our understanding of how formation and resorption are coupled, or linked, is very limited, but it is clear that bone loss must occur if resorption is greater than formation.

In general, there is agreement that the basic abnormality in osteoporosis is an increase in bone resorption. This fact has been established by kinetic studies in which calcium isotopes were used (6); morphologic studies showing an increased bone resorbing surface; and an increased urinary hydroxyproline, which reflects increased bone matrix breakdown (7).

Hormonal Factors

In addition to providing structural support, a major function of the skeleton is to maintain serum calcium and phosphorus concentrations in order to preserve nerve and muscle function. The movement of these minerals in and out of bone is, therefore, closely controlled by the healthy body. Three calcium-regulating hormones are largely responsible for this control, and a brief discussion of their functions is necessary for the understanding of their roles in the etiology and therapy of bone disease.

Parathyroid hormone (PTH) functions by raising serum calcium when necessary, by stimulating bone resorption, by increasing the amount of filtered calcium that is retained by the kidney, and by stimulating the production of the active metabolite of vitamin D so that calcium absorption is increased. PTH also causes an increased loss of urinary phosphate, a subsequent decrease in serum phosphate, and a reduced deposition of calcium and phosphorus in bone.

The most important function of vitamin D is to increase the intestinal absorption of calcium and phosphorus, so that these minerals are available for bone formation. The most active vitamin D metabolite in this respect is 1,25-dihydroxyvitamin D or calcitriol. Calcitriol is formed in three steps (8). In the skin, 7-dehydrocholesterol is converted to vitamin D_3, cholecalciferol. The next step is hydroxylation in the liver to 25-hydroxyvitamin D or calcifediol. Lastly, a 1-hydroxylase enzyme in the kidney adds a second hydroxyl group to calcifediol to form 1,25-dihydroxyvitamin D, calcitriol. Calcitriol increases the intestinal absorption of calcium and phosphorus, probably by inducing the synthesis of intestinal calcium-binding protein.

The third calcium-regulating hormone is calcitonin (produced by the thyroid gland), which has a smaller effect on bone metabolism. Calcitonin prevents bone resorption, thereby preventing hypercalcemia. This is probably most important in young animals who consume and absorb large amounts of calcium.

Several other hormones deserve brief mention because they affect bone and calcium metabolism. In particular, some of these hormones may be affected by the aging process and, therefore, may be implicated in age-related bone loss. The most obvious of these is estrogen; the rapid fall in serum levels of this hormone in postmenopausal women has been implicated in the onset of postmenopausal osteoporosis, as will be discussed later. Thyroxin and adrenal glucocorticoids can stimulate bone resorption, while insulin and growth hormone both stimulate skeletal growth. In some individuals, an altered secretion of these hormones could contribute to osteoporosis, but this explains only a small fraction of the incidence of this disease.

The Role of Dietary Calcium Intake

Intestinal calcium absorption occurs both by diffusion and by an active, energy-requiring process. The latter process probably involves an intestinal calcium-binding protein (CaBP), which requires vitamin D for its synthesis. The active process is most important when dietary calcium intake is low; in this event, there is an increased synthesis of CaBP and an increase in the percentage of dietary calcium that is absorbed.

Because the intestine can adapt to low calcium intakes by increasing the fractional absorption of calcium, some investigators believe that calcium deficiency cannot be caused by a low dietary calcium intake, except in a situation of extreme calcium deficiency. Evidence cited to support this view includes the fact that the calcium intake of many people in the world is considerably lower than that in the United States, without obvious harmful effects on growth, final height, tooth development, or bone composition (9).

In contrast, several more recent studies provide evidence of harmful effects of a low calcium intake. For example, children in South Africa consuming 125 mg calcium/day had hypocalcemia and elevated serum alkaline phosphatase levels; in contrast, those eating 337 mg/day had normal values (10). In a Yugoslavian study, investigators compared the bone status and fracture rates of two communities with different calcium intakes (11). The median intake of one group was 400 mg/day, while the other consumed 900 mg. The communities were similar in their ethnic background, exposure to sunlight, and physical activity. In the group with the low calcium intake, both men and women had less cortical bone mass between the ages of 35 and 80 years and a higher incidence of bone fractures.

The most commonly used method of measuring how much dietary calcium is needed is the calcium balance technique. Over a period of at least several days, calcium intake is kept constant and the amount excreted in urine and feces is measured. If intake is greater than excretion, the subject is in positive balance. However, if excretion is greater than intake, a negative balance exists and there is a net loss of calcium from the body.

In a review of 212 calcium balance studies conducted on 84 normal subjects in many countries, Marshall et al. found that most balances were negative at calcium intakes below 600 mg/day and positive above this level (12). Closer to 900 mg was required to meet the needs of 95% of the group. We can assume, therefore, that our calcium requirement is at least 600 mg/day on average. Below this intake, absorption does not increase sufficiently to maintain calcium balance.

In view of the above evidence, it is important to consider whether osteoporosis is the result of dietary calcium deficiency. There is sufficient evidence from studies on animals, including monkeys (13), that experimental calcium deficiency produces bone loss indistinguishable from human osteoporosis. However, most investigators have failed to show that calcium intake is lower in those subjects with clinical symptoms of osteoporosis (14–16) as compared to age-matched controls.

Effect of Aging and Menopause on Calcium Absorption

A more serious problem in the elderly in general, and osteoporotic patients in particular, is a reduced ability to absorb calcium. Ireland and Fordtran (14) studied this phenomenon after feeding older (average age 68 years) and young (average age 28 years) subjects a low-calcium diet (250 mg/day) and a high-calcium diet (2000 mg/day) for 4–8 weeks. They measured the absorption of calcium from a known quantity perfused into the intestinal lumen. During the low calcium diet, the young subjects absorbed about 45% more calcium than did the older ones. During the high calcium period, younger subjects absorbed 35% more. There was also a marked decrease in the ability of the elderly to adapt to the calcium-deficient diet; absorption increased by 66% when the young group was switched from the high to the low intake, but the older group increased absorption by only 50%.

Bullamore et al. (17) also found that men and women both absorbed less calcium in old age. This occurred at an earlier age in women than in men. The onset of menopause causes a change in calcium balance performance. In 207 studies, premenopausal women (42 years of age) were in negative balance of −20 mg/day, compared to a balance of −43 mg/day after menopause (47 years of age) (15). The daily intake at both ages was approximately 650 mg. The difference in balance was caused approximately equally by a reduced intestinal absorption and an increased urinary excretion of calcium. Marshall et al. (12) also reported that most 61-year-old postmenopausal women were in a negative balance of 50–70 mg/day.

Recently, evidence has been obtained that the negative calcium balance after menopause is caused by the reduction in estrogen secretion at this time. For several decades it has been known that estrogen therapy retards the loss of bone in osteoporotic women. In fact, the administration of estrogens improves calcium absorption in both normal postmenopausal women and those with postmenopausal osteoporosis (18, 19). The highest rates of bone resorption and the poorest absorption of calcium occur in those women with the lowest estrogen levels (20).

Estrogen treatment probably improves calcium absorption through its effect on vitamin D metabolism. Osteoporotic patients have a reduced ability to produce calcitriol. Gallagher et al. (21) studied 21 osteoporotic women before and after 6 months of treatment with estrogen or a placebo. The estrogen-treated group increased their calcium absorption by about 20%, and their serum levels of 1,25-dihydroxyvitamin D by 40%. There was a very strong correlation between the increases in calcitriol levels and calcium absorption. The rise in serum calcitriol was associated with a decrease in serum PTH.

The authors suggest that the most likely causal mechanism is an estrogen-induced decrease in bone resorption and, therefore, in serum calcium. Subsequently, PTH secretion would be stimulated; PTH stimulates the renal 1α-hydroxylase so that calcitriol production from 25-hydroxyvitamin D is increased. Calcitriol would then stimulate intestinal calcium absorption. It would also increase the renal tubular reabsorption of calcium, thereby reducing the urinary loss of calcium, which also contributes to negative calcium balance after menopause.

PATHOGENESIS OF OSTEOMALACIA

There is some disagreement among authors about the frequency with which osteomalacia occurs in the elderly. Some have described it as uncommon (22) while others found that approximately 25% of patients with bone loss and hip fractures had occult osteomalacia (23). Diagnosis is sometimes complicated by the occurrence of both osteoporosis and osteomalacia in the same individual. It has been suggested that some of the osteoporotic component may be due to a mild vitamin D deficiency, whereas osteomalacia is caused by a more severe deficiency (24).

Most cases of osteomalacia probably arise secondarily to other disease states or surgery. Examples include gastrectomy, intestinal resection, primary biliary cirrhosis, kidney disease, and diabetes. In the above situations, osteomalacia usually results from a reduced vitamin D absorption or, in the case of renal disease and diabetes, from a defect in the synthesis of active vitamin D metabolites. Therapy with vitamin D or its metabolites is generally effective.

The diet of Americans and Europeans contains relatively small amounts of vitamin D. In the United States, the major source is milk, which is fortified with 400 I.U. per quart. Other sources include eggs, fatty fish, liver, cheese, and butter.

Sunlight is a much more important source of vitamin D than is diet, even at northern latitudes or in cloudy regions. Ultraviolet radiation from the sun induces the synthesis of vitamin D_3 in the skin, and, apart from fish, this is the only important natural source of vitamin D_3. In 1973, vitamin D_2 was used in the United States to fortify foods such as milk. At this time, Haddad and Hahn (25) found that serum levels of 25-hydroxyvitamin D_2 were very low in the U.S. population; 84% of the circulating 25-hydroxyvitamin D was derived from D_3 synthesized in the skin, and serum levels of this metabolite increased markedly during summer months.

The elderly tend to have lower exposure to sunlight, especially if illness prevents them from spending time outdoors. The incidence of bone fractures has been reported highest at the end of winter and lowest at the end of summer. A British study showed that the most likely cause of osteomalacia in persons with partial gastrectomy was the reluctance of these patients to spend time outdoors (26). An additional problem for the elderly is a marked decrease in their capacity to synthesize vitamin D_3 in their skin when exposed to sunlight (23). Individuals over the age of 60 were found to have only half the amount of vitamin D_3 precursor in their epidermis as compared to 10–20-year-olds.

During the last few years, there has been considerable interest in the high incidence of osteomalacia in Asian immigrants to Great Britain. Early reports suggested that this was due to the tendency of Asian women to remain indoors and to wear traditional clothing. However, there is a high incidence of this disease even in those Asian women who wear Western dress, go out daily, and sunbathe. One current interpretation of its etiology is the adherence to traditional diets containing unleavened bread (which impairs calcium absorption due to its high phytate content) and low amounts of calcium (27).

In summary, several factors may be involved in the etiology of osteomalacia in the elderly. Alteration of vitamin D metabolism by illness or surgery is the most common. Low exposure to sunlight and a reduced capacity to synthesize vitamin D_3 in the skin are also important risk factors. Low dietary intakes of vitamin D and, perhaps, inadequate consumption or poor absorption of calcium may add to the risk of developing this disease.

THERAPY

Assessment of the effectiveness of various therapies is made difficult by the fact that most investigators have not included age-matched controls. Another problem is that bone loss is a slow and somewhat sporadic process, so that large numbers of patients must be followed for considerable lengths of time before the therapy can be accurately evaluated.

Most therapies have been attempted on patients who already have osteoporosis; no well-controlled study of prospective victims has been attempted comparing the efficacy of several treatments to prevent the onset of bone loss. The most common approach to slow the bone loss is recommendation of calcium and vitamin D supplements and an increase in exercise. Estrogen therapy is usually restricted to those women who are less than 10 years postmenopausal.

Estrogens

Estrogens effectively slow down bone loss for about 8 years after menopause (28). Treatment of postmenopausal women with estrogen reduces the rate of bone resorption until it is the same as that of premenopausal women (6). Calcium balance is also restored.

On the negative side, a number of complications may result from estrogen replacement therapy. These include hypertension, hypertriglyceridemia, stroke, and an increased risk of uterine cancer (29). The therapy is also expensive, and discontinuation results in a rapid resumption of bone loss. Estrogens are, therefore, best used in high-risk individuals. However, it is possible that the doses used in routine management of postmenopausal women are higher than is necessary to protect against bone loss (6).

Calcium

Nordin et al. (16) examined the effect of calcium therapy on postmenopausal women with and without osteoporosis. Bone loss was evaluated by sequential X-rays of the metacarpals and vertebrae and by measurements of height. The provision of calcium gluconate supplements increased the calcium intake of the osteoporotic women from 696 to 1756 mg/day. This resulted in a doubling of the amount of calcium absorbed and a change in calcium balance from negative to positive.

Albanese (30) demonstrated a cessation of bone loss, or an increase of up to 12% in bone density, in older females when their calcium intake was increased from 400 to 1000 mg/day and their vitamin D_2 intake, by 375 I.U. Similar results were obtained by Lee et al. (31), who provided cheese and supplements containing calcium, phosphorus, and vitamin D to elderly women (average age 70 years) for 6 months. All women had osteoporosis and low calcium intakes prior to supplementation and consumed 1150 mg calcium/day during the experiment. Within 6 months, supplementation caused a significant increase in bone density as judged from hand X-rays. It is not clear which supplemented nutrient was responsible for the improvement, but it is encouraging that beneficial effects of supplementation could be detected by simple techniques in a relatively short period of time.

Vitamin D

Relatively large doses of vitamin D_2 are used to improve calcium absorption in elderly calcium malabsorbers. In patients less than 70 years old, 1000 I.U. of vitamin D_2 results in increased calcium absorption (32). In contrast, over the age of 70, at least 10,000–20,000 units provide an equivalent response; this difference might be due to the reduced conversion to calcitriol. Alternatively, small doses (1 μg/day) of 1α-hydroxyvitamin D_3 or calcitriol (0.5 μg/day) are as effective as the large doses of D_2 in increasing calcium absorption (33).

Although vitamin D and its metabolites increase calcium absorption in the elderly (34, 35), it is not clear that bone loss is prevented. In one study, calcitriol administration to women with osteoporosis caused an increase in both the absorption and urinary excretion of calcium, so that balance was not improved (36). Nordin et al. (36) showed that vitamin D and its metabolite 1α-hydroxyvitamin D_3 did not reduce bone loss and may even have had a negative effect. However, they found that a combination of 1α-hydroxyvitamin D_3 with estrogen therapy may have the most beneficial effect, especially if calcium malabsorption is evident. Combining calcium and vitamin D produced conflicting results; this therapy did not improve calcium balance, but may have increased bone density; therefore, the usefulness of this combination is uncertain at this time.

Calcitonin

Since calcitonin is a potent inhibitor of bone resorption, several attempts have been made to study the effectiveness of this hormone as a treatment for osteoporosis. However, calcitonin given alone has not been proven to be completely effective. Although 75% of osteoporotic patients reported relief of bone pain with calcitonin therapy, only half of them showed an increase in body calcium, while the other half suffered a net calcium loss. A recent report suggested that combined calcitonin and phosphate therapy might increase bone calcium in osteoporotics (37). Although the effectiveness of calcitonin combined with other agents deserves further study, the use of this hormone might be limited by its side effects, such as anorexia, nausea, and vomiting. The only type of calcitonin currently available for therapy is salmon calcitonin to which humans can produce antibodies. It is also expensive and must be given by injection. The use of synthetic human calcitonin in the future might be more satisfactory.

Fluoride

The potential use of fluoride to treat osteoporosis was suggested by the observation that people who developed fluorosis by consuming large quantities of this mineral in their natural water supply had increased bone density. Although fluoride therapy does stimulate bone synthesis, this new bone is poorly mineralized unless supplemental calcium and vitamin D are administered at the same time (38). Even then, the new bone may be less strong than normal bone, and side effects such as joint pain and gastrointestinal symptoms occur in some patients. Prolonged therapy with fluoride does appear to prevent fractures, especially in those patients with increased bone density (39).

Summary of Available Therapies

From the above discussion of available therapeutic measures, it is obvious that further research is needed before we can identify the most effective treatment for osteoporosis. The most dramatic improvements are seen with estrogen therapy, although harmful side effects are of concern. A combination of estrogen and 1α-hydroxyvitamin D_3 may be even more beneficial. Calcium supplements are also of great benefit and have the advantages of less cost, less risk of harmful side effects, and probably a slower resumption of bone loss if they are discontinued.

NUTRITION IN THE PREVENTION OF METABOLIC BONE DISEASE

Although calcium deficiency produces osteoporosis in experimental animals, it has been relatively difficult to demonstrate that the adequacy of dietary calcium intake is important in the etiology of osteoporosis. This situation may have occurred because it is difficult to acquire an accurate estimate of "usual" calcium intake during the years prior to disease symptoms and because there are no good methods for assessing the calcium status of individuals.

In this context, the studies by Matkovic et al. and Heaney et al. are important in showing that dietary calcium adequacy affects bone mass even by 30 years of age, and that premenopausal women who select higher intakes have a more positive calcium balance (11, 40). Those individuals who consume or absorb inadequate amounts of calcium over a number of years are probably at greater risk of developing metabolic bone disease in older life, when absorption becomes even more difficult.

The current Recommended Dietary Allowance (RDA) in the United States for the adult is 800 mg calcium/day (41). There has been a considerable amount of discussion about whether this amount is too low to afford maximum protection against osteoporosis or whether it is higher than necessary (41). In the United States, about 60% of our calcium comes from milk and dairy products. The average calcium intake is probably close to 800 mg, although people who do not drink milk (which contains 300 mg/cup) tend to consume closer to 500 mg. Heaney et al. (40) found that closer to 1.2 mg/day was needed to produce calcium balance in 130 normal women, 30–35 years old, eating self-selected diets. A review of 212 balances in normal adults showed that balance was reached at an average intake of 578 mg, but that to cover the needs of 95% of the group, the dietary intake requirement would be 900 mg (12). It would appear, therefore, that the RDA for younger adults may be reasonable, but that requirements are substantially increased in older persons, especially postmenopausal women, because of their lessened capacity for calcium absorption and their increased urinary loss (6).

In addition to the amount of calcium in the diet, we should concern ourselves with other factors in foods that can greatly affect calcium absorption or retention in the body. On the average, about 30% of dietary calcium is absorbed. In the past, there was considerable concern about the presence of oxalic acid in some green leafy vegetables, and phytic acid in the seed coats of cereals, which might impair calcium absorption. However, these factors may not be of as much importance as the amount of fiber in the United States diet.

Whole grain products and bran have become popular in recent years because of reported health benefits of dietary fiber. This practice may have very harmful effects on calcium absorption. Cummings et al. (42) demonstrated that replacement of refined wheat products by similar products made from whole wheat caused a negative calcium balance to occur in young men, even though their calcium intake was 1302 mg/day. Kelsay et al. (43) fed adult men foods containing 1100 mg calcium daily, and showed that the addition of fiber from fruits and vegetables changed the balance from $+72$ to -122 mg/day. These studies suggest that intakes of calcium even greater than the RDA are not sufficient to prevent negative calcium balance if high fiber foods are consumed. James et al. (44) believe that the uronic acids in plant fiber are responsible for the inhibition of calcium absorption.

The lactose content of milk appears to increase the absorption of calcium. Those persons with lactose intolerance may be at greater risk of bone loss because their ability to absorb calcium from milk is reduced (45), and their intake of milk may be lower. Treatment of milk with the enzyme lactase—a practice sometimes used by lactose-intolerant individuals to reduce the lactose content of milk—also decreases the absorbability of calcium (45).

Contrary to popular belief, no adverse effect of high phosphorus intakes on calcium balance has been found in humans (46). The amount of fat in the diet does not reduce calcium absorption, unless a person has health problems that impair fat absorption. In this case, calcium forms unabsorbable complexes with fatty acids in the intestine.

It is now well established that an increase in the amount of protein in the diet results in a rapid increase in urinary calcium loss. Human subjects fed adequate or even high calcium intakes suffer a severe, continuous negative calcium balance when high protein diets are fed (47), because of an increase in their urinary calcium. The mechanism by which this occurs is a reduction of renal calcium reabsorption, probably mediated by the increase in serum insulin which occurs as a response to protein consumption (48). At this time it is not possible to set a safe level of protein intake that will prevent negative calcium balance. A more important issue may be the observation that some individuals lose more urinary calcium when protein intake is increased, while others do not. The degree of calciuric response appears to be proportional to the amount of insulin secreted after a protein meal, so that those individuals with a greater insulin response may be at more risk of developing bone loss in later life (48). At present, it would seem wise to avoid excessive consumption of protein; on the average, the protein intake of most adults in the United States is about twice the Recommended Dietary Allowance.

There is evidence that weight loss tends to be accompanied by negative calcium balance (31), and that fatter women have a lower risk of osteoporosis. This may be related to the ability of fatty tissue to produce estrogens.

Chronic alcoholism may cause skeletal demineralization in men and women even at a relatively young age (49). Alcohol impairs the intestinal absorption of calcium.

In summary, a calcium intake of 800 mg/day may be marginally satisfactory for younger, healthy adults. The requirement of older persons may be considerably greater. A recommended allowance of 1400 mg may be necessary for postmenopausal women and those elderly people who are less able to absorb calcium; calcium balance has been restored in postmenopausal women at this level of intake. Excessive consumption of whole grains and other high fiber foods should be avoided, as should excessive protein and alcohol intake. Consumption of milk, either whole or low fat, has the combined benefits of being a good source of calcium and lactose.

There is also less risk of osteoporosis developing in women who are nonsmokers, probably because of an earlier onset of menopause in smokers (50). Maintenance of physical activity by the elderly is important for preventing the bone calcium loss that occurs during inactivity and immobilization and for increasing the synthesis of vitamin D_3 through the action of sunlight on the skin.

REFERENCES

1. W. L. Dunn, H. W. Wahner, and B. L. Riggs, Measurement of bone mineral content in human vertebrae and hip by dual photon absorptiometry. *Radiology* **136**, 384 (1980).
2. P. S. Jensen, S. C. Orphanoudakis, E. N. Rauschkolb, R. Baron, R. Lang, and H. Rasmussen, Assessment of bone mass in the radius by computed tomography. *Am. J. Roentgenol.* **134**, 285 (1980).
3. J. E. Harrison, K. G. McNeill, A. J. Hitchman, and B. A. Britt, Bone mineral measurements of the central skeleton by in vivo neutron activation analysis for routine investigation of osteopenia. *Invest. Radiol.* **14**, 27 (1979).
4. R. Neer, G. Tully, P. Schatz, and D. J. Hnatowich, Use of stable ^{48}Ca in the clinical measurement of intestinal calcium absorption. *Calcif. Tissue Res.* **26**, 5 (1978).
5. A. M. Parfitt, Quantum concept of bone remodeling and turnover: implications for the pathogenesis of osteoporosis. *Calcif. Tissue Int.* **28**, 1 (1979).
6. R. P. Heaney, R. R. Recker, and P. D. Saville, Menopausal changes in bone remodelling. *J. Lab. Clin. Med.* **92**, 964 (1978).
7. A. Horsman, D. H. Marshall, B. E. C. Nordin, R. G. Crilly, and M. Simpson, The relation between bone loss and calcium balance in women. *Clin. Sci.* **59**, 137 (1980).
8. H. F. DeLuca, Some new concepts emanating from a study of the metabolism and function of vitamin D. *Nutr. Rev.* **38**, 169 (1980).

9. A. R. P. Walker, The human requirement of calcium: should low intakes be supplemented? *Am. J. Clin. Nutr.* **25**, 518 (1972).

10. J. Pettifor, P. Ross, G. Moodley, and E. Shuenyane, Calcium deficiency in rural black children in South Africa: A comparison between rural and urban communities. *Am. J. Clin. Nutr.* **32**, 2477 (1979).

11. V. Matkovic, K. Kostial, I. Simonovic, R. Buzina, A. Prodarec, and B. E. C. Nordin, Bone status and fracture rates in two regions of Yugoslavia. *Am. J. Clin. Nutr.* **32**, 540 (1979).

12. D. H. Marshall, B. E. C. Nordin, and R. Speed, Calcium, phosphorus and magnesium requirement. *Proc. Nutr. Soc.* **35**, 162 (1976).

13. H. J. Griffiths, R. D. Hunt, R. E. Zimmerman, H. Finberg, and J. Cuttino, The role of calcium and fluoride in osteoporosis in rhesus monkeys. *Invest. Radiol.* **10**, 263 (1975).

14. P. Ireland and J. S. Fordtran, Effect of dietary calcium and age on jejunal calcium absorption of humans studied by intestinal perfusion. *J. Clin. Invest.* **52**, 2672 (1973).

15. R. P. Heaney, R. R. Recker, and P. D. Saville, Menopausal changes in calcium balance performance. *J. Lab. Clin. Med.* **92**, 963 (1978).

16. B. E. C. Nordin, A. Horsman, D. H. Marshall, M. Simpson, and G. M. Waterhouse, Calcium requirement and calcium therapy. *Clin. Orthop. Relat. Res.* **140**, 216 (1979).

17. J. R. Bullamore, J. C. Gallagher, R. Wilkinson, and B. E. C. Nordin, Effect of age on calcium absorption. *Lancet* **2**, 535 (1970).

18. J. C. Gallagher and B. E. C. Nordin, Effects of oestrogen and progesterone therapy on calcium metabolism in postmenopausal women. *Front. Horm. Res.* **3**, 150 (1975).

19. R. Lindsay, J. M. Aitken, J. B. Anderson, D. M. Hart, E. B. MacDonald, and A. C. Clarke, Long-term prevention of postmenopausal osteoporosis by oestrogen. *Lancet* **1**, 1038 (1976).

20. B. E. C. Nordin, A. Horsman, R. Brook, and D. A. Williams, The relationship between oestrogen status and bone loss in post-menopausal women. *Clin. Endocrinol.* **5** (suppl.), 353S (1976).

21. J. C. Gallagher, B. L. Riggs, and H. F. DeLuca, Effect of estrogen on calcium absorption and serum vitamin D metabolites in postmenopausal osteoporosis. *J. Clin. Endocrinol.* **51**, 1359 (1980).

22. A. A. Albanese, The vitamins. In A. A. Albanese, ed., *Nutrition for the Elderly*, Alan R. Liss, New York, 1980, p. 145.

23. M. F. Holick and J. A. MacLaughlin, Aging significantly decreases the capacity of the human epidermis to produce vitamin D_3. *Clin.*

Res. **29**, 408A (1981).

24. J. Aaron, J. C. Gallagher, J. Anderson, L. Stasiak, E. B. Longton, B. E. C. Nordin, and M. Nicholson, Frequency of osteomalacia and osteoporosis in fractures of the proximal femur. *Lancet* **1**, 229 (1974).

25. J. G. Haddad and T. J. Hahn, Natural and synthetic sources of circulating 25-hydroxy vitamin D in man. *Nature* **244**, 515 (1973).

26. P. H. Pittet, M. Daire, and D. E. M. Lawson, Role of nutrition in the development of osteomalacia in the elderly. *Nutr. Metab.* **23**, 109 (1979).

27. M. G. Dunnigan and I. Robertson, Residence in Britain as a risk factor for Asian rickets and osteomalacia. *Lancet 1*, 770 (1980).

28. L. E. Nachtigall, R. H. Nachtigall, R. D. Nachtigall, and E. M. Beckman, Estrogen replacement therapy. I. A 10-year prospective study in the relationship to osteoporosis. *Obstet. Gynecol.* **53**, 277 (1979).

29. M. C. Weinstein, Estrogen use in postmenopausal woman: costs, risks and benefits. *N. Engl. J. Med.* **303**, 308 (1980).

30. A. A. Albanese, Calcium nutrition in the elderly. *Postgrad. Med.* **63**, 167 (1978).

31. C. J. Lee, G. S. Lawler, and G. H. Johnson, Effects of supplementation of the diets with calcium and calcium-rich foods on bone density of elderly females with osteoporosis. *Am. J. Clin. Nutr.* **34**, 819 (1981).

32. B. E. C. Nordin, R. Wilkinson, D. H. Marshall, J. C. Gallagher, A. Williams, and M. Peacock, Calcium absorption in the elderly. *Calcif. Tissue Res.* **215**, 442 (1976).

33. B. E. C. Nordin, Treatment of postmenopausal osteoporosis. *Drugs* **18**, 484 (1979).

34. A. Caniggia and A. Vattimo, Effects of 1,25-dihydroxycholecalciferol on ^{47}calcium absorption in post-menopausal osteoporosis. *Clin. Endocrinol.* **11**, 99 (1979).

35. S. Lawoyin, J. E. Zerwekh, K. Glass, and C. Y. C. Pak, Ability of 25-hydroxyvitamin D_3 therapy to augment serum 1,25- and 24,25-dihydroxyvitamin D in postmenopausal osteoporosis. *J. Clin. Endocrinol. Metab.* **50**, 593 (1980).

36. B. E. C. Nordin, A. Horsman, R. G. Crilly, D. H. Marshall, and M. Simpson, Treatment of spinal osteoporosis in postmenopausal women. *Br. Med. J.* **1**, 451 (1980).

37. H. Rasmussen, P. Bordier, P. Marie, L. Auquier, J. B. Eisinger, D. Kuntz, F. Caulin, B. Argemi, J. Gueris, and A. Julien, Effect of combined therapy with phosphate and calcitonin on bone volume in

osteoporosis. *Metab. Bone Dis. Relat. Res.* **2**, 107 (1980).

38. J. Jowsey, B. L. Riggs, P. J. Kelly, and D. L. Hoffman, Effect of combined therapy with sodium fluoride, vitamin D and calcium in osteoporosis. *Am. J. Med.* **53**, 43 (1972).
39. F. W. Reutter and A. J. Olaf, Bone biopsy findings and clinical observations in long-term treatment of osteoporosis with sodium fluoride and vitamin D_3. In B. Courvoisier, A. Donath, and C. A. Baud, eds., *Fluoride and Bone*, Hans Huker, Berne, 1978.
40. R. P. Heaney, R. R. Recker, and P. D. Saville, Calcium balance and calcium requirements in middle-aged women. *Am. J. Clin. Nutr.* **30**, 1603 (1977).
41. Committee on Dietary Allowances, Food and Nutrition Board, National Research Council, *Recommended Dietary Allowances*, 9th ed., National Academy of Sciences, Washington, D.C., 1980.
42. J. H. Cummings, M. J. Hill, H. Houston, W. J. Branch, and D. J. A. Jenkins, The effect of meat protein and dietary fiber on colonic function and metabolism. I. Changes in bowel habit, bile acid excretion, and calcium absorption. *Am. J. Clin. Nutr.* **32**, 2086 (1979).
43. J. L. Kelsay, K. M. Behall, and E. S. Prather, Effect of fiber from fruits and vegetables on metabolic responses of human subjects. II. Calcium, magnesium, iron, and silicon balances. *Am. J. Clin. Nutr.* **32**, 1876 (1979).
44. W. P. T. James, W. J. Branch, and D. A. T. Southgate, Calcium binding by dietary fibre. *Lancet* **1**, 638 (1978).
45. J. Kocian, I. Skala, and K. Bakos, Calcium absorption from milk and lactose-free milk in healthy subjects and patients with lactose intolerance. *Digestion* **9**, 317 (1973).
46. H. Spencer, L. Kramer, D. Osis, and C. Norris, Effect of phosphorus on the absorption of calcium and on the calcium balance in man. *J. Nutr.* **108**, 447 (1978).
47. L. H. Allen, E. A. Oddoye, and S. Margen, Protein-induced hypercalciuria: A longer term study. *Am. J. Clin. Nutr.* **32**, 741 (1979).
48. L. H. Allen, G. D. Block, R. J. Wood, and G. F. Bryce, The role of insulin and parathyroid hormone in the protein-induced calciuria of man. *Nutr. Res.* **1**, 3 (1981).
49. H. Spencer, L. Kramer, C. A. Gatza, and M. Lender, Calcium loss, calcium absorption, and calcium requirement in osteoporosis. In U. S. Barzel, ed., *Osteoporosis II*, Grune & Stratton, New York, 1979, p. 80.

50. O. Lindquist and C. Bengtsson, The effect of smoking on menopausal age. *Maturitas* **1**, 171 (1979).

ADDITIONAL RECENT REFERENCES

R. Marcus, The relationship of dietary calcium to the maintenance of skeletal integrity in man—an interface of endocrinology and nutrition. *Metabolism* **31**, 93 (1982).

L. H. Allen, Calcium bioavailability and absorption: a review. *Am. J. Clin. Nutr.* **35**, 783 (1982).

J. C. Gallagher, C. M. Jerphak, W. S. S. Lee, K. A. Johnson, H. F. DeLuca, and B. L. Riggs, 1,25—dihydroxyvitamin D$_3$: Short- and long-term effects on bone and calcium metabolism in patients with postmenopausal osteoporosis. *Proc. Natl. Acad. Sci USA* **79**, 3325 (1982).

H. McA. Taggart, C. H. Chestnut, J. L. Ivey, D. J. Baylink, K. Sisom, M. B. Huber, and B. A. Roos, Deficient calcitonin response to calcium stimulation in postmenopausal osteoporosis? *Lancet* **1**, 475 (1982).

Nutrition Policy and Food Advertising

14
Nutrition Policy Update

MARION NESTLE, Ph.D.
Associate Dean, School of Medicine

PHILIP R. LEE, M.D.
Professor of Social Medicine
Institute for Health Policy Studies
School of Medicine

ROBERT B. BARON, M.D.
Senior Medical Resident
Primary Care Internal Medicine Residency Program

University of California, San Francisco

Address correspondence to Marion Nestle, Ph.D., Associate Dean, School of Medicine, Director, Nutrition Curriculum Development Project, University of California, San Francisco, California 94143.

ABSTRACT

The U.S. government helps to assure an adequate food supply for Americans by sponsoring a wide variety of food, nutrition, and agricultural support programs. These federal activities were developed in the absence of a clearly articulated national policy, a situation that has resulted in the fragmentation of government programs and in their wide disbursement among numerous agencies and departments.

Federal food, nutrition, and agriculture programs include six key areas: food and nutrition surveys, food assistance, nutrition research, food industry regulation, agriculture support, and nutrition education. Some current programs have roots reaching back to the turn of the century, but it is just within the past 25 years that the government has begun to play an active role in policies that affect awareness of inadequate nutrition among the poor, of the function of diet in chronic illnesses, and of the importance of adequate nutrition in early child development.

The effect on the nation's health of food processing and other changes in the U.S. diet is controversial. Salt, sugar, fiber, saturated fats, alcohol, caffeine, calories, vitamins, and food additives—all elicit vigorous debate. In recent years a number of federal agencies have attempted to evaluate the evidence that links diet to health and to recommend dietary changes to improve nutritional status. Despite the controversy surrounding these and other recommendations, an apparent consensus emerges from among the various reports. Nevertheless, certain factors have acted as constraints against the formulation of a coordinated national nutrition policy that would implement these recommendations.

DEVELOPMENT OF A FEDERAL NUTRITION POLICY

The food system is the nation's largest industry. It employs more than 20 million workers and accounts for 16% of all personal expenditures—$218 billion in 1979 (1). Federal policies affect almost every phase and aspect of the food system, from basic research to the price of food in the market. During the past 25 years, national food and

286

agriculture policies have moved increasingly toward attention to the nutritional health of the population and away from their former emphasis on food production and the financial interests of agricultural producers.

Many of these policy changes occurred in response to altered patterns of American agriculture following World War II. Farm production per hour of farm labor increased almost threefold between 1950 and 1973, and labor use dropped almost 50% (2). These great increases in productivity brought on a variety of adjustments, including complex commodity price and income support programs for farmers (3).

Although the changes in American agriculture and in food and agriculture policies occurred rapidly in the postwar years, domestic nutrition policies have evolved slowly and in a piecemeal fashion. The first major step toward the establishment of current policies was the enactment of the Social Security Act in 1935. This act authorized federal grants-in-aid to the states for health services and for mothers and children, and it provided support for the application of nutrition principles to preventive and curative health care. In 1941, the Food and Nutrition Board of the National Research Council, National Academy of Sciences, issued its first Recommended Dietary Allowances (RDA). Updated periodically, these reports have been used as standards for nutritional adequacy in food assistance programs and for food labeling requirements.

One early policy development was the establishment of the National School Lunch Program in 1946. It was not until the 1960s, however, that the federal government assumed an active role in combating the problems of malnutrition among the poor. Even then, the commitment was piecemeal. The Food Stamp Act of 1965 initiated a small-scale program to meet what was perceived as a limited need. At its inception, the Child Nutrition Act of 1966 expanded the federal role only modestly.

With the 1968 report *Hunger USA* (4) and the 1969 White House Conference of Food, Nutrition and Health (5), national attention began to focus on the nutritional needs of the poor. As a result, the Department of Health, Education, and Welfare, now the Department of Health and Human Services (DHHS), began a major nutrition surveillance program in order to determine the extent of malnutrition in the United States. These surveys revealed substantial nutritional problems among poverty groups, and they contributed a great deal of information on nutritional problems and their impact on health.

Congress responded by expanding a number of food assistance programs in the 1970s—the Food Stamp Program, the School Lunch Program, the Child Care Food Program, and the Child Nutrition Program—and it established the Nutrition Program for the Elderly through an amendment to the Older Americans Act. These programs were greatly enlarged during the 1970s, serving millions of people and costing billions of dollars. Many of these programs appear slated for reduced federal support in the 1980s, as attention focuses on reducing government spending rather than assisting the poor.

In the late 1960s and early 1970s, the Senate Select Committee on Nutrition and Human Needs played a key role in the development of food assistance programs to meet the needs of the poor and to stimulate the evolution of a national nutrition policy. In 1974, the Select Committee issued Guidelines for a National Nutrition Policy (6) prepared by the National Consortium. The consortium defined five basic goals for national nutrition policy that have provided the framework for many subsequent developments. The goals were to:

1. Assure an adequate, wholesome food supply, at reasonable cost, to meet the needs of all segments of the population.
2. Maintain food resources sufficient to meet emergency needs and to fulfill a responsible role as a nation in meeting world food needs.
3. Develop a level of sound public knowledge and responsible understanding of nutrition and foods that will promote maximal nutritional health.
4. Maintain a system of quality and safety control that justifies public confidence in its food supply.
5. Support research and education in foods and nutrition with adequate resources and reasoned priorities to solve important current problems and to permit exploratory basic research (6).

Events entirely outside the fields of health and nutrition, however, have had the greatest impact on nutrition policy during the past decade. Poor harvest in many parts of the world and the extraordinary grain purchases by the Soviet Union in 1972, accompanied by rapid increases in domestic food prices, brought world food policy to the attention of the American public as never before. For the first time, the capacity of the United States to meet its own food needs, as well as its commitments to the rest of the world, was in doubt. The world food crisis arose at a time of extraordinary worldwide inflation and an energy crisis due to skyrocketing oil prices. These events profoundly altered the process of food policymaking (2, 7, 8).

Two major policy developments that followed these events were reflected in the Agriculture and Consumer Protection Act of 1973: (1) income support payments to farmers were continued by the U.S. Treasury Department in order to ensure a stable income for agricultural producers; and (2) the Food Stamp program was expanded to become the principal food assistance program in order to protect the poor from food price inflation (3).

Regulatory policies were also affected by these changes and by dramatic increases in the development and use of processed foods (9). The growing interest in nutrition influenced policies adopted by the Food and Drug Administration (FDA) that regulated the labeling of foods.

Another important nutrition policy of the 1970s was expressed in the Food and Agriculture Act of 1977, which included the Congressional declaration that "nutrition and health considerations are important to the United States agricultural policy" and which directed the U.S. Department of Agriculture (USDA) to establish human nutrition research as one of its distinct missions. As a result, the Department moved to strengthen and expand its human nutrition research programs.

These developments of the 1960s and 1970s changed the role of the federal government in human nutrition policy, and they helped to focus the public's attention on the relationship between nutrition and health.

FEDERAL FOOD, NUTRITION, AND AGRICULTURE PROGRAMS

This brief historical outline serves to demonstrate that federal food, nutrition, and agricultural support activities were developed in the absence of a clearly defined national nutrition policy. They were established in response to particular needs or problems at different times by discrete Congressional committees, and they were designed for highly diverse political constituencies. As a result, various related functions came to be fragmented among many agencies and departments. Because no single federal organization has been designated to oversee these programs, it becomes a formidable task to determine their scope and content or to evaluate their quality and effectiveness.

In response to Congressional concern about the diversity, possible duplication, rapid growth, and high cost of these programs, the General Accounting Office prepared an inventory of federal food, nutrition, and agriculture programs. By late 1979, the inventory had identified 359

Table 1. Various Domestic Food, Nutrition, and Agriculture Activities of the United States Government

Department	Agency	Food and Nutrition Surveys	Food Assistance	Nutrition Research	Food Quality Regulation	Agricultural Support	Nutrition Education
Agriculture	Animal and Plant Health Inspection Service				X		
	Agricultural Stabilization and Conservation Service					X	
	Agricultural Marketing Service					X	
	Agricultural Research Service			X			
	Economics, Statistics and Cooperatives Service			X			X
	Farmers Home Administration					X	
	Federal Crop Insurance Corporation					X	
	Food and Nutrition Service		X	X	X		X
	Food Safety and Quality Service				X		
	Nationwide Food Consumption Service	X					
	Office of Policy, Planning and Evaluation			X			
	Office of Governmental and Public Affairs						X
	Science and Education Administration			X			X
Commerce	National Oceanic and Atmospheric Administration			X		X	
Community Service Administration			X				
Defense				X			

Department	Agency	Food and Nutrition Surveys	Food Assistance	Nutrition Research	Food Quality Regulation	Agricultural Support	Nutrition Education
Environmental Protection Agency				X	X		
Federal Trade Commission				X			
Health and Human Services	Alcohol, Drug Abuse, and Mental Health Administration			X			X
	Center for Disease Control	X		X			
	Food and Drug Administration			X	X		X
	Health Resources Administration			X			X
	National Institutes of Health			X			X
	National Center for Health Statistics	X		X			X
	Office of Human Development Services		X				X
	Social Security Administration		X				
National Aeronautics and Space Administration				X			
National Science Foundation				X			
State	Agency for International Development			X			X
Treasury							X
Veterans Administration	Department of Medicine and Surgery			X			

separate programs distributed among 28 federal departments and agencies (10). The 1980 update of this inventory includes 1305 pages of computer listings (11). A partial listing of the agencies and their most important programs is provided in Table 1. Most activities are conducted by the Department of Agriculture and the Department of Health and Human Services, but a great many other government agencies are also responsible for portions of national nutrition policy.

The food, nutrition, and agriculture programs of the U.S. government include six key areas: (1) food and nutrition surveys, (2) food assistance, (3) nutrition research, (4) food industry regulation, (5) agriculture support, and (6) nutrition education.

No single agency has complete responsibility for any one area. Instead, many agencies are assigned partial responsibility for one or more major functions. The result of this shared responsibility is that lines of authority for program policies intersect and overlap.

The difficulties generated by multiple responsibility for specific functions are best illustrated by food assistance programs. The 13 most important food assistance programs are distributed among agencies in three separate federal departments. The organizational chart of administrative authority for these programs is as complex as a wiring diagram for a computer chip (12). It reveals that children of low-income parents may be eligible to receive food assistance from as many as 11 separate city, county, state, or federal agencies. This situation immediately suggests that at least some coordination of these programs might be desirable or necessary to ensure that they are effective in meeting federal goals.

FOOD AND NUTRITION SURVEYS

In order to develop a rational program that ensures an adequate nutrient intake for all U.S. residents, policymakers must identify standard food consumption practices and trends among the general population to determine the relationship between these practices and overall nutritional status, to establish the extent of malnutrition (whether from under- or overconsumption of nutrients), and to identify specific groups within the population that are most likely to be malnourished or to have special needs for food assistance or education.

As officials began to uncover vast amounts of hunger and malnutrition among U.S. citizens (4), the Department of Health, Education, and Welfare (now DHHS) conducted the Ten-State Nutrition Survey (1968–1970) and the Preschool Nutrition Survey (1968–1970), and the National Center for Health Statistics initiated periodic Health and Nutrition Examination Surveys (HANES) I

(1971–1974) and II (1976–1979). In addition, the Center for Disease Control established a program for gathering data that could be used to determine nutritional status. These surveys examined the extent of inadequate food intake among specially identified low-income groups (the Ten-State Survey), young children (the Preschool and Center for Disease Control surveys), and a representative sample of the general population over time (HANES I and II).

These surveys provided only limited data on the relationship of food consumption patterns to health. The federal nutritional surveillance program has been criticized for its duplication of effort, its inadequate population samples, its inability to identify high-risk groups or to relate food intake to health status, and its failure to use and to report the data in a manner that would reveal the groups most in need of assistance (13). Some of these problems occurred because of political pressures. Certain states did not want the federal government to reveal the extent of poverty and malnutrition within their boundaries (14). Some federal policymakers did not want to identify groups in need because federal funds would then be required to meet the needs. With many of these problems uncorrected, it has not been possible to identify with confidence the extent of malnutrition within the general population or within high-risk groups or to evaluate the success of federal nutrition intervention programs.

Even with these limitations, the results of the various surveys have been quite consistent. Malnutrition is associated with poverty. It is found most frequently among Blacks and least frequently among Caucasians. Young children, adolescents, pregnant women, and the elderly, especially those of low socioeconomic status, are the groups at highest risk (13). Thus, it is toward these groups that most federal food assistance efforts have been directed (12).

FOOD ASSISTANCE PROGRAMS

The federal government sponsors 13 major programs designed to increase the amount of food available to high-risk segments of the population (15). These programs and their sponsoring agencies are listed in Table 2. Most food assistance programs are administered by the Department of Agriculture. The DHHS is responsible for two food assistance programs and two cash assistance programs targeted to food needs. The Community Services Administration has one program that is designed to increase participation in all government food assistance programs.

These programs provide eligible households or individuals with meals, food, vouchers for food, or food stamps to buy food. The largest

Table 2. Federal Food Assistance Programs

Department of Agriculture
  Food Stamps
  Food Distribution
  National School Lunch Program
  School Breakfast Program
  Child Care Food Program
  Special Milk Program
  Summer Food Service Program for Children
  Special Supplemental Food Program for Women, Infants, and Children (WIC)

Department of Health and Human Services
  Headstart
  Nutrition Program for the Elderly
  Aid to Families with Dependent Children
  Supplemental Security Income

Community Services Administration
  Community Food and Nutrition Program

---

and most important programs are the Food Stamp Program, the National School Lunch Program, and the Special Supplemental Food Program for Women, Infants, and Children (WIC). By the late 1970s, these three programs served more than 43 million recipients at a cost of over $7.6 billion (12).

The cost of federal food assistance efforts has been of great concern to Congress. Between 1967 and 1976, federal expenditures for food assistance rose from $664 million to $8.5 billion and in 1981 they exceeded $11 billion (16). This 16.5-fold increase occurred in the early 1970s, at a time of relatively liberal eligibility requirements. Inflation and increased unemployment also contributed to the sharp rise in expenditures.

As the cost of food assistance programs increased, so did the controversy surrounding them. Various reports to Congress have noted their fragmentation and duplication of benefits, their inconsistent eligibility requirements and lack of common goals, and their failure to demonstrate improved nutritional or health status among recipients (12, 13).

The two largest and most expensive programs, Food Stamps and School Lunches, have been singled out for critical comment. The Food Stamp Program has been particularly controversial because of concern by Congress that it has been abused by its beneficiaries. Critics argue that the program fails to monitor food stamp recipients adequately, so that some people who receive stamps are not "truly" eligible. Also, because the program does not include a major nutrition education component, there is no guarantee that recipients are using stamps to purchase nutritious foods (13).

The School Lunch Program has also been scrutinized by Congress, particularly concerning the quality and acceptability of food served to eligible children. However, no effort has been made to evaluate the program's health benefits.

Fragmentation and lack of adequate evaluation of food assistance programs are weaknesses that have left the programs vulnerable to criticism and to attempts to reduce their budgets. As part of the Reagan administration's effort to reduce federal spending for domestic social programs, the Food Stamp and School Lunch programs were specifically targeted for major budgetary reductions amounting to over $3 billion in 1981 (16). In order to accomplish these reductions, application requirements have been modified to reduce the number of individuals who are eligible for benefits. Because attempts to limit these programs are likely to continue, the future of food assistance remains uncertain.

Throughout the arguments over the quality and cost-effectiveness of food assistance programs, the WIC Program has remained relatively untouched. Although Congress has noted some problems with WIC (13), the program has been both popular and successful. Perhaps one reason for its at least partial immunity from serious criticism and budgetary reduction is that it has been carefully evaluated. Several studies have documented WIC's effectiveness in improving the health of its recipients. WIC beneficiaries demonstrate improved infant survival and child growth rates (17). This information has been of value in protecting the program from attempts to eliminate it, and it suggests strongly that evaluation should be a major priority of the remaining food assistance programs.

In 1978, the Comptroller General reported to Congress that, in spite of the large number of federal food assistance programs and the large amount of money spent on them, it was not possible to state with certainty that all eligible persons receive benefits or that all U.S. residents receive adequate food intake (12). Because food assistance programs have been designated for expenditure reduction, it becomes especially important to identify high-risk groups and to document the effectiveness of intervention.

NUTRITION RESEARCH

Nutrition research is the responsibility of a large number of federal departments and independent agencies. In 1979, the major nutrition research agencies devoted nearly $200 million to basic research in nutrition, to nutrition research manpower development and training, and to nutrition education research (18). The need for coordination of these efforts has been an expressed recommendation of many federal reports during the past decade.

Because the Food and Agriculture Act of 1977 provided major roles for both the Department of Agriculture and the Department of Health and Human Services in human nutrition research, the White House convened the Nutrition Research Interagency Working Group to recommend coordinated priorities for nutritional research among the various agencies. This report was the first to reflect genuine cooperation among the federal agencies that support nutrition research. The Working Group proposed that primary responsibility for disease-related human nutritional research be assigned to the National Institutes of Health; for food sciences research and food consumption surveys, to the Department of Agriculture; and for health and nutritional status surveillance, to the National Center for Health Statistics (19).

The report classified human nutritional research into four essential areas: (1) studies of human nutrient needs, (2) food sciences, (3) nutrition education research, and (4) monitoring of diet and nutrition-related health status. The authors emphasized the importance of each of these areas and identified specific research needs within each category. They recommended four urgent research needs: (1) a rapid and relatively inexpensive food consumption survey capability, (2) more precise clinical and laboratory methods for measuring changes in nutritional status, (3) analysis of the HANES data, and (4) expansion of nutrition-related epidemiologic studies.

Within the next year, two additional reports supported these recommendations but also criticized federal activities for their lack of coordination and duplication of effort (20) and suggested specific options that Congress might follow to increase the coordination of federal research activities (21).

In response to these recommendations, the Director of the Office of Science and Technology Policy appointed representatives from nine federal agencies to form a Joint Subcommittee on Human Nutrition Research. This Subcommittee began meeting toward the end of 1978

". . . to ensure that the nutrition research efforts of the federal agencies be mutually reinforcing" (18).

In its December 1980 report (18), the Subcommittee commended the federal government for its increased support of nutrition research since 1977. It identified the many agencies that support nutrition research but it found little duplication of these efforts. In fact, it observed that many agencies had developed joint programs to coordinate research activities. The Subcommittee recommended increased support for research training and for several specific areas of applied nutrition research, but it emphasized that applied research must be ". . . conducted in close collaboration with basic biomedical and behavioral research so that these causal relationships and their modulating factors can be understood and precisely defined to prevent or ameliorate disease" (18).

FOOD INDUSTRY REGULATION

Three federal agencies—the Food and Drug Administration, the Department of Agriculture, and the Federal Trade Commission (FTC)—regulate food quality and food safety standards in manufacturing, interstate commerce, and food labeling and advertising. In addition, the Environmental Protection Agency is responsible for maintaining the quality of drinking water.

Standards of food sanitation, safety, contamination, quality, and labeling are enforced separately by the FDA and the USDA. The FDA ensures that all foods consumed by the American public are safe, sanitary, and labeled properly. Through its Food Safety and Quality Service, the USDA regulates these aspects of the meat and poultry industries. This agency also inspects food packing plants, condemns and destroys contaminated food, and regulates many additional aspects of the food industry (13). The Federal Trade Commission oversees food advertising.

Although federal regulation of the food industry dates back 75 years, the amount of regulatory activity has accelerated recently, largely as a result of advancing technology in food production and processing, in the increased use of pesticides and chemical fertilizers in crop production, and in the use of antibiotics and hormones to promote the growth of animals.

Food Standards

The FDA maintains standards of identity for more than 280 food products. These standards specify the ingredients and the method of processing that must be followed if a product is to be sold under its common name. Once a food product is standardized, its ingredients do not have to be listed on the label. This recipe format precludes deceptive modifications of a food, but it may prevent consumers from knowing what substances a food contains. More importantly, it prevents the elimination of unnecessary or potentially harmful ingredients. Thus, the FDA recently was required to propose regulatory changes in the standard of identity for cola-type soft drinks in order to allow manufacturers to remove caffeine as an ingredient (22).

Food Safety

The FDA and the USDA share responsibility for the safety of the food supply. Together they protect consumers from food-borne disease, environmental contaminants, food toxicants, and dangerous additives.

The food safety activities of the Department of Agriculture are conducted by its Food Safety and Quality Service. This agency inspects plant, animal, and poultry foods for disease or contamination, supervises meat processing, inspects facilities where animals are slaughtered, and controls plant and animal food pests. The role of the Department of Agriculture in food safety has always generated controversy (23). In the past, the Department of Agriculture has been accused of conflict of interest because it favored commercial over consumer interests in its meat inspection program. More recently, it has been accused of too much concern for the consumer and neglect of its primary constituency — agribusiness. Part of that concern arises because of its much more vigorous pursuit of food safety policies, particularly as they relate to carcinogens.

The FDA has an even wider range of responsibilities for food safety. Its programs range from control of food sanitation to regulation of food packaging and testing the safety of food additives. The agency is required to ensure that deficiencies in food safety control are corrected. This aspect of its responsibility has brought the FDA into conflict with consumer groups, who find its regulatory policies insufficient, as well as with leaders in the food industry who criticize it for overregulation. The inability of the FDA to prohibit the use of saccharin as an additive, due to Congressional action specifically exempting it from provisions of the Food, Drug, and Cosmetic Act, provides one recent example of the FDA's vulnerability to political pressure (24).

The most important food safety issue to be debated in the 1980s is the Delaney Amendment to the Food, Drug, and Cosmetic Act. This amendment prohibits the use in any form of a substance that is demonstrated to be carcinogenic. In permitting the marketing of saccharin, Congress made a specific exclusion to the requirements of the Delaney Amendment. Whether Congress will continue a case-by-case approach to the use of substances found to be carcinogenic or whether they will adopt a policy based strictly on safety and cost remains to be seen.

Food Advertising

The role of the Federal Trade Commission in regulation of food advertising is to prevent deception and to improve the reliability of advertisements, so that consumers may make informed choices (25). In recent years, the Commission has become increasingly concerned about the nutritional quality of the processed foods being advertised. A former chairman of the FTC observed that the great majority of food advertisements promote foods that are high in fat, cholesterol, refined sugar, salt, or alcohol (9).

The agency has long been handicapped in its regulatory efforts by inadequate funding; it spent less than $150,000 on nutrition advertising regulation in 1977 (25). By comparison, the 29 leading food, candy, chewing gum, soft drink, and alcoholic beverage advertisers worked with a combined advertising budget of over $3.5 billion in 1979 (26).

As the FTC has taken an increasingly active role in attempting to regulate claims made in food advertisements and to modify food commercials during children's television programs, it has come into conflict with the food industry and with Congress. Congress has withheld funding in order to force the Commission to modify its positions, and it now has the power to veto FTC rules. The deregulation policies espoused by the Reagan administration have left the future role of the FTC in question. Early in 1981, the Commission suspended an investigation into regulation of children's television advertising, largely in response to political pressures (27).

Food Labeling

The FDA requires that nutrition information be listed on food labels when nutritional claims are made in advertising or when certain additives, such as vitamins and minerals, are present. All additional food labeling is voluntary. According to FDA regulations, food labeling must include the following information: size of normal serving; grams of carbohydrate, fat, and protein per serving; calories per serving; and percentage of the U.S. Recommended Dietary Allowances for vitamins and minerals per serving. Currently, more than 60% of processed foods are labeled with this limited information, primarily on a voluntary basis (28).

In response to demands by consumer groups and by some members of Congress for compulsory, detailed food labeling legislation, the three major regulatory agencies developed two joint proposals for changes in food labeling regulations. Their proposals called for more complete information on food ingredients, greater federal control over food fortification, and nutrition labeling of more foods.

These proposals were considered by Congress, and they were supported by the Carter administration. They were opposed, however, by the food industry, which prefers a voluntary labeling program. Without strong public and Congressional support, it is unlikely that more rigorous, comprehensive labeling requirements will be instituted in the near future. This situation is especially unfortunate because improved food labeling is an essential part of any rational food policy. It provides consumers with information about food composition and the losses that occur during food processing. It enables consumers to control caloric intake and to avoid an excess of certain ingredients, such as fat, sugar, and salt. Adequate food labeling would help bring the country closer to the National Nutrition Consortium's 1974 goal of developing a level of public knowledge and understanding of nutrition and foods that will promote maximal health (6).

In the absence of comprehensive labeling reforms, however, important steps can be taken by the FDA to extend voluntary labeling, particularly with respect to sodium and sodium chloride. Millions of patients with hypertension might benefit from such labeling. Recent indications are that the FDA, with support by the Secretary of Health and Human Services, will move forward with such proposals.

AGRICULTURAL SUPPORT

The Department of Agriculture is the primary agency responsible for federal agricultural support programs. More than 50 separate programs ensure the adequacy and stability of the domestic food supply, regardless of national or international economic fluctuations. Agricultural support programs provide a remarkable variety of services to food growers and producers: pest control, commodity loans and purchases, income protection, indemnity payments, incentive payments, product grading, education, technical assistance, marketing information, crop insurance, grants, and loans (29).

The fact that these programs protect the specific interests of agricultural producers has brought the Department of Agriculture into conflict with consumer groups, who accuse it of strengthening the economic interests of U.S. agricultural businesses at the expense of the general population. Nowhere is this conflict more apparent than within the Department of Agriculture itself. For many years, the Agricultural Stabilization and Conservation Services protected sugarcane and sugarbeet growers through a complex system of price supports that guaranteed producers a minimum price per pound of sugar (30). Now, a different USDA agency advises the public to "avoid too much sugar" (31). The balance between these differing viewpoints, however, is not equal; the USDA's budget for agricultural support is far greater than that for consumer education.

NUTRITION EDUCATION

Individuals in the United States receive information about food, nutrition, diet, and health from a bewildering array of sources, only one of which is the federal government. Although nutrition education is a specified function of several federal agencies and an important minor activity of many more of them, the government has no central program for nutrition education. Instead, nutrition information is disseminated independently by the various agencies to their target population groups. Because these groups range from schoolchildren to professional scientists, educational materials produced by the government are exceptionally diverse; they include dietary advice to the public, nutrition information for consumers, technical materials for farmers, and research reports for professionals.

The Department of Agriculture produces many of these materials. In 1979, it made available 313 separate items for distribution to scientists and health professionals, the general public, and recipients of food assistance (32). In addition, it sponsors training programs, scientific conferences, and education programs for school teachers and workers in food service, procurement, and regulation. These activities accounted for an expenditure of more than $100 million per year in the late 1970s (25). Much of this funding supports cooperative extension services, which provide consumers with information to improve diets and to fight inflation, and the Expanded Food and Nutrition Education Program, which has taught improved dietary practices to more than 1.5 million families since 1969 (32).

The need to provide more and better nutrition instruction to the general public, to food assistance recipients, and to health professions' students and practitioners has been a major recommendation of a great many federal reports. One of these reports notes that government educational materials are often ". . . uninteresting, simplistic, repetitive, or irrelevant," and that whether or not they make a difference in the health of the American people is simply not known (13). This report also emphasizes that, no matter how effective current federal efforts might be, they cannot possibly counteract the enormous educational impact of televised food advertising on young children.

Yet another report comments that federal nutrition education activities are neither coordinated nor evaluated. In order to direct education efforts toward "the common good of the consumer," the government must develop a clear statement of educational goals; a systematic process for developing, evaluating, and disseminating nutrition information; and a coordinated mechanism to ensure that all necessary areas are covered and that duplication of effort is avoided (25).

DIETARY RECOMMENDATIONS AND NUTRITION POLICY

Although the federal government plays an important part in nutrition education, its role is minor when compared to the activities of a multitude of other sources of nutrition information, particularly the food industry. Major changes are occurring both in the sources of information and in the nutrition information communicated to the public. In the past 5 years alone, more than 20 public and private organizations have produced nutrition reports and dietary recommendations for the U.S. population (33). These recommendations generally have focused on the relationship between diet and chronic diseases, such as heart disease, stroke, cancer, diabetes mellitus, arteriosclerosis, and cirrhosis—six of the nation's 10 leading causes of death. The most important of these reports and their recommendations are summarized in Table 3.

The recent emphasis on diet and chronic diseases represents a major change in focus for nutrition education, information, and policy. Prior to the mid-1970s, adequate nutrition was considered to be the absence of undernutrition, and nutrition education centered on micronutrients (vitamins and minerals) and nutrition deficiency diseases. The major sources of nutrition information for the public were advertisements by industry, books and articles, and a few government publications, particularly the Basic Four Food Groups, published by the Department of Agriculture in 1957 (34), and the Recommended Dietary Allowances, published and updated periodically by the Food and Nutrition Board of the National Academy of Sciences (35). By the mid-1970s, however, a growing body of epidemiologic and clinical evidence suggested a relationship between diet and a number of degenerative diseases. Nutritional adequacy was redefined to emphasize the role of macronutrients (fat, carbohydrate, and protein) and overnutrition in the prevention of these diseases.

The publication of policy statements reflecting these new findings represented a major change in the United States government's nutrition policy. Formerly, government policies paid relatively little attention to

Table 3. Dietary Advice to the Public by Various U.S. Reports[a]

Group	Maintain Ideal Body Weight	Reduce Total Fat	Reduce Saturated Fat	Increase Polyunsaturated Fat	Reduce Cholesterol	Reduce Sugars	Increase Starches	Increase Fiber	Reduce Salt
Dietary Goals, 2nd ed. 1977 (36)	yes	yes (30%)	yes	yes	yes (300mg)	yes	yes	yes	yes (~5g)
American Heart Assoc., 1978 (38)	yes	yes (30-35%)	yes	yes	yes (300mg)	yes	yes	no	yes
Healthy People, 1979 (37)	yes	yes	yes	no	yes	yes	yes	no	yes
American Diabetes Assoc., 1979 (41)	yes	yes	yes	no	yes	yes	yes	yes	yes
American Medical Assoc., 1979 (39)	yes	yes, if at high risk	yes, if at high risk	yes, if at high risk	yes, if at high risk	moderate	no	no	yes (<12g)
National Cancer Inst., 1979 (40)	yes	yes	no	no	no	no	no	yes	no
USDA Guidelines DHEW, 1980 (31)	yes	yes	yes	no	yes	yes	yes	yes	yes
Food & Nutrition Board, *Toward Healthful Diets*, 1980 (42)	yes	adjust to calorie need	no	no	no	adjust to calorie need	yes for diabetes	no	yes (3-8g)

[a] This table was adapted from one designed by Dr. Kristen McNutt (33).

meeting the public's need for nutrition information. That situation changed with the work of the Select Committee on Nutrition and Human Needs, chaired by Senator George McGovern. In 1977, after extensive hearings, extending over several years, that examined the relationship between nutrition and health, the Select Committee issued its controversial report, *Dietary Goals for the United States* (36). Although a Congressional committee report, *Dietary Goals* was perceived by much of the U.S. public as official government policy. The government has since issued two official publications containing dietary advice: *Healthy People: The Surgeon General's Report on Health Promotion and Disease Prevention* (37) and *Nutrition and Your Health: Dietary Guidelines for Americans* (31), published jointly by the USDA and the DHHS.

These reports stimulated widespread discussion. There are those who question whether the government should be making such recommendations at all. Others debate the merits of specific recommendations. Fueling the controversy in recent years have been the sometimes contradictory recommendations from organizations such as the American Heart Association (38), the American Medical Association (39), the National Cancer Institute (40), the American Diabetes Association (41), and the Food and Nutrition Board of the National Academy of Sciences (42). Additionally, numerous foreign governments have issued major nutrition policy statements (43–45).

Increasing Consensus and Ongoing Debate

The controversy generated by these reports has obscured the gradual emergence of an apparent consensus among nutrition experts on many important nutritional issues. Most nutrition experts agree that the present U.S. dietary recommendations should be modified to emphasize the importance of variety in food intake, to urge an increase in the consumption of complex carbohydrate foods (starch and fiber), and to advocate a restriction in the consumption of fats, sugars, alcohol, and salt. In addition, breast feeding of infants now receives broad support. While specific details of these recommendations may differ, they generally support the proposals outlined in the *Dietary Goals* It is noteworthy that, on the basis of evidence linking diets high in starch and fiber to increased control of blood insulin, glucose, and lipid levels (46), the American Diabetes Association now recommends for patients with diabetes mellitus a diet with proportions of fat, carbohydrate, and protein paralleling those outlined in the *Dietary Goals*

Despite the increasing consensus in dietary recommendations, much public attention has been directed toward differences among the various reports. The most controversial recommendations are those that describe dietary intake of total fat, saturated and unsaturated fat, and cholesterol. Many of the reports urge a decrease in the percentage of total calories derived from fat (31, 36—40). As indicated in Table 3, however, they differ in specific percentages of caloric intake, proportion of polyunsaturated to saturated fat, limitation in amounts of cholesterol, and whether the recommendations should be directed to everyone or only to individuals in special high-risk groups.

At the heart of this dispute is the controversial relationship between dietary lipids and coronary heart disease. In a careful analysis of the problem, Hulley et al. argue that the data clearly support dietary intervention for individuals with certain risk factors for coronary heart disease, but that "to be effective, public health measures should be applied uniformly to the entire population" (47). Thus, these authors support the recommendations set forth in *Dietary Goals* and stress the importance of informative nutrition labeling regarding fat and cholesterol. At the same time, they urge clinicians to suggest dietary interventions tailored to the particular needs and beliefs of individual patients.

Recommendations for fiber intake are also controversial. Despite an increasing consensus in the medical literature about the importance of dietary fiber in the prevention of certain diseases of the intestines, such as appendicitis, diverticulosis, and, perhaps, colon cancer (48, 49), and the maintenance of normal blood sugar (46) and blood lipid levels (50), several groups omit recommendations for dietary fiber intake in their recommendations (38, 39, 42).

Most reports simply avoid the subject of food additives or present the issue without a conclusion (37, 40). Similarly, the effects of food processing on nutrient content receive little attention other than the recommendation for "decreased consumption of refined sugars" (31) or "increased attention to the nutritional quality of processed food" (37). *Dietary Goals* does recommend "decreased consumption of refined and processed sugars and foods high in such sugars" (36). The Surgeon General notes that increased attention needs to be paid to the nutritional qualities of processed food (37).

Implications for Nutrition Education Policy

The apparent inability of different groups of nutrition "experts" to reach agreement on specific recommendations, although agreeing on the need to modify the American diet, underscores several major problems in formulating national nutrition policies. Who should develop a national policy? How should the policy be developed? What is the nature of the evidence required for nutrition policy? How should the policy be implemented?

Who Should Develop Nutrition Education Policy?

Federal policy may be made by Congress, by federal agencies implementing the laws enacted by Congress, or by the courts in interpreting Congressional intent. Experts often play a key role in advising policymakers, particularly in areas such as health and nutrition where there is a large body of scientific evidence germane to public policy.

Few areas have generated more difference of opinion, scientifically and politically, than nutrition policy. Nearly all of the authors of the various nutrition/dietary recommendations in recent years have been criticized for bias, self-interest, or possible conflict of interest. Although the U.S. Senate's *Dietary Goals* was prepared in response to testimony by a large number of food and nutrition experts, the Select Committee's motivation for producing the report was criticized as a political document designed by lawyers rather than nutritionists. It was suggested that if diet did affect chronic disease morbidity and mortality, costs for National Health Insurance would decrease, aiding the legislative program and generating votes for its advocates (51). A second example is the Food and Nutrition Board's controversial decision in a recent report, *Toward Healthful Diets*, to make no recommendation regarding dietary intake of saturated fat and cholesterol. Board members have been accused of lack of expertise in this area and of potential conflict of interest, because several of them have ties to various food industries, particularly the meat, egg, and dairy industries (52).

The USDA/DHHS report *Dietary Guidelines* (31) has also been criticized for a potential conflict on the part of USDA, since its "political raison d'être . . . is to make it easier for farmers to make money" (53). In contrast to the Surgeon General's report *Healthy People* (37), the USDA/DHHS report makes little mention of the potential danger of food additives, the growing consumption of processed foods, or the role of advertising and the media in formulating food preference (53).

Scientific Research Findings as a Basis for Policy

Although consideration of who should develop a national policy influences how that policy is developed, additional controversy surrounds the transformation of scientific data into health policy. Some groups demand established proof of benefit while others feel that the recommendations should reflect the best available evidence even without proof of benefit. The Food and Nutrition Board goes even further, demanding proof that the recommendations themselves will not be harmful (42). Other authors point out that nutritionists and other health professionals historically have made recommendations based upon the best available scientific knowledge without such proof (54).

The Food and Nutrition Board has been further criticized for applying a sliding scale of scientific standards to its various recommendations (55). In support of its decision to omit recommendations for reduced intake of fat and cholesterol, the Board reviewed seven intervention trials that failed to demonstrate a decrease in overall mortality. Yet, in the same report, the Board strongly recommended weight reduction and salt restriction, despite the lack of adequate clinical trials to demonstrate decreased mortality for these interventions.

Many authors emphasize the technical difficulties involved in conducting a well-designed clinical trial to test the role of dietary factors in cardiovascular mortality (47, 56). Yet, numerous groups that support reduction in dietary fat and cholesterol note that clinicians often must make decisions in the absence of proof, and that current dietary recommendations are prudent (47). Furthermore, it is likely that we will never have sufficient proof (47), and that decisions must be made on the basis of the best possible scientific judgment (57).

Application of Dietary Recommendations

Even with agreement on the content of a national nutrition policy, major controversy remains on the application of the policy. In concluding *Dietary Goals for the United States,* for example, the Senate Select Committee recommended that Congress support a public education program in nutrition, require more extensive food labeling for all foods, sponsor research on the effects of food processing on health, coordinate human nutrition research undertaken by the Department of Agriculture and the Department of Health and Human Services, and consider the implications of nutritional health concerns on agricultural policy. Unfortunately, few of these proposals have been implemented in the 6 years since their publication. Powerful interest groups within the food industry have actively opposed them, as have some influential farm-state Representatives and Senators, as well as nutrition scientists. Congress abolished the Select Committee that made the recommendations.

The recent political victory of anti-big-government forces in the 1980 national elections may signal the formal end of the efforts of the past decade to develop a comprehensive, consumer-oriented federal nutrition policy. The effect of governmental withdrawal from leadership in dietary recommendations and nutrition information for the public is likely to turn the responsibility for nutrition education back to private industry. The potential effect of such a change in leadership is controversial. While some experts believe that a more active role by the food industry would be highly beneficial (5), others are concerned that the food industry's profit motivation and enormous capacity to alter the dietary habits through processing and advertising will have increasingly deleterious effects on U.S. diets. To avoid this catastrophe, it has been proposed by consumer advocates that the federal government support a "comprehensive federal program to change the American diet" (58).

Such programs are already in place in other countries, most notably Norway and Sweden. Interestingly, these countries and others with less comprehensive programs are primarily those in which the government has assumed major fiscal responsibility for the population's health care. Thus, in the same way that it is in the self-interest of a prepaid health plan to reduce health care costs, it has become in the self-interest of these national governments to change eating habits to minimize risk of widespread chronic diseases. Whether these programs will accomplish their goals has yet to be proven, but they hold great promise for the future efficacy of federal nutrition intervention.

NUTRITION POLICY RECOMMENDATIONS

The lack of coordination of federal food and nutrition activities does not necessarily doom them to failure. Indeed, programs may flourish under a flexible and responsive organizational structure. It does, however, subject the government to charges that it is not adequately meeting the nation's needs for food and nutrition services. More important, the lack of coordination leaves individual programs open to criticism that they are redundant and dispensable. Without a coherent national policy and clearly defined departmental and agency responsibility within this policy framework as vital parts of a coordinated national effort, the specific programs are vulnerable to budgetary reductions and restrictions. The most urgent need for the 1980s is the development of a coherent national nutrition policy.

A coordinated policy and administrative structure, coupled with stronger evaluation procedures, would help to ensure that federal food and nutrition programs are meeting national needs, thus protecting them from the vagaries of political fortune. These policy changes would go a long way toward ensuring maximum nutritional health for all residents of the United States.

REFERENCES

1. U.S. General Accounting Office. *Food, Agriculture and Nutrition: Issues for Planning,* U.S. Government Printing Office, Washington, D.C., 1980.
2. M. Chou, Changing food policies. In M. Chou and D. Harmon, eds., *Critical Food Issues of the Eighties,* Pergamon Press, New York, 1978, p. 103.
3. W. Boehm, A U.S. food policy. *Natl. Food Rev.* (USDA) 6, 34 (Winter 1979).
4. Citizens Board of Inquiry. *Hunger USA,* Beacon Press, Boston, 1968.
5. *White House Conference on Food, Nutrition and Health. Final Report.* Government Printing Office, Washington, D.C., 1970.
6. U.S. Congress, Senate, Select Committee on Nutrition and Human Needs. *National Nutrition Consortium Guidelines for a National Nutrition Policy,* U.S. Government Printing Office, Washington, D.C., 1974. [Reprinted in *Nutr. Rev.* 32, 153 (1974).]
7. P. Lee, Nutrition policy—from neglect and uncertainty to debate and action. *J. Am. Diet. Assoc.* 72, 581 (1978).
8. T. Warley, *Agriculture in an Interdependent World: U.S.–Canadian Perspectives,* National Planning Association, Washington, D.C., 1977.
9. T. H. Stafford and J. H. Wills, Consumer demand increasing for convenience in food products. National Food Review (USDA) 6, 15 (Winter 1979).
10. Comptroller General of the U.S. Inventory of federal food, nutrition and agriculture programs. CED–79–125. U.S. Government Printing Office, Washington, D.C., 1979.
11. U.S. Department of Agriculture. *Federal Food, Nutrition, and Agriculture Programs, Prototype Inventory: 1980 Update,* U.S. Government Printing Office, Washington, D.C., 1980.
12. Comptroller General of the U.S. *Federal Domestic Food Assistance Programs: A Time for Assessment and Change,* CED–78–113. U.S. Government Printing Office, Washington, D.C., 1978.
13. U.S. General Accounting Office. *National Nutrition Issues,* CED–78–7. U.S. Government Printing Office, Washington, D.C., 1977.
14. U.S. Congress; Senate, Select Committee on Nutrition and Human Needs. *Nutrition and Health II,* U.S. Government Printing Office, Washington, D.C., 1976.
15. U.S. General Accounting Office. *Food, Agriculture, and Nutrition: Issues for Planning,* U.S. Government Printing Office, Washington, D.C., 1980.

16. Anon., Reagan food cuts would cost recipients at least $4.3 billion, *CNI Weekly Report* 11 (11), 1, March 12, 1981.
17. J. Berkenfield and J. B. Schwartz, Nutrition intervention in the community: The WIC program. *N. Engl. J. Med.* **302**, 579 (1980).
18. U.S. Congress, Joint Subcommittee on Human Nutrition Research, Federal Coordinating Council on Sciences, Engineering, and Technology. *Federally Supported Human Nutrition Research, Training, and Education: Update for the 1980s.* I. *Human Nutrition Research and Training,* U.S. Government Printing Office, Washington, D.C., 1980.
19. Executive Office of the President, Office of Science Technology Policy, Nutrition Research Interagency Working Group. *New Directions in Federally Supported Human Nutrition Research,* U.S. Government Printing Office, Washington, D.C., 1977.
20. Comptroller General of the U.S. Report to the Congress of the U.S., *Federal Human Nutrition Research Needs a Coordinated Approach to Advance Knowledge,* PSAD—77—156—A, U.S. Government Printing Office, Washington, D.C., 1978. 2 vols.
21. Office of Technology Assessment. *Nutrition Research Alternatives,* OTA—F—74, U.S. Government Printing Office, Washington, D.C., 1978.
22. *Federal Register.* October 21, 1980, and December 23, 1980.
23. M. Chou, The preoccupation with food safety. In M. Chou and D. Harmon, eds., *Critical Food Issues of the Eighties,* Pergamon Press, New York, 1978, p. 18.
24. R. J. Smith, Latest saccharin tests kill FDA proposal. *Science* **208**, 154 (1980).
25. Comptroller General of the U.S. Report to Congress of the U.S., *Informing the Public about Nutrition: Federal Agencies Should Do Better,* CED—78—75, U.S. Government Printing Office, Washington, D.C., 1978.
26. M. Elmquist, Top 100 advertisers spend $11.7 billion. *Advertising Age,* September 11, 1980, p. 1.
27. A. O. Sulzberger, A bleak mood pervades F.T.C. *The New York Times,* 25 May 1981, business section, p. 1.
28. J. Weimer, Nutrition labeling: the unresolved issue. *Natl. Food Rev.* (USDA) 11, 20 (Summer 1980).
29. U.S. Office of Management and Budget. *Catalog of Federal Domestic Assistance: 1980,* U.S. Government Printing Office, Washington, D.C., 1980.

30. W. Robbins, I. Conflicting interests over sugar create unwanted U.S. surpluses. (14 Jan., p. 1) II. Lobbyists worked off stage to shape sugar laws. (15 Jan., p. 1) III. Powerful rivals clash over sugar price supports. (16 Jan., p. 1) *The New York Times,* 1979.

31. U.S. Department of Agriculture and U.S. Department of Health, Education and Welfare. *Nutrition and Your Health: Dietary Guidelines for Americans,* U.S. Government Printing Office, Washington, D.C., 1980.

32. U.S. Department of Agriculture. *Food and Nutrition in the 1980s: Moving Ahead. Comprehensive Plan for Implementing the National Food and Human Nutrition Research and Education and Information Programs,* U.S. Government Printing Office, Washington, D.C., 1979.

33. K. McNutt, Dietary advice to the public: 1957 to 1980. *Nutr. Rev.* **38**, 353 (1980).

34. U.S. Department of Agriculture, Agricultural Research Service. *Essentials for an Adequate Diet. Home Economics Research Report No. 3.* U.S. Government Printing Office, Washington, D.C., 1957.

35. Committee on Dietary Allowances, Food and Nutrition Board, National Research Council. *Recommended Dietary Allowances,* 9th ed., National Academy of Sciences, Washington, D.C., 1980.

36. U.S. Congress, Senate, Select Committee on Nutrition and Human Needs. *Dietary Goals for the United States,* 1st and 2nd eds., U.S. Government Printing Office, Washington, D.C., 1977.

37. U.S. Department of Health, Education, and Welfare. *Healthy People: The Surgeon General's Report on Health Promotion and Disease Prevention,* U.S. Government Printing Office, Washington, D.C., 1979.

38. American Heart Association, Committee on Nutrition, Diet and Coronary Heart Disease. *Circulation* **58**, 762A (1978).

39. Council on Scientific Affairs, American Medical Association, Concepts of nutrition and health. *J. Am. Med. Assoc.* **242**, 2335 (1979).

40. National Cancer Institute. *Statement on Diet, Nutrition and Cancer,* National Cancer Institute, Washington, D.C., 1979.

41. American Diabetes Association, Committee on Food and Nutrition. Principles of nutrition and dietary recommendations for individuals with diabetes mellitus: 1979. *Diabetes* **28**, 1027 (1979).

42. Food and Nutrition Board, National Research Council. *Toward Healthful Diets,* National Academy of Sciences, Washington, D.C., 1980.

43. G. T. T. Molitor, National nutrition goals: How far have we come? In M. Chou and D. Harmon, eds., *Critical Food Issues of the Eighties*, Pergamon Press, New York, 1979, p. 134.
44. Canada, Department of National Health and Welfare. *Recommendations for Prevention Programs in Relation to Nutrition and Cardiovascular Disease*, Bureau of Nutritional Sciences, Health Protection Branch, Ottawa, Canada, 1977.
45. B. Winikoff, ed., *Nutrition and National Policy*, MIT Press, Cambridge, Mass., 1978.
46. J. A. Anderson and K. Ward, High carbohydrate, high fiber diets of insulin treated men with diabetes mellitus. *Am. J. Clin. Nutr.* **32**, 2312 (1979).
47. S. Hulley, R. Sherwin, M. Nestle, and P. Lee, Epidemiology as a guide to clinical decision. II. Diet and coronary heart disease. *West. J. Med.* **135** (7), 25–33 (1981).
48. D. P. Burkitt, A. R. P. Walker, and N. S. Painter, Dietary fiber and disease. *J. Am. Med. Assoc.* **229**, 1068 (1974).
49. W. S. Worthington–Roberts, Dietary fiber. In W. S. Worthington–Roberts, ed., *Contemporary Developments in Nutrition*, C. V. Mosby, St. Louis, 1981.
50. D. A. Jenkins, Dietary fiber, diabetes and hyperlipidemia. *Lancet* **2**, 1287 (1979).
51. R. W. Olson, The U.S. quandary: Can we formulate a rational nutritional policy? In M. Chou and D. Harmon, eds., *Critical Food Issues of the Eighties*, Pergamon Press, New York, 1979, p. 119.
52. J. Turner, We feel compelled to break relations. *CNI Weekly Rep.* **10** (24), 4 (1980).
53. D. S. Greenberg, Nutrition: A long wait for a little advice. *N. Engl. J. Med.* **302**, 535 (1980).
54. D. M. Hegsted, Rationale for change in the American diet. *Food Technol.* **32** (9), 44 (1978).
55. P. Hausman, Academy gets egg on its face. *Nutr. Action* **7** (7), 10 (1980).
56. R. Sherwin, Controlled trials of the diet–heart hypothesis: some comments on the experimental unit. *Am. J. Epidemiol.* **108**, 92 (1978).
57. A. E. Harper, Dietary goals: A skeptical view. *Am. J. Clin. Nutr.* **31**, 310 (1978).
58. L. Brewster and M. Jacobson, *The Changing American Diet*, Center for Science in the Public Interest, Washington, D.C., 1978.

ADDITIONAL RECENT REFERENCES

Committee on Diet, Nutrition, and Cancer, National Research Council, National Academy of Sciences. *Diet, Nutrition, and Cancer,* National Academy Press, Washington, D.C., 1982.

S. M. Grundy, Chairman, Nutrition Committee of the American Heart Association, Rationale of the Diet—Heart Statement of the American Heart Association: Report of Nutrition Committee. *Circulation* **65**(4), 839A (1982).

Comptroller General of the U.S., *Progress Made in Federal Human Nutrition Research Planning and Coordination: Some Improvements Needed.* CED—82—56. U.S. Government Printing Office, Washington, D.C., 1982.

Multiple Risk Factor Intervention Tri. l Research Group, Multiple risk factor intervention trial: risk factor changes and mortality results. *J. Am. Med. Assoc.* **248**, 1465 (1982).

15

Dietary Recommendations and Policy Implications

THE U.S. EXPERIENCE

JOHANNA DWYER, D.Sc.

Associate Professor
Departments of Medicine and Community Health
Director, Frances Stern Nutrition Center
Tufts Medical School
and
New England Medical Center Hospital

Boston, Massachusetts

Address correspondence to Johanna Dwyer, D.Sc., New England Medical Center Hospital, 171 Harrison Avenue, Box 783, Boston, Massachusetts 02111.

ABSTRACT

Dietary recommendations and their policy implications depend not only on developments in the science and art of nutrition but on larger social, political, and economic events. Therefore, it is important to understand the background from whence they come.

This chapter reviews the developments that have been involved in bringing about changes in American nutrition policymaking, the recommendations that have resulted, and their likely effects. First, the scientific, social, and political contexts from which various recommendations have emerged in the past few years are reviewed.

Second, basic questions having to do with dietary recommendations are raised and addressed. These include a consideration of whether dietary recommendations are necessary and, if they are, who should make them, by what process, what they should consist of, and to whom they should be addressed.

Third, several different sets of recommendations that are in use today and their alternative policy implications are examined.

Finally, conclusions are drawn that may be useful to nutrition scientists in considering other dietary recommendations and their policy implications in the future.

Although experience only on domestic issues in the United States is discussed, nutrition scientists who are involved in making dietary recommendations in other countries may find similarities to processes in their own countries.

PROGRESS

The decade of the 1970s was a time of extraordinary growth both in fundamental knowledge of the biologic and behavioral sciences undergirding nutrition and in the extension of these findings through practical applications to better the lives of Americans. A detailed description of the fruits of this activity would itself fill a book, but since it was in this context that the dietary recommendations of the later 1970s developed, it is important to recall here the highlights of the period.

316

Two events began the long process of coordination and refinement of government, private sector, and voluntary activity to focus attention more sharply on the nutrition-related challenges facing the country. The White House Conference on Food, Nutrition and Health, which was held late in 1969, set the agenda for problems that needed to be addressed in later years. It energized those in government to address these issues, and drew together those in the public, private, and voluntary sectors who needed to become involved in their solution (1). Dozens of hearings held by the Senate Select Committee on Nutrition and Human Needs and other Congressional committees throughout the late 1960s and early 1970s (2) played a similar catalytic role in Congress. While the Committee had no authorizing or appropriating authority, it was successful in focusing the attention of those on the nine major Senate committees and 12 major House committees and the myriad subcommittees under them to take a more active interest in this area. Heightened interest in both the executive and legislative branches soon stimulated changes in government.

Until the 1970s the hundreds of food and nutrition programs involving at least 12 cabinet-level departments and 21 independent agencies had gone their separate ways with little sense of overall direction and purpose. Gradually greater coordination was achieved, and the area was increasingly viewed as a whole rather than as a mass of incoherent and unrelated component parts. Public interest in nutrition also increased during the period, so that private sector and voluntary groups devoted increasing attention and resources to improving the nutritional status of populations. The end result of these efforts by all sectors of society was gratifying and is briefly summarized in Table 1. For all of these issues, multisectoral involvement of all of the stakeholders (e.g., professionals, those in the food industry, consumers, and government) was common. Stakeholders also were able to agree about the existence of a problem, the need for a solution, and the desired ends, although there was often considerable disagreement about the means by which those ends should be met.

CONTROVERSIES

Until the late 1960s, nutrition was a relatively noncontroversial topic in comparison to the enormous attention it received from the public and the media in subsequent years. Disputes among nutritionists rarely came to public attention. In the late 1960s, nutrition became increasingly politicized, and controversy between nutrition scientists frequently erupted on the front pages of newspapers, on television screens, in hearing rooms of Congress and the courts, rather than solely

Table 1. Progress and Problems Involved In Nutrition Policy and Programs at the Federal Level During the 1970s

Progress	Problems
Improved surveillance and evaluation of nutritional status	Definitions, prevalence, causes, remedies, responsibility, and costs of alleviating poverty-related malnutrition
Nutrition component added to the National Health and Nutrition Examination Survey	
Preschool nutrition examination survey of representative samples of children completed	
Ten-State Nutrition Survey documented nutritional status of poor and near poor in 10 low or high income ratio states	
Improved food consumption survey completed by U.S. Department of Agriculture	
Surveillance system to monitor growth and iron nutritional status of infants enrolled in WIC programs in several states launched by Center for Disease Control of U.S. Public Health Service	
Special growth surveys of refugee children from Southeast Asia living in the United States begun by Center for Disease Control	
Improved standards for evaluation of diet and nutritional status	
Updated tables of food composition with more complete analyses issued by U.S. Department of Agriculture	
Better test and standards for biochemical and anthropometric measurements of nutritional status developed	
More specific data recommendations developed on nutritional needs of especially vulnerable groups within the population	
For example, pregnant and nursing mothers, young infants, children, adolescents, adults at high risk or with already apparent chronic degenerative diseases, the sick who require dietary therapy, and various groups for which the federal government has special responsibility	

Progress	Problems
Growth of food programs for poor and other vulnerable groups	
Rapid growth of research on human nutrition problems	Extent to which diet is involved in the consumption and/or prevention of certain chronic degenerative diseases
Development of large-scale trials of the effects of multiple risk factor interventions, including diet, in modifying risks for premature coronary artery disease	
Elucidation of dietary measures for nutritional support and therapy in various diseases	
Improved food safety policy	
Review of GRAS (generally recognized as safe) lists of components added to foods	Regulations governing the sale of vitamin, mineral, and other other dietary suplements, the advertising and sale of "organic," "natural," health foods, and permissible doses for over-the-counter sales of vitamins and minerals
	Magnitude and scope of risks to human health posed by various direct and indirect food additives, how best to monitor the food supply for their occurrence, and how best to regulate or control their occurrence in foods
Better nutrition education	
More nutrition education at elementary and secondary levels under the Nutrition Education and Training Act and local initiatives	Appropriate types of dietary recommendations for various groups of consumers and how best to develop different sources of information to provide consumers with tools for making informed decisions about food choices
Improved nutrition education for professionals	
More consumer information and education programs involving nutrition	
More relevant guides for food choices	
Nutrient labeling of processed foods grows in popularity; better ingredient labeling and more unit pricing	

within professional circles. Table 1 also summarizes the major issues that generated controversy during the 1970s. All of these problematic issues had several characteristics in common, including a relatively weak knowledge base, consumer informational and educational dimensions, and a crosscutting nature that involved issues broader than those within the competence of nutrition scientists alone. They were also all politically volatile issues with ideological implications which were likely to engender public policy debate on the appropriate role of government.

DIETARY RECOMMENDATIONS: BASIC QUESTIONS

Are Dietary Recommendations Necessary?

Long ago, the American federal establishment found it necessary to have nutrient standards and nutrition principles for its own operations. For example, guidance was required for feeding personnel in the armed forces, those in federal hospitals, and, in times of war, for making decisions about rationing. Other sectors in society also needed such guidance, but they lacked the resources and expertise necessary to develop them on their own. Therefore, nutrient recommendations of an authoritative nature were viewed as necessary; they were developed and periodically revised by a quasigovernmental body, the National Research Council, and, later, the National Academy of Sciences; and they were adopted for government use. Dietary recommendations for the public, such as the food guides using the seven food groups or the basic four food groups publicized by various federal agencies and other groups, were usually based upon them.

The dilemmas and difficulties in this process were few until the mid-1960s, when some biomedical scientists began to suggest that authoritative guidance might also be necessary and appropriate for dietary components that were not dealt with specifically in the Recommended Dietary Allowances, such as the type and amount of some macronutrients, sodium, and cholesterol. By the mid-1970s enough sentiment had grown that such topics needed to be dealt with more definitively than they had been in the recommended allowances of the time, but members of the Food and Nutrition Board apparently did not believe that the evidence was sufficient to do this.

In 1977, the staff of the Senate Select Committee on Nutrition and Human Needs issued a widely publicized set of dietary recommendations entitled *Dietary Goals for the United States* (3). These covered food constituents that were not quantitatively specified in existing federal recommendations, and suggested upper limits for intakes. In 1980, *Dietary Guidelines for Americans* (4), addressing the same issues in less quantitative terms by specifying only directions for changes in intakes of these constituents, was disseminated by the U.S. Department of Agriculture and the U.S. Department of Health, Education and Welfare. The guidelines were preceded by a series of other reports, also funded from federal sources, on the advisability of dietary and other health-related changes in promoting health and delaying the onset of certain chronic degenerative diseases. Several months later, recommendations which conflicted with these reports in several respects were issued by the Food and Nutrition Board of the National Academy of Sciences in a short publication entitled *Toward Healthful Diets* (5).

These diverse reports led to much confusion. It was not clear whether the recommendations of the Department of Health and Human Services (formerly, Department of Health, Education and Welfare) and the Department of Agriculture, as embodied in the *Dietary Guidelines for Americans* (4) or the somewhat disparate recommendations in *Toward Healthful Diets* of the Food and Nutrition Board (5) were authoritative or whether several other sets of recommendations proposed by other bodies were more appropriate. Nevertheless, some progress in the direction of dealing with concerns having to do with guidance about excess as well as sufficiency in diets had been made. This was evident in the ranges provided for intakes of certain micronutrients, such as sodium, in the newly revised 1980 edition of the *Recommended Dietary Allowances* (6). However, a number of basic questions had been raised by these developments. These included issues of what kinds of dietary recommendations were necessary, of what they should consist, who should make recommendations, how they should be implemented, and the role of government in their dissemination. These will be discussed below.

Of What Should Dietary Recommendations Consist?

Opinions about what dietary recommendations to the general public should consist of have changed rapidly over the past decade. Ideally, complete dietary recommendations for the public should be formulated to include all of the desiderata listed in Table 2. We shall see later that very few of the recommendations extant today address all of these issues; when they do, the dietary components that are singled out for attention often vary markedly.

The most striking feature of the popular dietary recommendations prior to the 1970s, in contrast to those of today, is that only the first four issues were covered; that is, translating statements of nutrient needs into common food usage, achieving adequate but not escessive

Table 2. Desirable Components in Dietary Recommendations to the Public

---

1. Translate statements of nutrient needs into terms of common food usage.

2. Achieve appropriate but not excessive energy intakes.

3. Assure sufficiency of intakes of micronutrients, protein, and calories to decrease risk of undernutrition and deficiency disease.

4. Specify any special dietary considerations relevant to a certain age or physiologic group.

5. Increase intakes of dietary components which are thought to have positive health promotional effects.

6. Avoid excessive intakes of macro- or micronutrients or other substances which are judged to be imprudent and to increase risks of ill health.

7. Emphasize closely associated health promotion and disease prevention measures which may also be helpful (e.g., exercise) and de-emphasize those which are not (e.g., megadoses of vitamins and minerals, "health" foods, etc.).

8. Urge those with special diseases or risk conditions to seek appropriate and individualized dietary guidance.

---

energy intakes, assuring sufficiency of intakes of micronutrients and protein, and adjusting these as necessary for various ages and physiologic groups. For example, the Basic Four Food Groups covered only these points. It is little wonder, given the fact that four new issue areas are now being addressed in some recommendations that complete consensus is not always apparent among various sets of guidelines.

Most professional nutritionists have little difficulty in reaching agreement on the desirability of including advice that deals with all of the issue areas. The problems revolve around what is to be said with respect to excessive consumption of certain dietary components, the association of diet with chronic degenerative diseases, and other aspects of health beyond consideration of diet in the prevention of deficiency diseases and obesity, and are not concerned with whether the issues need to be dealt with at all.

Once what is to be recommended in each of these issue areas has been determined, it is possible to develop recommendations for

Table 3.   **Groups That Have Published Dietary Recommendations at the National Level from 1970–1980**

Type of Organization	Names of Recommendations
1. Federal government and related agencies	
One executive agency or cabinet-level department	Basic Four (USDA), Five Food Groups (USDA, 1979), Menus for Dietary Guidelines (USDA, 1980), *Healthy People* (HEW, 1979), National Cancer Institute Prudent Interim Principles (1979)
Two or more cabinet-level departments	USDA–HEW Dietary Guidelines (1980)
Legislative committee staff reports	*Dietary Goals for U.S.*, 1st ed. (1977) *Dietary Goals for U.S.*, 2nd ed. (1977)
Food and Nutrition Board	*Toward Healthful Diets* (1980)
2. Professional associations	American Heart Association Recommendations (1973, 1978), American Medical Association Recommendations (1979)
3. Voluntary or private groups	American Council on Science and Health Report (1980), Center for Science and the Public Interest Recommendations (1977), National Dairy Council Food Guide (1977), General Foods Corporation's Guide (1980–81), American Health Foundation (1978)

subgroups within the population and to provide them with more specific information on food choices and to modify these further in line with other considerations, such as food preferences, food availability, and money available for food. As the 1980s opened, a consensus had not been reached, so that age-specific guidelines could not be developed and generally endorsed.

Who Should Make Dietary Recommendations?

During the past decade at least 16 sets of dietary recommendations for the general public have been popularized by various groups in this country. These are listed in Table 3 and discussed in greater depth by McNutt elsewhere (7). Groups within the legislative or executive branches of the federal government or related agencies account for eight of the recommendations, professional associations for three, and private or voluntary groups for five. Surprisingly, only recently has any consistency been apparent in the pronouncements of government agencies. No clear patterns with respect to uniform recommendations are apparent among professional associations and voluntary or private groups, in contrast to those of the federal government.

The fact that all of these groups have generated dietary recommendations reminds us that various alternatives exist for providing dietary guidance. At least three different types of organizations presumably have the expertise to make dietary recommendations since they have done so in the past: professional organizations of scientific experts, the food industry or other privately sponsored groups, and governmental agencies. The strengths and weaknesses of each will now be considered.

One alternative for the making of dietary recommendations is to leave such recommendations up to scientists. Individuals or groups of scientists could issue dietary recommendations and influence food consumption directly through their professional associations or the mass media or by serving as advisors, consultants, or employees of the food industry, other privately sponsored groups, or quasigovernmental agencies which issue such recommendations.

Several professional associations and various private nonprofit groups of scientists have issued dietary recommendations over the past few years. Individual scientists have also made dietary recommendations and communicated them over the mass media directly to consumers. Other scientists have served as consultants or advisors to food companies, trade associations, or other groups and have assisted in developing and endorsing dietary recommendations issued by these bodies. Although the recommendations developed by some of these groups have been helpful, they often contradict each other, and the bodies making them are too narrowly constituted to be regarded as authoritative and to generate widespread support from the wider scientific community, let alone in the larger society.

Nutrition scientists can also make dietary recommendations by serving as consultants, advisors, or employees of government. This alternative will be considered under the government option in the succeeding discussion. However, the special case of the role of scientists as advisors or consultants to quasigovernmental agencies deserves discussion here, since these agencies, while they enjoy a special advisory relationship with government, presumably do not operate under the same constraints and political pressures that governmental agencies are subject to. The major agency of this type that is relevant in discussions of nutrition is the National Academy of Sciences and its various constituent entities, such as the Food and Nutrition Board of the National Research Council, the Institute of Medicine, and special committees which may be developed for specific purposes. Depending on the issue to be dealt with, various committees may be requested by government to study the problem, make recommendations in specific areas, and issue public reports. The federal government is free to accept or reject the advice proffered, but the Academy's stature is such that its reports receive a good deal of publicity and usually receive widespread scientific and public credence.

The most well known of the reports by the National Academy of Sciences dealing with diet are the Recommended Dietary Allowances (6). These were first established during World War II by the Food and Nutrition Board.

In subsequent years the Recommended Dietary Allowances were revised as new scientific information became available. Publications have also been issued by the Food and Nutrition Board and other committees, as well as by the Institute of Medicine of the Academy, which deal with food, diet, or nutritional issues. Two recent examples of interest to the present discussion are *Toward Healthful Diets*, issued by the Committee on Dietary Allowances of the Food and Nutrition Board (5) and *Healthy People: The Surgeon General's Report on Health Promotion and Disease Prevention* (8), which was prepared by the staff of the Institute of Medicine of the Academy and published by the Department of Health and Human Services. The authoritative nature of an Academy report derives not from the fact that it has official status but from the quality of the staff and consultants involved. Therefore, it is important when advisors are selected that acknowledged experts be chosen who represent the entire range of legitimate viewpoints within the scientific community on the questions to be addressed, and that these views be considered in deliberations and processes for review, revision, and comment. If this is not done, the authority of the Academy and the weight accorded its advice by policymakers could fall by the wayside.

A second alternative is to leave the task of making dietary recommendations to those in the food production sector. Such persons could consult with scientists and others who have special expertise in the area, and draw upon their own knowledge of consumer eating habits to do so. In the past few years, dietary recommendations and food guides have been produced by groups such as the National Dairy Council or adopted from the other guides by the General Foods Corporation, and these groups have used this approach. The major difficulties of this approach are that these industry-sponsored modifications or elaborations of recommendations are not viewed as being objective by some observers, and, thus, they lack authority.

The third alternative is for dietary recommendations to be made by government. In the United States, the federal government has traditionally played a role, albeit often a relatively minor one, in informing citizens about nutrition principles, providing authoritative guidance to reduce consumer confusion, and assisting consumers in making decisions about nutrition. If history can be used as a guide, it would seem that this has been viewed as an appropriate role for government. The federal government has been actively involved in research and dissemination of information about food since at least the turn of the century. Dietary guidance on food selection to meet nutrient needs has been provided by the federal government to consumers for well over 50 years (9, 10). For example, the U.S. Department of Agriculture has disseminated guides for good eating, suggested menu plans for those on different food budgets, and provided food growing, preparation, safety, budgeting, and buying information. For several decades it has also provided monies for advertising certain food commodities.

Other government agencies, especially the state and federally supported cooperative extension programs, have produced and disseminated a great deal of informational and educational material about foods and diet (11). The federal government has also promulgated regulations or standards for diets and foods provided in certain settings. Examples include regulations specifying permissible foods, patterns of foods at meals, or minimum nutrient contents of meals served in certain federally sponsored feeding programs; the master menu for the nutrient content of the U.S. armed forces' daily rations; nutritional standards for diets served in federal hospitals; and the like. Scientists and food producers as well as government officials are usually involved in formulating these recommendations. Periods of public comment to obtain the views of consumers, the food industry, and other interested parties are also utilized. Government agencies have also contracted with professional and other groups to develop authoritative statements about issues associated with diet for dissemination to professionals and from them to the public.

There is considerable reluctance on the part of those who believe that federal powers are already far too great to have the government generate dietary recommendations. This is true in spite of the facts that government traditionally has made dietary recommendations, that the data necessary to formulate such recommendations are generated and to a certain extent controlled by the federal government, and that government has access to the expertise to do so. The root cause of the ideological malaise appears to be a deeply seated fear that, if the federal government issues recommendations about diet, it may use its power to influence unduly what its citizens eat by forcing or coercing them to follow the recommendations. Oddly enough, the more fundamental question of whether the many other food-related activities the federal government is presently engaged in constitute even more powerful influences on consumption is rarely raised. We will return to this point later.

Arguments about the power of government are not the only reasons why many Americans appear to be reluctant to have government make dietary recommendations. Some believe that government is not to be trusted to make balanced judgments. Ideally, dietary recommendations would best be made by the government's making good use of those in the professions, the food sector (e.g., producers, marketers, and distributors), and consumers, since all of these parties stand to gain or lose by the decisions that are reached. However, we live in an imperfect world, and, when government makes decisions and recommendations about diet, there is no guarantee that all of these groups will be represented or utilized. Some observers, such as Payne and Thomson (12), claim that government decisionmaking is more heavily influenced by the food production sector than it is by consumers or scientists, because the former groups have more formalized and frequent associations and influence within government than do the latter. They argue that government must make special efforts to include the other stakeholders if it is to develop balanced recommendations.

How Should Dietary Recommendations Be Implemented?

Perhaps the most controversial question of all is how dietary recommendations should be implemented. Presumably, dietary recommendations, if followed, will sometimes involve changes in practices of food consumption, and the issue is how these changes will come about.

Usually is is assumed that when a sufficient number of consumers want to change their food consumption practices, they will influence the food production sector to change the types and amounts of food that are available through the choices they make in the marketplace. However, the free marketplace philosophy may not operate perfectly, for a number of reasons. For example, information may be lacking. Although a good deal of progress has been made in the past few years in the labeling of processed foods for nutrients, a great number of foods remain unlabeled, and even those which are labeled may not provide all the information that is relevant to the consumer who attempts to choose foods in line with dietary recommendations. Those consumers who wish to do so do not have information at the point of purchase. This makes it difficult to express preferences which are based upon nutritional considerations. Payne and Thomson argue that the dietary choices consumers are able to make are also under a considerable number of other constraints (12). Consumers are free to choose, but only among those products which are available. Consumers cannot register preferences for products which are not available in the marketplace. Usually, if market research shows a sufficient demand for a product, it will be produced, but the nature of the food production system still influences the type of product that is most likely to result. Products which involve a high degree of processing, low levels of direct labor input, and a high potential appeal to mass markets tend to be favored because the production, marketing, and distribution system is best suited to producing them. Moreover, consumers may sometimes lack the power to alter the environment within which they make choices. This lack of consumer power vis-à-vis that of other, better organized groups to influence what is available means that consumer "sovereignty" or the opportunity for the consumer to have free choice operates only at a very superficial level.

Other observers believe that additional steps must be taken to implement nutrition recommendations besides a simple reliance on consumer sovereignty, because, although dietary considerations and nutrition may be given some attention, these factors are clearly not dominant in making production decisions. Commercial considerations such as short- and long-term profitability remain the driving objectives. Also, food advertising often influences consumer decisions along lines other than nutritional ones. The purpose of advertising is to stimulate the development of mass markets and of consumer perceptions of product differences as being unique, usually for individual, branded products, thereby increasing the market share and returns to investment that a particular product enjoys. Nutritionally based appeals are subject to government regulations and, in any event, have not been found to be as effective as appeals based on other product attributes. Although there is no inherent reason why advertising and marketing techniques cannot be employed to influence consumers to buy products more in line with dietary recommendations, neither is there necessarily any stimulus for most food producers to undertake such campaigns in the present competitive environment. Incentives must be provided if they are to do so.

Consumers might also influence government through their elected representatives to implement changes in government-sponsored feeding programs and to bring them more into line with dietary recommendations. Since the government buys a great deal of food, changes in what it purchases would be a potent force in the marketplace toward encouraging food producers to alter the types of products which they make available. Some measures of this type, such as making low-calorie options available in some government-sponsored feeding programs, have been attempted, but they have often met with a great deal of criticism. Among the obstacles to doing this are consumer preferences, availability of low-cost acceptable products, and fierce resistance on the part of those who produce foods that do not fit well with such recommendations.

More extensive government involvement in implementing dietary recommendations might be contemplated in some countries. But in the United States and most other Western countries, the notion of the government's dictating or compelling citizens to eat in a certain way is anathema. "Government may inform, remonstrate, reason, persuade or entreat citizens to follow certain dietary habits, but it must not attempt to compel them to do so or punish them if they choose otherwise" (12). These are the limits that clearly must not be exceeded by government action. Within these limits there are a number of steps that the government can take, and has taken over the years, to disseminate dietary guidance. It has played a direct role through programs funded by federal dollars for nutrition education or information activities and health promotion or disease prevention programs which include dietary guidance. It has promulgated regulations which govern the nutrient profiles and, in some cases, the types of foods that will be paid for by federal funds. Such regulations govern programs, such as the Special Supplemental Food Program for Women, Infants, and Children (WIC), school lunches, and meals served to those in the armed services. The effect of these regulations is to alter the possible choices which can be made by the eater. Government has also played an indirect role by serving as a convener or catalyst for stimulating other institutions in society to undertake such activities. Whether government plays a direct or indirect role depends on ideologies concerning the proper role of government and the support for these views in the legislative, executive, and judiciary arms of the government.

Should Government Play a Role in Disseminating Dietary Recommendations?

The legislative and executive branches of government exert powerful influences on all the stakeholders in the areas of food and nutrition. Government is the patron of the nutritional sciences, funding the vast majority of research that is conducted in the food, nutrition, biomedical, and agricultural sciences. Government regulates and influences food production in myriad ways. It also influences what food products and information about food are available to consumers. The government provides food directly or indirectly to many consumers through food distribution programs to the military, to government-operated hospitals, to schoolchildren, and to federally sponsored feeding programs. Finally, and perhaps most importantly, government collects the information on diet and health status of the population which is vital for making dietary recommendations and for assessing the extent to which they are followed. Therefore, it comes as no surprise that food guides and dietary recommendations have long been disseminated by the government (13–17).

DIETARY RECOMMENDATIONS TODAY

Although the Recommended Dietary Allowances serve many important functions for nutrition professionals, they are not simple enough for the average consumer to comprehend easily, nor do they provide guidance for all substances in the diet about which consumers want advice. There is good evidence that many American consumers are confused about their diets as well as about broader questions having to do with nutrition (18). They want objective and authoritative information about these subjects, and some among them want advice and guidance about what to eat. While there is little disagreement among nutrition scientists that the Recommended Dietary Allowances are useful and necessary in developing food guides and dietary guidance for the public, the allowances are not sufficient in themselves to fulfill all of the purposes to which guides must be directed, nor are they geared to individuals. In the past few years, repeated calls have been made for the development of better food guides to translate for the consumer the Recommended Dietary Allowances and other scientific knowledge about diets into information that the consumer can use.

The rationale for such guides is that they will help consumers to develop diets that satisfy the Recommended Dietary Allowances and nutrition guidelines and that they will address current nutrition concerns regarding food components, lifestyle factors, diet, and health (19–22). The need for information and education, in addition to food guides alone, which deal with more general topics involving food safety, nutrition, diet, and health is often mentioned (23, 24).

Table 3 above lists the major recommendations to the American public from U.S. sources over the past decade. Table 4 summarizes the most widely publicized recommendations of governmental and professional associations (3–5, 25–32). Virtually all of them stress appropriate energy intakes, maintenance of desirable body weight or loss of excess body weight, increased intakes of dietary components thought to have positive effects upon health, and the avoidance of those thought to have negative effects. Also usually included are special considerations necessary for certain age or physiologic groups, related health promotion and disease prevention measures, and the need for those with special risks or those who are already ill to seek appropriate medical guidance.

Turning to specific items, further analysis reveals that most of the recommendations agree about certain general principles of diet selection, such as balance, variety, and moderation. Also, desirable directions for altering intakes of dietary constituents are usually similar, although the extent of changes suggested and the nutrients singled out for attention vary.

Table 5 summarizes my views on both the areas of consensus and the major areas of controversy which continue today. Since the recommendations were formulated by different kinds of bodies, it is not possible to regard this summary as a "vote," nor is it necessarily the case that, when scientists agree, the matter upon which they agree is scientifically valid. Note that the issues upon which consensus is evident greatly outnumber those upon which controversy is apparent. In four out of the seven issue areas, no major controversy exists at all. Several of the recommendations neglect to provide guidance to assure sufficiency of micronutrient and protein intakes. Moreover, they differ on the specific dietary components that are singled out for attention for inclusion or avoidance, recommended intake levels for the types of recommendations given for certain age or physiologic groups, related nondietary health promotion and disease prevention measures (when mentioned), and those within the population who are regarded as being in need of individualized medical guidance on diet.

The large number of recent publications that discuss the various dietary recommendations or the data and underlying principles used to formulate them testify to the fact that, if nothing else, a vigorous intellectual debate has been generated (30–59). The controversies are many. They are important since it is highly unlikely that until they are resolved any major public or privately sponsored efforts to provide dietary recommendations to the public will meet with widespread success.

The reasons for the disagreements and controversy are several, and these are highlighted below (47). The first major reason for disagreements about dietary recommendations concerns the type and strength of scientific evidence available on the effectiveness of dietary measures for the prevention of certain chronic degenerative diseases. The strength of evidence on the associations between dietary components and these diseases varies from solid to weak, depending upon the substance and disease of interest. Also, the diseases in question are recognized by all the contending parties as being multifactorial in their etiology, pathogenesis, and in their treatment.

Table 4. Elements Covered in Various Dietary Recommendations for the Public

Source	Elements Included						
	Stress on Adequate but not Excessive Caloric Intakes	Guidance to Assure Sufficiency of Intakes of Micronutrients and Protein	Increase Intakes of Dietary Components Thought to Have Positive Effects	Avoid Excessive Intakes of Dietary Components Thought to Have Negative Effects	Specifies Special Dietary considerations for Certain Ages or Physiologic Groups	Emphasizes Other Related Health Promotion or Disease Prevention Measures	Urges Those with Special Risks or Diseases to Seek Other Medical Guidance
Basic Four of USDA, 1970	Yes	Yes	No	No	Yes	No	No
American Heart Association, 1978	Yes	No	Complex carbohydrates, polyunsaturated fat	Total fat, saturated fat, cholesterol, simple sugars, sodium, alcohol	Yes	Yes	Yes
Dietary Goals, 1st ed., 1977	No	No	Fiber, complex carbohydrates, polyunsaturated fat	Total fat, saturated fat, cholesterol, sodium, simple sugars	No	No	Yes
Dietary Goals, 2nd ed., 1977	Yes	No	Fiber, complex carbohydrates, polyunsaturated fat	Total fat, saturated fat, cholesterol, sodium, simple sugars, alcohol	Yes	Yes	Yes
Healthy People, 1979	Yes	No	Complex carbohydrates	Total fat, saturated fat, cholesterol, sodium, simple sugars	Yes	Yes	Yes
USDA Five Food Groups, 1979	Yes	Yes	Yes	Yes	Yes	Yes	No

Elements Included

Source	Stress on Adequate but not Excessive Caloric Intakes	Guidance to Assure Sufficiency of Micronutrients and Protein	Increase Intakes of Dietary Components Thought to Have Positive Effects	Avoid Excessive Intakes of Dietary Components Thought to Have Negative Effects	Specifies Special Dietary considerations for Certain Ages or Physiologic Groups	Emphasizes Other Related Health Promotion or Disease Prevention Measures	Urges Those with Special Risks or Diseases to Seek Other Medical Guidance
American Medical Association Recommendations, 1979	Yes	Yes	Fiber, complex carbohydrates — Yes	Fat, alcohol, simple sugars and food high in energy but low in protein nutrients — Yes	Yes	Yes	Yes
National Cancer Institute Prudent Interim Principles, 1979	Yes	No	Fiber, complex carbohydrates — Yes	Yes	No	Yes	Yes
USDA-DHEW Dietary Guidelines, 1980	Yes	Yes	Fiber — Yes	Total fat, alcohol — Yes	Yes	Yes	Yes
Food and Nutrition Board, *Toward Healthful Diets,* 1980	Yes	Yes	Fiber, complex carbohydrates — No	Total fat, saturated fat, cholesterol, sodium, simple sugars, alcohol — Yes	Yes	Yes	Yes

Alcohol

Table 5. Areas of Consensus and Controversy in Current Dietary Recommendations to the Public

Issue Area	Consensus	Controversy
General	More research is needed on the role of diet in health promotion and disease prevention	
	Balance, variety, and moderation should guide diet choices	
	"Health," "natural," and organic foods have no unique or special advantages, nor do processed foods have disadvantages for health promotion or disease prevention	
Stress energy intakes which are adequate but not excessive	Maintenance or achievement of desirable weights appropriate to one's physiologic state promotes health	Levels of underweight or overweight that pose health risks and the association of weight levels with other interactive risk factors
	Physical activity is advisable	Benefits of vigorous physical activity with respect to disease prevention
Guidance to assure adequacy of protective nutrient intakes	Intakes of protein, energy, and micronutrients should be adequate	
	Vitamin-mineral supplements are necessary only for specific physiologic states and are not uniformly required	
	Megadose intakes of vitamins or minerals are potentially hazardous	
	Until intakes of basic foods high in essential nutrients are assured, consumption of foods that are high in calories but low in essential nutrients (such as fats, oils, alcohol, and sweets) should be moderate	
Increase intakes of dietary components thought to have positive effects	Complex carbohydrate intake should be increased in the diets of some persons	Benefits of increased intakes of complex carbohydrate for nondiabetics
		Benefits of increased intakes of dietary fiber
Decrease intakes of dietary components thought to have negative effects if consumed in excess	For persons in certain age groups, reductions in intakes of one or more of these nutrients is advisable: total fat, simple sugars, sodium	Benefits, risks, and effectiveness of reductions in total fat, simple sugars, and sodium for all groups in the population and appropriate levels for these if they are desirable
	Alcohol intake is unnecessary, and moderation is essential if it is used	Definition of excessive alcohol intake

Issue Area	Consensus	Controversy
	Reduction in risk factors or prevention of chronic degenerative disease cannot be assured on an individual basis by these measures	Advisability of mass measures involving decreased intakes of fat, saturated fat, cholesterol, sodium, and simple sugars for entire population
		Advisability of reduced intakes of saturated fat and cholesterol and appropriate levels for these
		Risks posed by caffeine, certain additives
Special dietary considerations for certain ages or physiologic groups	During pregnancy, moderation is necessary in alcohol intakes; iron supplements are advisable; weight gain should be monitored and adjusted to recommended levels; and intakes should be of especially high nutrient density, with increased intakes of protein, calories, and most micronutrients	
	Breast feeding is desirable	
	During lactation, maternal intakes should be increased in nutrient density and energy, and the infant may need supplements of vitamin D, iron, and fluoride (Note: similar examples from other age groups can also be cited.)	
Emphasizes related health promotion and disease prevention measures	Moderate physical activity and exercise are helpful in maintaining and achieving appropriate weight levels	
	Measures such as not smoking, weight control, good oral hygiene and temperance in alcohol use may affect risks for certain degenerative diseases	
Urges those with special risks or already ill to seek medical guidance	Those who are known to be at high risk and those who are already ill may require special dietary measures	Who is at high risk, how this should be determined, and whether dietary measures should be undertaken before rather than after a risk assessment

For most of the dietary components which are currently causes of controversy, definitive clinical trials of the efficacy of dietary measures in preventing early onset of these conditions are not available, and the practical difficulties and expense involved in mounting such trials are so great that they are unlikely ever to be done. Given these realities, some scientists argue that other evidence —epidemiologic, animal experiments, and human metabolic studies —must be relied upon. They feel that dietary recommendations should be made, based upon what evidence is available; and when new information becomes available, the recommendations should be changed if warranted. Other scientists insist upon more rigorous standards of proof and counsel silence until such standards of proof have been met, regardless of how long it takes. They argue that knowledge of the field is insufficient to provide practical advice, in ordinary language, to the public on intakes and types of fatty acids (saturated, mono- and polyunsaturated) and carbohydrates (sugar and starch), and on amounts of sodium, cholesterol, dietary fiber, and alcohol which are healthful. Thus, while the abstract proposition that excesses of several nutrients may be associated with disease processes is one with which most nutrition scientists can readily agree, a number of disagreements arise on specifics. These disagreements have made it difficult to formulate dietary recommendations with which all parties can agree. The most controversial issue area involves recommendations to decrease intakes of dietary components thought by some of the expert groups to have negative effects upon health if they are consumed in excess.

The substances upon which dissension with respect to recommendations is sharpest are dietary fat and cholesterol. The guidelines of the Food and Nutrition Board and of the American Medical Association do not recommend moderation in fat consumption for all but suggest reductions from current levels only for those who are sedentary or overweight. They argue that the data are inadequate to justify general dietary recommendations for disease prevention, but that, for those with metabolic problems of lipid and carbohydrate metabolism, a treatment offering some possibility of benefit is justifiable even if its effectiveness cannot be assured. In contrast, other reports suggest overall reductions for most adults on the grounds that such modifications will be of benefit to those who are uniquely susceptible to such disorders and that they will not do harm to others. They argue further that the number of persons at risk of disorders of carbohydrate and lipid metabolism is a significant proportion of the total population and that not all of those who are at risk have been identified. The cholesterol reductions are endorsed by fewer groups, and are generally limited only to those in the population whose plasma lipid profiles indicate that they are at risk.

The desirability of other suggested reductions for most adults and the appropriate decreases to be suggested are also debated. In most cases it is not the desirable direction which is at issue, but the extent of limitation which should be called for, if any.

At the crux of these arguments about dietary components are the associations between them and pathology, and what kinds of mathematical models best fit these relationships. Nutrition scientists have usually assumed that these relationships fit a linear model, but the evidence to buttress this contention is not great. Other hypothetical relationships might also exist: exponential models, asymptotic models, or any of these with different slopes depending upon genetics or some other intervening factor (43). Let us assume that we can identify evidence of pathology in the population which is to be avoided, that we can describe the distribution of intakes for a given dietary constituent, and that we can observe the effects if different models prove to be true. With the asymptotic model, the level of intake above which pathology occurred would be lowest; the linear model would suggest a somewhat higher level of intake; and the exponential model, the highest. The predicted incidence of pathology in the population will depend on the number of people who eat more of the dietary component than is necessary to produce pathology, and these numbers, in turn, will be affected by the model chosen. If the population alters its intake upward or downward, the numbers of persons affected will vary, but the extent to which these changes will affect the incidence of pathology will vary depending upon which model is correct. Obviously, a great deal more work needs to be done on these issues before dietary guidance can reach a firm footing.

The second major area for disagreement about dietary guidelines is to whom dietary recommendations should be directed. Should they be made only to those who are known to be at high risk or to the entire population? It is well known that genetics and other factors unrelated to diet affect individual responses to similar levels of a substance in the diet. Thus, there is every reason to suspect that some people will be more affected by intakes above a certain level in the diet than will others. The practical problem is that we do not always know how to identify these persons in advance. If we could do this with perfect accuracy by identifying characteristics or risk factors which especially predisposed people to disease, we could then concentrate on advising them to change their diets and leave others who had high intakes but lesser chances of developing pathology for later. Theoretically, it would be possible to do this for some disorders associated with diet if everyone could be screened for these characteristics. But this is unlikely to happen. Moreover, none of the risk factors or risk factor constellations are totally predictive on an individual basis, and, for some forms of pathology, we do not even know what these other characteristics that predispose to risk are.

All these difficulties are well known. Attitudes toward what to do vary. Some advocate mass measures to reduce consumption of dietary components associated with pathology. Others prefer a screening approach to find those at high risk and then targeting dietary advice only to them. A combination approach—mass measures to reduce consumption, other measures that people can take on their own to reduce risks, and emphasis on screening with special steps for high risk groups—is urged by others. Still other professionals are convinced that no mass measures directed toward either reducing consumption or screening are necessary and that the whole issue is handled best at the individual doctor-patient level.

The third major reason for disagreement about dietary guidelines is the fear that suggestions about dietary changes will alarm the public, downgrade its faith in the many positive aspects of current American diets, and lend support to the proponents of various unorthodox dietary measures. Most nutrition scientists agree that little merit, indeed, harm from the health standpoint derives from the wholesale adoption of such practices as the use of "health foods," "natural" or "organic" foods, megadoses of vitamin-mineral supplements, or extreme vegan types of vegetarianism, especially when these are used as an alternative to more conventional and effective measures for the prevention or treatment of disease. Some believe that provision of dietary recommendations similar to the Dietary Guidelines performs a positive function in that it helps those in the public who wish to make dietary alterations to focus on changes which are more likely to be of benefit within an overall framework of prevention-oriented, health-related behaviors.

Thus, many professionals think the guidelines play a positive role. They believe that the way to deal with issues such as health foods, natural-organic foods, vegetarianism, and the like is to provide consumers with objective information on the pros and cons of these eating styles, letting consumers make up their own minds. However, other equally sincere authorities say that dietary recommendations should be eschewed by government unless there is virtually 100% unanimity on the effectiveness of the measures, that silence is to be preferred; and even the discussion of pros and cons about various dietary practices may be taken as official endorsement of questionable practices by some consumers in the population, and that it is better simply to condemn these practices.

The fourth reason for disagreement about dietary guidelines concerns the disruption involved in implementing dietary changes and how such changes should be brought about. Proponents of dietary recommendations argue that consumer education can be a more potent force than it is today in changing the foods available and food habits for the better. Opponents argue that authoritative dietary recommendations sponsored by government might lead to coercion or undue governmental regulation, based on misguided or premature conclusions. They favor more individualized advice provided by a physician or another orthodox health counselor for topics which have to do with the associations of dietary components and chronic degenerative diseases. Therefore, proponents and opponents of dietary recommendations not only disagree on whether recommendations should be made and what they should be, but whether the government should make or endorse them.

The final reason for disagreement about dietary guidelines relates to views of when advice or recommendations to the public should be given. Nutrition scientists today are asked to give advice and guidance on issues when often evidence is incomplete or where consensus with respect to interpretation of the data is lacking. Neuberger (44) has emphasized that this problem is not exclusive to nutrition research but that it is one faced by all of the sciences as they attempt to relate to the problems and demands of the larger society. He further points out that although scientists are loath to give advice until full consensus has developed within the scientific community and the evidence upon which their advice is based amounts to virtual certainty, those in other fields, such as economists, have taken a different path. Governments usually rely upon and take the advice of economists who are generally in agreement with their political thinking rather than acting only when consensus involving the entire discipline can be obtained. Most scientists would regard such a state of affairs as undesirable, but it is not entirely inconceivable that, as nutrition becomes increasingly politicized, similar practices may evolve in the arena of nutrition policy.

POLICY IMPLICATIONS

Even those who know better often assume that when the government endorses a series of dietary recommendations, everything will fall into place immediately and food consumption will change. In fact, such a scenario is highly unlikely, and the implications of policy pronouncements on diet by government are difficult to predict for at least three reasons. First, political rhetoric at the policymaking levels and programmatic realities at the operating levels within government are often disparate. Second, high-level policy pronouncements often change rapidly, and only rarely are they the controlling force in actual program implementation. Rather, policy tends to be made from the programmatic level upward. Finally, by the time policy is actually implemented, groups outside of the government have exerted considerable influence upon what will actually be done. Let us examine each of these issues more closely.

Rhetoric and Programmatic Realities

When an official agency of the federal government enunciates a policy, a number of possible effects may be intended since the word policy has many different nuances as it is employed in politics (60). Some policies are no more than political rhetoric; that is, symbolic statements by those in power, which involve little commitment of resources and the administrative apparatus of government toward reaching the stated goal. Others are simply prophetic policies, which are nothing more than statements of intent or aspirations about personnel and resources. Many policy statements made by politicians are of the symbolic or prophetic variety and are, thus, not intended for actual implementation. The final type of policy statements actually constitute forward plans for action and implementation of personnel and resources to achieve the goal through politics and administrative means. These, too, can be tempered or fall by the wayside as they clash with political and administrative realities. Only rarely is it possible for policies enunciated even by those in the highest positions within the federal government to be implemented in precisely the manner in which they were originally envisioned or within the time frames which were originally contemplated.

Fragmentation of Government Policymaking Power

Most of us assume that American government policy is made by a logical process which begins by a leader's enunciating goals, quickly followed by a clear statement of purposes and objectives, which then proceeds as soon as agreements on means as well as ends have been obtained regarding the establishment and ongoing funding of programs which are essential to achieve that policy. In fact, the process is quite different (61, 62).

In actuality, high federal officials in this country have relatively little power to control the specific steps which will be taken in implementing their decisions, although they may be able to determine general directions. This is because the actual centers of power for making decisions are much more complex, fragmented, and interdependent than are those which are outlined in organizational charts or described in civic textbooks. The actualities of federal decisionmaking in the United States have been more realistically described as "cooperative feudalism," in which executive and also legislative and judicial branches of government at the federal, state, and local level as well as private and voluntary sector groups all play a part (63). Most of the important actions and decisions of government involve the "iron triangle" of subgovernments comprising civil servants at the program level, staff of the authorizing and appropriating committees in Congress, and lobbyists for the special interest groups at the federal level. In comparison to these subgovernments, the power at higher levels of the executive branch is relatively weak and fragmented. The end result of these actualities of political power is that policy usually ends up being made less by a rational and comprehensive analysis than by an incrementalist approach, which is more attuned to past experience, the inertia of bureaucratic organizations, politics, and legal realities. This process is sometimes referred to as "muddling through" (63).

Policy Implications of the Dietary Guidelines

Given the actualities of policymaking and implementing in the United States, what are the implications for a government-sponsored set of dietary recommendations such as the USDA-USHHS Dietary Guidelines, or for that matter, any government-sponsored guidance?

We can assume that, since the administration which originally promulgated the Guidelines was voted out of office in 1980, the decision makers in the new administration have a number of options at their disposal with respect to this particular policy. The two extremes would involve outright repudiation or enthusiastic embrace, but neither of these is likely. A more realistic option from the political standpoint is that the Guidelines will be relegated to the realm of a symbolic policy statement, with a minimum commitment of federal resources to their implementation; and that they will be revised so that they are more in line with the recommendations embodied in the report *Toward Healthful Diets* (4). For purposes of discussion, let us examine in a stepwise fashion the likely implications on food consumption of each of these three scenarios.

Outright Repudiation: The Basic Four Reborn. First let us imagine a minimum possible impact scenario in which the executive branch puts implementation of the guidelines on the back burner and the guidelines into the category of symbolic statement only, with no commitments of personnel or other resources for their implementation. At the same time, assume that other policies of deregulation by the federal government were pursued in other spheres, so that price supports and target prices for basic commodities were eliminated. Whenever possible, control over federally sponsored food programs would be returned to the states. Nutrition education and information effects, which were mounted under federal auspices, would emphasize only the Basic Four; that is, achieving recommended levels of the protective nutrients (e.g., protein, vitamins, and minerals) and achieving or maintaining desirable body weight, although governmental bodies at the state and local level or private and voluntary groups might continue to promulgate other messages.

Under such circumstances, it is probably realistic to predict that existing long-term trends in food consumption practices would continue in the same directions as they do today, with the most powerful effects upon consumption over the short term continuing to be income, the overall price of food, and relative prices of foods. These trends can be estimated from per capita food consumption data collected by USDA. They compare quite well to estimates of these same trends predicted in 1969, long before the Dietary Goals or Guidelines were visible on the nutritional horizon (1).

Most observers and analysts predict that food prices will continue to rise over the next few years and that they may remain a problem for the rest of the decade (64, 65), and this factor is likely to be extremely significant in altering food consumption. In 1981, food price rises were expected to be steepest for meats (18%), poultry (18%), eggs (17%), and sugars and sweets (22%). In contrast, fruits and vegetables (8%) are expected to rise at rates lower than the general inflation rate. Other foods, such as fish and seafood (10%), dairy products (11%), nonalcoholic beverages (12%), and other prepared foods (10%) were thought to be closer to predicted inflation rates (64, 65). Consumers can be expected to respond to these price signals and to alter their food consumption somewhat in line with these realities of the marketplace. The outcomes upon consumption might, in fact, be in line with some of the Dietary Guidelines in spite of the de-emphasis upon them. For example, refined sugar consumption may decrease and complex carbohydrate consumption might increase, simply in response to relative prices.

Enthusiastic Embrace: Dietary Guidelines Reborn. Now let us project the scenario for the maximum possible impact of the Guidelines. Assume an executive branch that was dedicated to their implementation by every educational means at its disposal which did not violate the Constitution and the tenets of consumer sovereignty, and a Congress that was supportive of these objectives. Finally, assume that food choice alternatives more in line with the Dietary Guidelines would be offered along with other choices in government meal programs.

In order to predict the probable effects of a federally sponsored consumer information and education campaign coupled with changes in government food assistance and feeding programs, a number of assumptions are crucial (66, 67). First, estimates of the actual changes which are likely to be made are needed. One person may select very different foods from another to achieve a given dietary objective. Second, the speed with which these changes are likely to be made must be estimated. Third, the projected changes in food consumption must be calculated on a national basis. Fourth, these must be converted into estimates of agricultural products necessary to produce these foods. Fifth, adjustments must be made for waste or food that is not eaten. Finally, the estimates of changes in production must be compared with current production and considered, giving due regard to the biological nature of the agricultural production process which cannot be turned on or shut off at will.

Unfortunately, we only have imperfect estimates of the actual changes which consumers are likely to make in their food consumption practices as a result of dietary advice. But, from what we do know about changes in food consumption practices, it is likely that they would be adopted initially only by a small proportion of the total population, and that changes would be gradual rather than sudden. Moreover, intakes of some constituents, such as those of added sugar or salt exclusive of those in foods or of cholesterol which is high in relatively small numbers of foods, would be easier to modify than would intakes involving the type and amount of fat, carbohydrates, or protein, which would involve changes in consumption of many foods. Finally, the major factors influencing food consumption would continue to be availability and price and would be related more to the food preferences of consumers than would nutrition information or education from any source.

Nevertheless, if the Dietary Guidelines were implemented, even given the fact that only slight changes in consumption on a per capita basis would be likely, the economic impact on demand for certain commodities could be considerable. Actual impact upon demand would depend upon the ways in which consumers would chose to reduce or increase their consumption of certain nutrients or constituents in the diet. However, decreases in consumption of certain commodities, such as sugar, eggs, butter, other fats and oils, and, to a lesser extent, meat, might ensue. In contrast, consumption of grain products might increase. Obviously, the trade associations and producers of basic agricultural commodities which might stand to lose and which can only alter their production very gradually could be expected to be opposed to any actions that would encourage the implementation of the Guidelines. Food processors, who have somewhat more latitude to alter the nutrient composition of recipes and formulated foods, might also find these trends troublesome because of the difficulties involved in achieving those nutritional goals from the standpoint of food technology, taste, and acceptability.

Simply for purposes of explication, let us examine the unlikely outcome of the immediate adoption on the part of the entire adult population of food consumption practices that would approximate recommendations in the Dietary Goals (i.e., within a few percent of calories for each of the energy-providing nutrients and close to those suggested for sodium and cholesterol), while also achieving nutrient intakes in line with the Recommended Dietary Allowances. Estimates of this kind were made in one recent study, in which it was assumed that the types of foods available would be similar to those on the market in 1977 (67).

Comparisons to actual (1977) food consumption were used, and it was assumed that approximately 20% of the calories purchased at retail was wasted. It was assumed that the Dietary Goals were met with a slight relaxation of the goals for protein (it was held at 15% of calories instead of 10−14%) and that all of the Recommended Dietary Allowances were met. Consumption would increase for grain products (23%), vegetables (5%), fruits (5%), and potatoes (5%). In contrast, consumption would decrease for sugars and sweeteners (42%), butter (20%), fats and oils (20%), eggs (15%), and meat (3%). That of other food groups would remain unchanged from levels then current. Other patterns of change in food consumption could also be calculated that would involve slightly different changes. Such changes could probably be accepted by many people. In actuality, alterations in consumption would probably be slow, occurring over many years, and would undoubtedly be accepted only by portions of the population, since even with massive educational campaigns food habits change very slowly. Therefore, in this sense, the predictions were based upon unlikely assumptions. Nevertheless, it is easy to see that some producers would stand to gain a great deal and others to lose a great deal if, in fact, such a scenario became an actuality, and that it would be in the interests of those who would be adversely affected to object to government-sponsored campaigns that would seek to implement the Dietary Guidelines and the Recommended Dietary Allowances.

Muddling Through: Toward Healthful Diets? The American political system is such that it encourages a new administration to set aside or at least restate the previous administration's policies, especially if they were controversial. Therefore, continuity in federal policy with respect to the Dietary Guidelines can hardly be expected.

The most likely development in the next few years is that the federal departments will leave the task of developing consensus on dietary recommendations to the National Academy of Sciences or other groups, and will act as a convener rather than as an initiator of actions itself. Over the long term, government recommendations will probably be brought in line with those enunciated by the Food and Nutrition Board. Government is also likely to request that more specific recommendations be developed for groups which, by virtue of their physiologic condition (e.g., pregnancy, lactation, infancy, childhood, adolescence, old age) or risk status, need specific attention. However, federal involvement in implementing such dietary recommendations is likely to be indirect rather than direct. In essence, the general approach is likely to be very little different from the activities in nutrition that are related to health promotion and disease prevention which were laid out in the Forward Plans for Health during the Ford administration, except that they will be implemented 5 years later than originally scheduled.

Given this scenario, whither the Dietary Guidelines, which were endorsed by two cabinet-level departments of the federal government only two years ago? At this juncture, the postures of these two departments appear to have reversed themselves: the enthusiasm of the Department of Health and Human Services has waxed, while that of the Department of Agriculture has waned from that exhibited in the Carter administration.

In July 1981, a committee, consisting of representatives of the Department of Health and Human Services, the Department of Agriculture, and the Food and Nutrition Board, was convened to review dietary recommendations.

The most likely course for the future is that the Dietary Guidelines will become a policy statement enunciated by officials in the Department of Health and Human Services within the broader context of health promotion and disease prevention programs (68). The Guidelines are broad enough and vague enough to permit a great deal of flexibility in their interpretation. Therefore, it is unlikely that they will be specifically repudiated, but neither will they be publicized. Rather, specific guidelines, which are in accordance with the Food and Nutrition Board's publication *Toward Healthful Diets* (5), will probably be given special emphasis. In areas where consensus is high, such as the guidelines on variety in the diet, control of body weight, reduction in sodium levels in the diet, and moderation in the use of alcohol, operational policy statements and follow-through are more likely. For example, voluntary labeling of processed foods for sodium has already been enthusiastically endorsed by the Food and Drug Administration, so broader labeling initiatives may also be initiated.

The future paths to be taken by the U.S. Department of Agriculture are not so clear. The enthusiasm exhibited by top policymakers toward the Dietary Guidelines during the Carter administration is gone (43), and early policy pronouncements from officials in the Reagan administration emphasize concerns about agricultural productivity, food scarcity, and inflation. Some high officials in the Department of Agriculture repudiated the Dietary Guidelines, then repudiated their repudiation, and now have reiterated their original negativism toward them. If nothing else, this signifies a certain lack of unanimity between the major cabinet-level departments with respect to a posture on the Guidelines.

The balance which is finally struck will probably see the USDA returning to its food production emphasis of earlier decades and being content to overlook whatever leads emerge from other branches of government on the health aspects of diet. Nutrition information for the general public will probably be downplayed, and that which is produced will emphasize information about the nutrient content of foods, wise buying, dietary adequacy, and the making of informed choices when buying food, such choices taking into account nutrition, health, and economic value. State initiatives may receive increased emphasis for dealing with dietary questions. Steps taken in the nutrition area are likely to be along the lines of those specified in recent publications from the Department, which are in line with state initiatives (69).

Within the Department of Agriculture, it currently appears likely that constriction, rather than broadening, of the agency's mission in the areas of nutrition, food assistance, feeding programs, and consumer affairs will occur. In the long run, however, the Department cannot afford to ignore new nonagricultural voices representing urban and other interests, even if they challenge the comfortable policy triangle that once existed between representatives of agricultural districts in Congress, the USDA, and agricultural interest groups (69). Too narrow an interpretation of its role may jeopardize political support for the

Department among urban constituencies and, secondarily, threaten older, more entrenched programs (69).

Larger Nutrition Policy Issues

In a larger sense, the battles over what the government's role should be vis-à-vis choice and dissemination of dietary recommendations is a tempest in a teapot. The role of government with respect to the much more pervasive influences on supply and demand for food that it already exerts is the more important issue.

Even a passing familiarity with American food policies over the past 50 years indicates that, in fact, government policies have exerted, and continue to exert, very powerful influences over what we eat. Government policies such as subsidies and price supports to regulate farm food output and food prices have influenced consumer behavior in the marketplace for over 50 years. Commodities that are the favored recipients of government benevolence in the form of subsidies to farmers or certain groups of consumers have advantages of availability and price that can heavily influence consumer choice. Federal regulations assure that minimum food safety standards are maintained. The vast bulk of monies spent by the government for consumer-related food and nutrition purposes goes to various social welfare or public assistance programs which provide food or money for food to certain consumers. These food and feeding programs influence the proportion of income that is spent on food as well as, in some instances, the types of foods or meals which are eaten. But the mechanisms by which these government policies have wielded these influences were by modifying factors such as supply and demand, rather than by attempts to alter consumer tastes and preferences for food directly by making dietary recommendations. That is, the vast bulk of federal expenditures that influence what we eat are not devoted to promulgating and publicizing dietary recommendations but rather to controlling the supply and demand for food by other, far more potent means.

Thus, a more salient question than whether the government should issue or disseminate dietary recommendations is whether the federal government should exert these *other* influences over the food supply. The current administration appears to be committed to a more laissez-faire approach than has existed over the past decade, but it remains to be seen what constraints will be imposed on these plans by the political process (70–72). The most likely outcome is probably a gradual shift in the direction of less direct government intervention in the food production sphere and of less stringent regulation. However, even inaction constitutes an influence, and, therefore, the government will still exert a considerable role even if it takes this course. Willy-nilly then, the federal government does and will continue to influence what consumers eat. The question is how this should be done. The form this involvement has taken over the years has varied, and it is likely to continue to do so in the future. The great challenge to nutrition policymakers is to assure that powerful claims on the public purse be made from the standpoint of merit rather than by that of powerful clients representing powerful interests. It remains to be seen how the executive and legislative branches of government rise to this important challenge.

CONCLUSIONS

Science can never take the place of political responsibility, executive leadership, and politics in making public policy that involves nutrition. But politicians and administrators can make better public policy by making more adequate use of the expertise of scientists (62). The difficulties lie partly in the organizational structure and processes of government as opposed to those of scientific institutions and, in part, in the characteristics of the personnel in each of these systems.

Consider the difficulties posed by institutional structures. Theoretically, government operates in a hierarchical fashion, with those at the top of the pyramid making very broad decisions on very general goals and with those at the bottom implementing them. The actualities are, in fact, very different from this, with decision-making power actually being much more decentralized and fragmented, as has already been discussed. But the fact remains that even at the lowest level of government, the administrator must deal with and control problems that cannot be reduced to precise and objective terms. These controlling decisions involve values and probabilities rather than absolutes. Decisions about whether or when things should be done and how much effort or money is to be spent on them constitute the main business of the administrator. Only at the lowest reaches of the government pyramid are the problems narrow enough to require the highly specialized training of scientists and the highly specialized structure of the sciences.

We must also consider the shortcomings of scientists in dealing with public policy issues. Price sees their limitations to include the following (62):

1. Competence. Most government decisions involve value judgments and entail very complex problems of a human and social nature. Scientists are not trained for (nor do they necessarily enjoy) working on issues that cannot be reduced to precise, objective terms. Some tend to shy away from the totalities of the problems

that must be dealt with by administrators on a daily basis. Others venture into areas outside their expertise and think that their approach is scientific and undiluted by personal bias when, in fact, it is not.

2. Ignorance of policy. Scientists often fail to recognize when they have gone beyond the bounds of what is provable by research, and speak *ex cathedra* on matters upon which their judgments are as personal and biased as those of a layman.

3. Tunnel vision. Scientists often regard their particular specialty as being the most important aspect of the total problem, ignoring the broader considerations of policy involved. Some of the more misguided believe that their tools and methods, which only give them a partial glimpse of the real nature of these complex problems, permit them, and them alone, to arrive at "truth."

4. Double dipping. Scientists serving as advisors may work at the same time for private industry, educational institutions, and the government in situations where conflicts of interest may arise, and they may fail to recognize this situation.

5. Institutional interest. Currently the scientific enterprise in universities is so heavily supported by federal funding that the views of scientists from these institutions on scientific programs may not be objective. This very problem led Seidman to observe that "grave risks are run when public power is exercised by agricultural, scientific and educational elites who are more concerned with advancing their own interests and the interests of the institutions they represent than the public interest. Serious distortions and inequities may occur in the allocation of funds among those eligible for assistance. Vested interests are created which are resistant to change and reordering of priorities to meet new national needs" (61).

6. Abuse of confidentiality. Some scientists want both the confidential ear of responsible officials and the right to tell the academic world all about the relationship.

7. Timing. Scientists often cannot deal with the time frames within which public policy decisions must be made. They fail to recognize that some questions call for immediate answers, and that delay itself is an answer of the worst kind. Since each question or problem which is answered by formal research leads to another question, the possibilities for infinite regression and study are always present, and scientists sometimes seem to be unaware of the fact that this is often politically unacceptable.

8. Distrust of politicians and administrators. Some scientists distrust those they must advise in the public policy arena, or they insist

that actions should be taken not only after their advice has been given, but preferably only in accord with their advice.

9. Failure to understand the political aspects and implications of research. Most scientists do not regard issues such as who frames research questions, funding of one study over another, or the like as involving politics, although they frequently do. Indeed, the major point of control which generalists have over the scientific enterprise is the control of the nature of the scientific planning and advisory system and the selection of its top personnel. Scientists also fail to understand that, in any society, the implications of scientific findings may be politically volatile and occasionally unacceptable. These issues can create friction with administrators, who are very much aware of these problems.

What can nutrition scientists learn from the successes and failures of the 1970s to strengthen nutrition policies in the 1980s? Three lessons are crucial. First, they must capitalize on the characteristics of issues which have been successfully resolved in the past and avoid the hallmarks of those which have generated controversy. Second, they must critically examine their role as advisors to the government and overcome their shortcomings in this role. Finally, and most important, they must continue to study those aspects of the still-unresolved problems that may yield to the scientific method and, thereby, provide decisionmakers with some of the information that they must have to make wise decisions.

REFERENCES

1. *White House Conference on Food, Nutrition and Health. Final Report.* Government Printing Office, Washington, D.C. , 1970.
2. K. Schlossberg, Government policy in the United States. In B. Winikoff, ed., *Nutrition and National Policy,* MIT Press, Cambridge, Mass., 1978, pp. 325–360.
3. U.S. Congress, Senate, Select Committee on Nutrition and Human Needs. *Dietary Goals for the United States,* 2nd ed., Government Printing Office, Washington, D.C., 1977.
4. U.S. Department of Agriculture and U.S. Department of Health, Education and Welfare. *Nutrition and Your Health: Dietary Guidelines for Americans,* U.S. Government Printing Office, Washington, D.C., 1980.
5. Food and Nutrition Board, National Research Council. *Toward*

Healthful Diets, National Academy of Sciences, Washington, D.C., 1980.

6. Committee on Dietary Allowances, Food and Nutrition Board, National Research Council. *Recommended Dietary Allowances*, 9th ed., National Academy of Sciences, Washington, D.C., 1980.

7. K. McNutt, Dietary advice to the public. *Nutr. Rev.* **19**, 570 (1980).

8. U.S. Department of Health, Education and Welfare. *Healthy People: The Surgeon General's Report on Health Promotion and Disease Prevention*, U.S. Government Printing Office, Washington, D.C., 1979.

9. J. T. Dwyer, Consumer needs for the translation of the recommended dietary allowances in human nutrition. In G. R. Beecher, ed., Beltsville Symposia in Agricultural Research [4]: Human Nutrition Research, pp. 237–252. Allanheld, Osmun, Granada, 1981.

10. L. Light and F. J. Cronin, Food guidance revisited. *J. Nutr. Ed.* **13**, 57 (1981).

11. J. T. Dwyer, *Nutrition Education and Information: Better Health for Our Children*, Report of the Select Panel for the Promotion of Child Health to the U.S. Congress and the Secretary of Health and Human Services, Vol. 4, Background papers, Publication no. 79–55071. U.S. Department of Health and Human Services, Public Health Service, Washington, D.C., Office of the Assistant Secretary for Health and Surgeon General DHHS (PHS); 1981.

12. P. Payne and A. Thomson, Food health: Individual choice and collective responsibility. *R. Soc. Health J.* **99**, 185 (1979).

13. U.S. Department of Agriculture, War Food Administration. *National Wartime Nutrition Guide*, Pamphlet no. NFC 4, U.S. Department of Agriculture, Washington, D.C., 1943.

14. L. Page and E. Phipard, *Essentials of an Adequate Diet: Facts for Nutrition Programs*, Home economics research report no. 33, U.S. Department of Agriculture, Washington, D.C., 1957.

15. Agricultural Research Service. *Food for Fitness: A Daily Food Guide*, U.S. Department of Agriculture leaflet no. 424, Consumer and Food Economics Research Service, U.S. Department of Agriculture, Washington, D.C., 1958.

16. M. M. Hill and L. E. Cleveland, Food guides: their development and use. *Nutrition Program News, July–October.* U.S. Department of Agriculture, Washington, D.C., 1970.

17. A. A. Hertzler and H. L. Anderson, Food guides in the U.S. *J. Am. Diet. Assoc.* **64**, 19 (1974).

18. Comptroller General of the United States. *What Foods Should Americans Eat: Better Information Needed on the Nutritional Quality of Foods,* CED 80–68, U.S. General Accounting Office, Washington, D.C., 1980.
19. E. B. Staats, *Recommended Dietary Allowances: More Research and Better Food Guides Needed,* CED 78–169, U.S. General Accounting Office, Washington, D.C., 1978.
20. H. Eschwege, *Recommended Dietary Allowances,* U.S. General Accounting Office, Community and Economic Development Division, Washington, D.C., 1978.
21. U.S. General Accounting Office. *National Nutrition Issues,* CED 78–7, U.S. General Accounting Office, Washington, D.C., 1977, pp. 26–36.
22. *A Summary Report on U.S. Consumers' Knowledge, Attitudes, and Practices about Nutrition, 1980,* General Mills, Minneapolis, 1980.
23. U.S. General Accounting Office. *Food, Agriculture and Nutrition Issues for Planning,* Staff study, CED–80–94, U.S. General Accounting Office, Washington, D.C., 1979, 1980, pp. 18–25.
24. E. B. Staats, *Informing the Public about Nutrition: Federal Agencies Should Do Better,* CED 78–75, U.S. General Accounting Office, Washington, D.C., 1978.
25. American Heart Association, Committee on Nutrition. Diet and coronary heart disease. *Circulation* **58**, 762A (1978).
26. U.S. Congress, Senate, Select Committee on Nutrition and Human Needs. *Dietary Goals for the United States,* 1st ed., U.S. Government Printing Office, Washington, D.C., 1977.
27. U.S. Department of Agriculture, Science and Education Administration. *Food,* Home and Garden bulletin no. 228, U.S. Department of Agriculture, Washington, D.C., 1979.
28. American Medical Association, Council on Scientific Affairs. American Medical Association concepts of nutrition and health. *J. Am. Med. Assoc.* **242**, 2335 (1979).
29. A. C. Upton, Statement on diet, nutrition and cancer. Hearings of the Subcommittee on Nutrition, Committee on Agriculture, Nutrition and Forestry, U.S. Congress, Washington, D.C., 1979.
30. E. H. Ahrens and W. E. Connors, cochairmen. Symposium report of the task force on the evidence relating six dietary factors to the nation's health. *Am. J. Clin. Nutr.* **32**, 2621 (1979).
31. R. Whitehead, Dietary goals: past and present. *R. Soc. Health J.* **101**, 58 (1981).
32. M. C. Latham and L. S. Stephenson, U.S. Dietary Goals. *J. Nutr. Ed.* **9**, 152 (1977).

33. U.S. Congress, Senate, Select Committee on Nutrition and Human Needs. *Dietary Goals for the United States: Supplementary Views*, U.S. Government Printing Office, Washington, D.C., 1977.
34. A. E. Harper, Nutritional regulations and legislation: past developments, future implications. *J. Am. Diet. Assoc.* **71**, 601 (1977).
35. B. Winikoff, Nutrition and food policy: The approaches of Norway and the United States. *Am. J. Public Health* **67**, 552 (1977).
36. D. M. Hegsted, Priorities in nutrition in the United States. *J. Am. Diet. Assoc.* **71**, 9 (1977).
37. G. A. Leveille, Recommendations for rational changes in the U.S. diet. *Food Technol.* **32**, 75 (1978).
38. C. T. Foreman, Address to the Food and Nutrition Board. *Nutr. Today*, May–June, pp. 18–21 (1978).
39. D. M. Hegsted, Rationale for change in the American diet. *Food Technol.* **32**, 44 (1978).
40. A. E. Harper, Dietary Goals: A skeptical view. *Am. J. Clin. Nutr.* **31**, 310 (1978).
41. P. R. Lee, Nutrition policy—from neglect and uncertainty to debate and action. *J. Am. Diet. Assoc.* **72**, 581 (1978).
42. R. E. Olson, Are professionals jumping the gun in the fight against chronic diseases? *J. Am. Diet. Assoc.* **74**, 543 (1979).
43. R. G. Whitehead, Dietary Goals: their scientific justification. *R. Soc. Health J.* **99**, 181 (1979).
44. A. Neuberger, General considerations on the future of nutrition and its social aspects. *Proc. Nutr. Soc.* **38**, 233 (1979).
45. A. Simopoulos, The scientific basis of the Goals: what can be done now? *J. Am. Diet. Assoc.* **74**, 539 (1979).
46. W. J. Broad, Jump in funding feeds nutrition. *Science* **204**, 1060 (1979).
47. W. E. Connor, Too little or too much: the case for preventive nutrition. *Am. J. Clin. Nutr.* **32**, 1975 (1979).
48. W. E. Connor, Diet, nutrition, disease and the dietary goals. *Health United States, 1979*, DHEW publication no. (PHS) 80–1232, U.S. Department of Health, Education and Welfare, Washington, D.C., 1979.
49. W. H. Stewart, The use of government to protect and promote the health of the public through nutrition. *Fed. Proc.* **38**, 2557 (1979).
50. H. Orlans, On knowledge, policy, practice and fate. *Fed. Proc.* **38**, 2553 (1979).
51. J. P. Habicht, Translation of scientific and nutrition findings to social policy. *Fed. Proc.* **38**, 2551 (1979).

52 P. White, Nutrition in the 1970's. *J. Am. Med. Assoc.* **243**, 2220 (1980).

53. D. S. Greenberg, A long wait for a little advice. *Nutr. Today*, March–April, pp. 20–21 (1980).

54. D. S. Greenberg, Nutrition. *Health United States, 1980 with Prevention Profile*, DHHS publication no. (PHS) 81–1232, U.S. Department of Health and Human Services, Hyattsville, Maryland, 1980.

55. E. M. Whelan and K. A. Meister, The pitfalls of shortcut science. *ACSH News and Views* **2** (2), 1 (1981).

56. P. Hausmann, *Jack Sprat's Legacy: The Science and Politics of Fat and Cholesterol*, Richard Marek Publishers, New York, 1981.

57. V. Herbert, Epidemiology, diet and killer diseases. *Am. J. Clin. Nutr.* **34**, 592 (1981).

58. A. E. Harper, Dietary guidelines for Americans. *Am. J. Clin. Nutr.* **34**, 121 (1981).

59. J. Thomas, The place of education in a national nutrition policy. *R. Soc. Health J.* **99**, 189 (1979).

60. D. A. Strickland, L. L. Wade, and R. E. Johnston, *A Primer on Political Analysis*, Markham Publishing, Chicago, 1968, p. 65.

61. H. Seidman, *Politics, Position, and Power: The Dynamics of Federal Organization*, Oxford University Press, New York, 1970, pp. 136–139.

62. D. K. Price, *Government and Science: Their Dynamic Relation in American Democracy*, Oxford University Press, New York, 1972.

63. C. E. Lindblom, The science of muddling through. *Pub. Admin. Rev.* **19**, 79 (1959).

64. P. C. Westcott, ed., 1981 Food price outlook. *Agricultural Outlook 1981*, U.S. Congress, Senate, Committee on Agriculture, Nutrition and Forestry, Washington, D.C., 1981, p. 21.

65. T. E. Young, Outlook for food prices. *Agricultural Outlook 1981*, U.S. Congress, Senate, Committee on Agriculture, Nutrition and Forestry, Washington, D.C., 1981, p. 30.

66. J. L. Jones and I. J. Abrams, Relating diet-health concerns to food choices. *Natl. Food Rev.* (Fall), p. 26 (1979).

67. C. LeBovit and W. T. Bochin, Changes to meet dietary goals. *Natl. Food Rev.* (Fall), p. 24 (1979).

68. U.S. Department of Health and Human Services. Prevention profile. *Health United States, 1980*. U.S. Government Printing Office, Washington, D.C., 1981, pp. 265–319.

69. D. E. Bowers, The setting for new food and agricultural legislation. *Agricultural—Food Policy Review Prescriptions for the 1980's*, No.

AFPR–4, U.S. Department of Agriculture, Economics and Statistics Service, Washington, D.C., 1981.
70. E. J. McAllister, ed., *Agenda for Progress: Examining Federal Spending*, The Heritage Foundation, Washington, D.C., 1980.
71. C. L. Heatherly, *Mandate for Leadership: Policy Management in a Conservative Administration*, The Heritage Foundation, Washington, D.C., 1980.
72. Executive Office of the President, Office of Management and Budget. *Fiscal Year 1982 Budget Revisions: Additional Details on Budget Savings*, U.S. Government Printing Office, Washington, D.C., 1982.

ADDITIONAL RECENT REFERENCES

Committee on Diet, Nutrition, and Cancer, National Academy of Sciences. *Diet, Nutrition, and Cancer*, National Academy Press, Washington, D.C., 1982.

A. Wretlind, Standards for nutritional adequacy of the diet: European and WHO/FAO viewpoints. *Am. J. Clin. Nutr.* **36**, 366 (1982).

Anon., Nutrition and the food industry: Ninth Annual Marabou Symposium. *Nutr. Rev.* **40**, 1 (1982).

U. S. General Accounting Office. *Food in the Future: Proceedings of a Planning Symposium*, U.S. General Accounting Office, Washington, D.C., 1981.

U. S. General Accounting Office. *Food, Agriculture and Nutrition Issues for Planning*, U.S. General Accounting Office, Washington, D.C., 1982.

U. S. General Accounting Office. *Informing the Public About Food—A Strategy Is Needed for Improving Communication*, U.S. General Accounting Office, Washington, D.C., 1982.

16
Food Advertising

KATHERINE L. CLANCY, Ph.D.
Syracuse University

DEBORAH L. HELITZER
Network for Better Nutrition
Washington, D.C.

Address correspondence to Katherine L. Clancy, Ph.D., Associate Professor, Department of Human Nutrition, Syracuse University, Syracuse, New York 13210.

ABSTRACT

As nutritionists have explored the factors that affect people's food choices, food advertising has assumed a prominent role. Nutrition educators and many others who have examined food advertising have wondered what its impact might be on the dietary habits of the public. They have attempted to secure access to the media in which advertising appears, for the purpose of providing food and nutrition information to the public.

Very little research has been conducted on the subject of food advertising, its intricacies and effects. In this chapter, we discuss both the research that has been reported and a wide range of public documents. We first give a descriptive and historical overview of food advertising in the United States. We then discuss the effects of food advertisements; the way in which advertising is regulated; the unique area of children's advertising; the questions about nutrition information and its place in food advertising; and end with a discussion of various proposals by which the mass media might be utilized for dissemination of information about food and nutrition.

WHAT IS ADVERTISING?[1]

According to the dictionary, advertising is the "action of calling to the attention of the public—especially by means of printed or broadcast announcements" (1), and "the art of announcing or offering for sale in such a manner as to induce purchase" (2). It has also been called "the lifeblood of the press," the virtual total support of commercial television programming (3), and a major economic tool of American industry (4).

Advertising is actually only one component of a number of different marketing techniques used by food product manufacturers to promote their products (some of the others are packaging, pricing, promotions, and coupons) (5). But ads are among the most visible of the marketing

---

[1]Much of the information in this section is based on material in Howard and Hulbert (3), pp. 7—45.

mix and have been the subject of a great deal of attention in the last 10 to 15 years.

Since much of what a food marketer has to sell consists of new products [50% of most companies' sales come from products introduced in the last 10 years (3)] and since advertising is essential to new product success, in many instances new food product development goes hand-in-hand with development of an advertising strategy. The two basic components of advertising are the creative production of the ad and the media selected to disseminate it. Ads are developed by advertising agencies or in-house advertising departments. Media are chosen on the basis of their ability to reach intended target groups, now often "segmented" through the use of complicated surveys that measure different social and psychological characteristics of the total audience. Media also have price differentials. In general, only widely consumed products with large profit margins can afford ongoing multimedia advertising expenditures (5, 6).

The major objective of advertising by a food company is growth, with profit as a secondary but necessary corollary. The working goal is to increase the share of a brand within its own market (6). Through advertising, manufacturers wish to (1) create awareness of and interest in the company's products, and (2) increase sales. Advertisements are crafted initially to attract the consumer's attention and then to transmit information about the product (a discussion on information can be found later in this chapter). Many persons in the advertising business believe that ads operate by associating in the consumer's mind his/her various needs with the advertiser's brand name. Others have argued that ads "create" needs by playing on consumers' emotions. It is accepted by all that ads appeal to consumers' attitudes and self-concepts in order to induce purchase decisions (3, 7).

There are various theories of how advertising works. These arise out of behavioral theory and psychology and posit that several things must occur if an ad is to have its intended effect. First, the attention of the audience must be directed to the key message in the ad. Then the viewer or reader must link the concepts of the ad to his/her personal cognitive structure. Depending on whether the creators of the ad are behaviorists or cognitivists, they will either (1) repeat the message to bring out a conditioned response or (2) rely on the viewers or readers to make the connections in their own minds. If the ad is successful, the consumer at some point will make a conscious or unconscious decision to buy the product (3, 8).

HISTORICAL PERSPECTIVE[2]

Although one could probably trace food advertising back to the invention of the printing press, or before, a useful perspective on the changes in food advertising is provided by following the advertising trends since just before the turn of the twentieth century.

Most of the food advertising before that time was of a local retail nature. The first food advertisers of national proportion were mass producers of low-priced, semiperishable, packaged products, and processors of perishable products for national markets, including flour (Pillsbury), breakfast cereals (Quaker), and canned goods (Heinz; Campbell; Libby, McNeil, and Libby). By the 1920s, advertising by large firms producing fluid milk, ice cream, cheese, and dry grocery products was common; and, by 1930, there were large firms in nearly every food line that engaged in national advertising (9).

During the years of the Depression and Second World War, advertising budgets decreased sharply, but they rose again quickly in the late 1940s. By the early 1950s, there were 50 large food companies who were million dollar advertisers. National advertising accounted for 51% of all food advertising in 1935 and 55% in the 1970s. Of this, 77% was for specific brand promotion. In 1948, food advertising expenditures were $428,000,000; by 1975, they had reached $3,092,000,000 (9).

Although the earliest general advertising medium was newspapers, magazines were used increasingly for promotional purposes from the Civil War through the 1890s. By 1898, there were 152 different food and drink advertisers regularly using periodicals. Other media used were handbills, signs, car-cards in streetcars, and posters. In the 1920s, national brands dominated advertising space. By the 1940s, newspaper retail ads (including copy on quality, service, price, and dependability) had garnered a much greater share of advertising expenditures (10). In 1927, food advertising accounted for approximately 17% of national advertising in newspapers, magazines, radio stations, and outdoor advertising (11) and, by 1975, this figure had risen to 21%. In summary, by 1975, 16% of all food advertising (including retail ads) was placed in magazines and newspaper supplements; 44% on television; 15% on radio; and 22% in other media (12).

---

[2]Much of the information in this section is based on material in Manchester (9).

Table 1.   Six Media Advertising Expenditures, 1978

Food Items	Advertising Expenditures (million $)	Total Six Media Advertising (%)
Breakfast cereals	186	8.8
Flour mix products	57	2.7
Ice cream, candy, desserts	277	13.0
Oils and salad dressing	152	7.2
Soups, baby foods, and prepared foods	176	8.3
Soft drinks	284	13.3
Seasonings and spices	63	3.0
Cookies, crackers, chips, and other snacks	92	4.3
Coffee	136	6.4
Sugar, syrup, jellies	17	0.8
Bread and rolls	72	3.4
Rice and pasta	17	0.7
Canned and processed meats, poultry, fish	93	4.4
Restaurants	363	17.1
Milk, butter, cheese	75	3.5
Fruits and vegetables	66	3.1
Unprocessed meat, poultry, fish and eggs	1	0.1
Total	2127	100.0

SOURCE: Leading National Advertisers.

A. Gallo, J. Connor, and W. Boehm, Mass media food advertising. *Natl. Food Rev.* (Winter) (1980).

WHAT IS ADVERTISED?

It has been stated that the advertising expenditures of the food and beverage industry have had a collective impact on the public's attitude toward food, nutrition, and dietary practices (13, 14). Table 1 lists the advertising expenditures and percentage of six media advertising for 17 food product categories, including restaurants, for 1978 (12).

As shown in the table, soft drinks, ice cream, candy, and desserts together account for more than 25% of all expenditures. Highly processed foods account for a large part of total media advertising, approximately 56%. Perishables or relatively unprocessed foods take a very small portion of advertising dollars. The categories with the lowest expenditures include unprocessed meats, poultry, fresh eggs, dairy products, fruits, and vegetables. Combined advertising expenditures in 1978 for these products were $140 million, or one-half of what was spent on soft drinks alone, accounting for 8% of total food advertising. It should be noted that restaurant expenditures listed are primarily those of fast food establishments.

A 1977 study that compared the content of food commercials to the then newly published Dietary Goals (15) showed that 25% of total food advertising time was devoted to foods in the basic four food groups; 75% was for nonnutritive beverages, wine, beer, baked goods, oil, fat, margarine, snack foods, sweets, and sugar substitutes (16). More recently, the author of a study of the content of both commercials and programming surmised that the television "diet" was weighted heavily toward consumption of nonnutritious foods (17).

WHAT ARE THE EFFECTS OF FOOD ADVERTISEMENTS?

Ten years ago, Gifft, Washbon, and Harrison stated that the degree of impact that food advertising had had on food consumption and buying practices could only be estimated (18). That statement is still true and the following points, among others, help to explain why.

1. There is no single, defined, tested structure of advertising research that provides a model for replicable studies (3, 8). Many advertisers function in an intuitive way, and useful concepts are reinvented in different agencies rather than being codified.

2. Although advertisers do undertake many different kinds of research—for example, on the psychosocial characteristics of their target groups, product sales, or reactions to products by consumers (3, 8)—little research is conducted on how advertisements themselves actually affect the response of the consumer. Research that reveals how an ad works is expensive, not well-defined, and may not be as valuable as research that answers the question "Does the ad work?"

3. Research done by manufacturers to test the efficacy of advertising campaigns is proprietary information and is not available outside of the individual companies.

4. Academic researchers are interested in generalized theories of how advertising works, rather than in the effects of specific isolated ad campaigns. There has been very little money available from government or private sources to finance this research.

In spite of these drawbacks, the following types of empirical evidence can be used to examine the effectiveness of food advertising:

1. Advertising has been shown in various studies to aid in the introduction of new products and to help shift market shares among brands (19, 20). At this time, it would appear to be quite difficult to introduce a new product successfully without advertising support.

2. Research conducted by or for government agencies on nonbranded food products has shown that demand is affected by advertising. The United States Department of Agriculture (USDA), which oversees the marketing orders for agricultural products, has completed studies of milk, butter and cheese, lamb, and orange juice sales, which show that sales increase when these foods are advertised (21−24).

3. A number of studies have shown that advertising has an impact on the food choices of children (25−28). Although the findings from these studies are not directly applicable to adults, there are no logical reasons not to believe that effects are comparable.

4. In an elegant, controlled study reported recently, data were presented that suggested that, under some conditions, television food commercials stimulate greater eating behavior in obese subjects than in normal-weight subjects (29).

5. As pointed out earlier, over two billion dollars was spent in 1978 to advertise food products (12). Companies could not afford to spend that amount of money unless they knew that the expenditure could be justified by an increase in sales.

HOW IS ADVERTISING REGULATED?

Truthful food advertising provides people with the information they need to understand nutrition, and better nutrition unquestionably will benefit our people immensely. On the other hand, incorrect or fraudulent advertising works immeasurable harm (30).

In the United States today, the government is not permitted to suppress speech except in limited instances not applicable to this discussion. The freedom the advertiser possesses, combined with the convincing quality of advertising, has created the need for regulation. The Supreme Court has ruled in Virginia State Board of Pharmacy v. Virginia Citizens Consumer Council, Inc., that under the First Amendment, commercial speech, while performing an indispensable role in the allocation of resources in a free enterprise system, can be regulated if it is deceptive, but otherwise should be protected from unwarranted or unjustified regulation (31). Therefore, the burden of proof of deception lies upon the regulatory institutions (government or industry) that attempt to limit commercial speech. Those regulatory activities are discussed below.

Government Regulation

In 1914, pursuant to the Clayton Anti-Trust Act (32) and the Federal Trade Commission Act of 1914 (33), the Federal Trade Commission (FTC) was organized as an independent regulatory agency, its original mission being to protect businessmen from dishonest competitors. In 1938, the Wheeler—Lea Act (34) amended the original statute to include the protection of consumers, specifying that unfair or deceptive acts and practices were illegal and giving the Commission new enforcement powers to deal with violations. It specifically gave the FTC control of food advertising, removing this control from the Food and Drug Administration (FDA) and USDA, whose jurisdiction remains over most other regulations concerning food, drugs, and cosmetics (35).

Congress conceived of the FTC primarily as a law-enforcement agency rather than as a mere information-gathering or advice-giving agency. Further, Congress over the last 40 years has increasingly emphasized protection of consumer interests when prescribing the Commission's duties (35). Among other things, the Commission can restrict dissemination of false, misleading, deceptive, or unfair advertisements of food whenever it finds that such restriction would be in the public interest. In addition, the Commission has the authority to prosecute the disseminators of "false advertisements" (as defined in Section 15 of the FTC Act) (33) of food, where the use of the commodity advertised may be injurious to health or where there is intent to defraud or mislead (36).

The Magnuson-Moss Warranty-Federal Trade Commission Improvement Act of 1975 (37) gave the FTC the power to regulate entire industries through rules that have the same legal effect as law. In accordance with this Act, the Commission initiated a rulemaking proceeding in 1974 in an attempt to regulate unfair and deceptive claims made in food advertisements on an industry-wide basis (38).

The proposed trade regulation rule (TRR) was, in part, a response to American dietary problems brought to light at the 1969 White House Conference on Food, Nutrition and Health (39). These problems included the finding that consumers are injured by misinformation as well as by lack of information, and that nutritional problems could be attributed more to this fact than to a shortage of available nutrients in the food supply.

Therefore, the TRR emphasized the public interest in remedying deception and unfairness in food advertising, and addressed the issues of the materiality of nutrition information and the failure to disclose nutrition information in advertising (38).

The original *Federal Register* notice outlined the Commission's proposed rule, which covered eight types of voluntary claims made in food advertisements. The original notice also contained a staff proposal to require affirmative disclosure of information found on food labels in food advertising.

In March 1976, the Commission gave notice that the proceedings would be divided into three phases (40). Phase I consisted of sections dealing with natural and organic food claims; energy and calorie claims; fat, fatty acid, and cholesterol claims; and health and related claims. Phase II covered primarily emphatic nutrition claims, nourishment claims, and claims for foods intended to be combined with other foods. Phase III involved the issue of mandatory affirmative disclosure of nutrition information in food advertising.

As of this writing, none of the three phases of the rule has been promulgated. After hearings and several sets of public comments, in December of 1982 the Commission decided to discontinue consideration of Phase 1. In April of 1980, the Commission asked for public comments regarding the suggestion that phases II and III be terminated (41). (For further discussion of the notice, see p. 372.)

Self-Regulation of Food Advertising

Since early in the twentieth century, three different bodies have been organized to carry out self-regulatory activities, two of which are still functioning. The Council on Foods and Nutrition was organized in 1929 to evaluate nutritional claims for foods for the guidance of the medical profession. The American Medical Association decided that some authoritative body was needed that could pass judgment on food products and food advertising in the same way that the Association's Council on Pharmacy and Chemistry had functioned in the field of drugs. At the time, the pages of popular magazines and newspapers were filled with advertisements of food products, many of which contained health appeals (30). The Council operated by releasing a statement of general information on the advertising and labeling of foods. When advertising copy was submitted to the Council for approval and was found to be satisfactory, permission was granted for it to display the following statement (42):

> The nutritional statements in this advertisement have been reviewed by the Council on Foods and Nutrition of the American Medical Association and found consistent with current authoritative medical opinion.

Over a period of 25 years, a number of food products were reviewed. The program ended in the late 1950s.

When the Better Business Bureau (BBB) came into existence in 1915, its main function was to combat false and misleading advertising (43). Local BBBs, working closely with the National Bureau, policed the vast amount of advertising and helped to correct fraudulent and misleading practices. In 1970, a new BBB structure, called the Council of Better Business Bureaus (CBB), was created out of a consolidation of the National Better Business Bureaus and the Association of Better Business Bureaus. At the same time that the CBB was formed, a decision was made by a number of advertisers to establish a program by which the advertising community would undertake to regulate the truth and accuracy of advertisements. The CBB was chosen to administer the industry's self-regulation agencies, the National Advertising Division (NAD) and the National Advertising Review Board (NARB).

The NARB's purpose is to achieve and sustain "high standards of truth and accuracy in national and regional advertising" (43). NARB is directed by the chairmen and presidents of the major advertising trade associations and consists of 50 members, 30 whose principal affiliation is with an advertiser, 10 whose principal affiliation is with an advertising agency, and 10 public members. The chairman of the NARB is responsible for appointing review board panels to hear and decide complaints. The five-member panels review complaints coming from the NAD or from advertisers and attempt to get advertisers to change misleading messages. If the advertiser does not agree to change, the matter is referred to the FTC.

NAD is the investigative arm of the NARB, developing evidence, negotiating with advertisers, and making initial decisions on complaints prior to their review by NARB (43). NAD also reviews questioned advertising, evaluates substantiation, and consults on advertising prior to production and use. In its 10-year history, NAD has investigated more advertising claims related to food than any other category, including complaints in the areas of wine, bakery products, cereals, baby foods, sugar, candy, vitamins, dairy products, fruit juices, sodas, and, most recently, the claim that a product is "natural."

NAD has not developed rules or guidance to cover advertising claims that might be considered misleading. Instead, all ads are judged on a case-by-case basis. They have, however, released a broad statement of ad review policy to be used as a general guide for NARB panels. Monthly reports are also released that explain the rationale for decisions and resultant actions by advertisers.

There are, in addition, various other industry groups that attempt to offer guidance to advertisers, including the National Association of Broadcasters (NAB), American Advertising Federation (AAF), American Association of Advertising Agencies (AAAA), and others.

CHILDREN'S ADVERTISING

Advertising that is aimed at children has become a separate area of interest in recent years. Children in the United States spend a considerable amount of time watching television; the figure appears to be almost double the amount of time that was spent listening to radio immediately before the advent of television (44). The quantity of commercials viewed by children between the ages of 2 and 11 is correspondingly high and numbers about 20,000 per year (45).

Issues about advertising of food products to children fall into two areas: (1) how much advertising affects children's consumption patterns and their attitudes toward nutrition, food preferences, and so on, and (2) how consumption of certain specific food products (i.e., sugared cereals and candy) affects children's dental health.

Both concerns stem from the fact that the majority of all food products advertised to children are sugared foods. One content analysis of weekend commercial children's programs showed that 68% of all commercials were for food products, including eating places. Of these commercials, 64% were for sugared foods. Dairy products, fruit, bread, and other prepared food accounted for less than 5% of all commercial announcements and for less than 7% of all commercials for edibles (46).

The impact of advertising for sugared food products is heightened by the techniques and appeals used in the marketing of those products. Advertisers have long been aware of the fact that children's receptivity to special versions of food products makes them an attractive market. With the direct medium provided by television, manufacturers of food, especially those who produce candies, gums, and sugared cereals, advertise and sell as directly and effectively to these youngsters as they do to adults (47). When the code of the National Association of Broadcasters (NAB) was in effect certain techniques, such as animation, were still available to food advertisers even though prohibited to toy advertisers (48).

Special solicitude by regulatory agencies for the protection of children has been in evidence since 1934, when the Supreme Court sustained a Federal Trade Commission order prohibiting the marketing of penny candy to children through a gambling device (49). During the period between 1974 and 1977, public questioning of advertising practices aimed at children prompted industry to encourage responsibility in children's advertising through voluntary self-regulation. The Children's Advertising Review Unit (CARU) was established in 1974 by the NAD to conduct an ongoing review and evaluation of advertising directed at children under 12 years. The Children's Advertising Guidelines were published by CARU to provide a basis for the investigation of child-related advertising (50). The CARU guidelines, while not directly addressing the issue of possible adverse effects of advertising of sugared products to children, do include sections on food advertising. Those sections provide that commercials for breakfast-type products include "at least one audio reference to and one video depiction of the role of the product within the framework of a balanced regimen," and that advertising for snacks, candy, gum, and soft drinks "shall not suggest or recommend indiscriminate and/or immoderate use of the product." In 1977, the NAB published the Children's Advertising Statement of Principles pursuant to the NAB code, which included provisions on the advertising of food in children's commercials (51).

Despite these efforts by industry, public concern was not abated and was reflected in the 1977 petitions to the Federal Trade Commission by Action for Children's Television (ACT) and the Center for Science in the Public Interest (CSPI). They requested that an investigation be conducted to explore whether the advertising of candy or sugared food products to children should be restricted because of its possible adverse effects on their nutritional and dental well-being.

In response to these petitions, the FTC in February 1978 initiated a full-scale rulemaking proceeding to attempt to remedy the problems associated with advertising directed at children (52). In extensive hearings, arguments for both sides were presented by dentists, nutritionists, psychologists, and others. At the same time, a tremendous amount of pressure to stop the proceedings was exerted in the media and the Congress by the manufacturers and advertisers whose advertising would be affected by the FTC proposals. The law was amended, which contributed to the finding by the staff in March 1981 that, even though minors constitute an especially vulnerable and susceptible group, making children's television advertising a legitimate cause for public concern, "the record establishes that the only effective remedy would be a ban of all advertising oriented toward young children. Such a ban, as a practical matter, cannot be implemented" (53).

Undoubtedly, interested parties will continue to engage in activities that could lead to changes in advertising practices of the manufacturers and the networks. In the meantime, educational programs can assist parents and children in understanding what the effects of those practices may be.

FOOD ADVERTISING AND NUTRITION INFORMATION

Within a free-market economy, advertising is considered to be essential. It is an important aid in "optimizing consumer choice," because it informs potential purchasers of a product of its existence and attributes (3).

It is an axiom of nutrition education that people choose foods for a multitude of reasons, including cost, habit, and convenience. We also know that they pay attention to advertising for various reasons (e.g., the appearance of the food, personalities in the ad, layout designs). (54). But consumers are also interested in the nutrient content of food (55), which information is rarely found in food ads. It has been argued that, because nutrition information is so material to the food purchaser, she or he is not able to make a truly informed choice unless that information is provided. This would appear to be especially true as food prices increase, spending power decreases, and people need to receive the best diet they can for their food dollar.

There is, of course, an available source for some of this information and that is the food label. However, many foods do not carry nutrition labels and food choices are often made before the consumer arrives at the supermarket. Many people believe that advertising could complement labeling by making nutrition more salient in food choice and by directing consumers to use label information (38).

The types of information that are provided in food ads can be analyzed in two different ways. First, there are several implicit messages in food advertising. The primary communication is that the product advertised should be purchased and consumed. A second message is implied by the fact that only some foods are advertised with any great frequency. As mentioned earlier, the least advertised products include unprocessed meats, poultry, fish, eggs, fruits and vegetables, milk and cheese (12). There are two major reasons for this. Fresh products, including those named above, are produced and marketed by a very large number of independent farmers and cooperatives. The products are not identified by brand name and are quite undifferentiated. If someone wants to advertise one of those products, the dollars they spend will accrue to the benefit of all producers of the commodity, whether or not they paid for the advertising. Therefore, the individual producer benefits less for his advertising dollar than do advertisers of branded products (56). At the same time, the products that are most advertised are, in general, those which have the highest profit margins (5, 6). These are mainly foods that have been highly processed in order to differentiate them. They carry brand names and those names are advertised to ensure that the advertising dollar returns to the manufacturer (advertiser) and not to a competitor.

The explicit messages found in food advertising have been the target of regulatory activity as well as of reform measures pursued by many critics of food ads. Data are scarce but a recent study of television advertising by Resnik and Stern found that less than half of the food ads contained any information at all, and only some of the information given was on nutrition (57). A 1971 study reported that the overwhelming emphasis in the food ads reviewed was on sensory pleasure (58). Similarly, an analysis of the content of magazine food ads for the period of 1900–1959 showed that 58% of the ads contained no nutrition information at all (59).

The nutrition claims that food ads do contain have been described as being of two types: vague statements regarding health, nutrition, or bodily welfare; and specific statements about the relationship of the food product to the health, welfare, or general functioning of the human body (59). Specifically, the most frequent nutrition claims now found in ads appear to fall into the major categories of (1) no cholesterol, (2) natural, (3) low calorie, diet or light, (4) fiber, and (5) vitamin C. Some of these claims are expressed in a truthful, accurate, and complete manner. It is difficult, however, to portray a food accurately by providing information about a single substance or nutrient in the food. In fact, over 50 years ago, Dr. Louise Stanley, Chief of the Bureau of Home Economics at USDA, told advertisers to "quit emphasizing vitamins so much" (60). She called it exploitation and suggested that consumers were becoming prejudiced against excessive advertising of nutrition values. Recently, one study found that nutrition claims did create more favorable impressions of food products even when nutrition claims were not the most potent attention-getting devices in food ads (54). Some claims presently being made are truthful but incomplete (e.g., the "no cholesterol" claims that are not accompanied by information about fat). And still other claims may be false or misleading and subject to legal remedies. There is no quantitative measure of what percentage of claims falls into each of the above categories. It is clear, however, that the number of fully informative ads that do not address only a fad or that do not give incomplete information is very small. This is because manufacturers do not often include information in their ads that will not function as a selling point (5, 6, 14). Therefore, nutrition messages either are not present at all in the ads or they become truncated and subjective. Problems arise when consumers do not have the knowledge to evaluate claims involving complex and controversial medical and nutritional issues (61); and it is these problems which have been addressed by the FTC's proposed Food Advertising Trade Regulation Rule (38) and by the Commission's actions in individual cases.

PROPOSALS TO UTILIZE MASS MEDIA FOR DISSEMINATION OF FOOD AND NUTRITION INFORMATION

The problems of the lack of food and nutrition information in ads and the imbalance of information in the mass media as a whole have been addressed by a number of individuals and organizations.

For over 40 years, a steady stream of hearings, statements, speeches, resolutions, and notices has piled request upon request to advertisers and the government that the dissemination of food and nutrition information to the public be increased via the mass media. This vehicle has been characterized as the simplest, most economical, and most effective way by which food and nutrition messages might be disseminated to a large number of.people in a short time (62).

In 1938 Dr. Wilder, speaking for a committee of the American Medical Association, stated that if the tremendous power of advertising could be turned to the socially useful purpose of disseminating truthful information about foods, it might be possible to make the citizens of the United States the healthiest people on earth (30). Just over 30 years later, the White House Conference on Food, Nutrition and Health brought forth a recommendation that 10% of all broadcast time be set aside over various time periods for public service communications (39). Between 1972 and 1973, speakers in several different fora urged advertisers to use nutrition information in advertising and to take more responsibility for providing nutrition information to consumers (63–65). In 1974, voices on both sides of the Atlantic were heard expressing similar opinions. The notion was advanced in Britain that sections of the food industry ought to contribute money to a government nutrition information organization to allow it to experiment with the use of mass-media advertising to raise the level of public understanding of nutrition (66).

In the United States, hearings on National Nutrition Policy were held by the Senate Select Committee on Nutrition and Human Needs. The Subpanel on Popular Nutrition Education recommended that a "specific and increased allotment of the public service time in the electronic media be devoted to nutritional matters, and that this time be based on some definite fraction of the time devoted to commercial messages for food and beverages" (67).

In 1977, Congressman Frederick W. Richmond, Chairman of the House Subcommittee on Domestic Marketing, Consumer Relations, and Nutrition, held hearings on the role of advertising in food marketing (68). The results of a questionnaire sent to a number of food companies were compiled by the staff of the subcommittee. They reported that the industry respondents felt it was the government's responsibility to disseminate basic information about nutrients. At the same time they believed it was the industry's responsibility to communicate information to the public about the principles of good health and the importance of a balanced diet. In their response, General Foods Corporation put forth the idea of developing a Nutrition Education Council, composed of public, private, and voluntary groups, to coordinate and focus nutrition education activities. As a follow-up to the hearings, a bill entitled the National Consumer Nutrition Information Act was introduced (69). It did not advance beyond the Committee.

In 1978, several industry representatives urged their colleagues to help reduce the confusion and to clarify serious nutritional misinformation through a concerted industry effort of consumer education, including packaging, promotion, advertising, and public relations (70, 71). In the ensuing months, a number of other people urged manufacturers to "balance the information environment" (72–75), which culminated in a resolution adopted at the National Nutrition Education Conference. It proposed that the Office of Consumer Affairs of the White House (or another appropriate organization) develop a task force to design strategies for increasing the quality and quantity of public access time for nutrition messages in the commercial media (76). In April 1980, the Federal Trade Commission published a *Federal Register* notice in which it stated that it believed claims being made in food ads were not readily susceptible to across-the-board remedies being proposed in the TRR. The Commissioners were not certain that a TRR represented the ideal solution for remedying deceptiveness and unfairness, and they requested comments on the idea of exploring a wider range of options with respect to the problems of food advertising, the mass media, and nutrition information. In response to this notice, in 1981 a group representing various sectors of the food system met to discuss the feasibility of developing an organization to increase the amount of food and nutrition information available to the public. At about the same time, the General Accounting Office (GAO) was researching the possible organization of a committee established by law to implement a national food information policy (77).

The reluctance of food advertisers to provide nutrition information to the public, either in ads or through messages delivered in the same media as advertisements, has been attributed to many factors. Underlying all the concern is the fact that people can only eat a certain amount of food in a year (60, 78), but the major implicit message in every food ad is that the product should be consumed. Accompanying this contradiction is the fact that many nutritionists and several government agencies have said that it would be prudent for the public to decrease their intake of certain nutrients and classes of foods (79). Many of these foods are among the most heavily advertised. At the same time, the lack of consensus in the scientific community about certain dietary practices confuses advertisers (80), and the lack of guidance from regulatory agencies about nutrition claims (70) makes them reluctant to work to change. There are, in addition, inherent technical difficulties in putting nutrition information into ads, especially in the electronic media (81). There is also disagreement among both advertisers and nutrition educators about the amount of information that viewers can absorb from a 30-second message (82, 83).

One option open to government agencies and consumers is the development of public service announcements (PSAs). Many such nutrition messages have been prepared and aired by local television and radio stations. However, there are drawbacks to this source. PSAs are often aired when audience numbers are low (84); they are often prepared by people who have far less expertise in communication than do advertising agencies; local stations choose which messages will air and, in general, are less likely to accept controversial messages; nutrition and health messages are in competition with other public interest messages for scarce PSA time; and the entire system is dependent on dwindling requirements of the Federal Communications Commission that local stations must meet public affairs responsibilities (85, 86). One source of PSAs, the Ad Council, has been fairly successful in placing announcements. However, due to the fact that all industry interests in the council must agree to a campaign (87), the ads the Ad Council will accept also tend to be noncontroversial.

In summary, although many nutritionists believe that the achievement of parity with food advertisers would require access to the mass media, especially radio and TV, there appear to be many forces, both structural and economic, that are working against that goal. Even if some type of representative organization were to be formed to increase the amount of accurate, useful food and nutrition information in the mass media, nutrition educators must remember that the information will serve as a necessary but probably not sufficient means to produce changes in dietary patterns. The most extensive mass media campaign ever undertaken was most successful when combined with individual counseling (88). Food and nutrition information campaigns can sell good nutrition, but, like advertisements for brand name products, such campaigns will probably require extensive budgets and exposure in order to change health-related behavior (89, 90).

REFERENCES

1. *Webster's Third New International Dictionary*, G. & C. Merriam Co., Springfield, Mass., 1967.
2. *Funk and Wagnall's New Standard Dictionary of the English Language*, Funk and Wagnall's, New York, 1946.
3. J. Howard and J. Hulbert, *Advertising and the Public Interest: A Staff Report to the Federal Trade Commission*, Crain Communications, Chicago, 1973.
4. R. Bauer and S. Greyser, *Advertising in America: The Consumer View*, Harvard University Press, Boston, 1968.
5. R. Manoff, The new politics of nutrition education. In Proceedings, National Conference on Nutrition Education. *J. Nutr. Ed.* **12**(2), 112–115, Suppl. 1 (1980).
6. R. Manoff, Refocusing advertising and marketing. CNI/FMI Third Annual Conference on Nutrition and the American Food System, Community Nutrition Institute, Washington, D.C., 1979.
7. A. A. Achenbaum, Advertising doesn't manipulate consumers. *J. Adv. Res.* **12**, 3 (1972).
8. K. O'Bryan, Advertising: the science of the art. Report on the techniques of media use in advertising, Prepared for the Federal Trade Commission, 1978.
9. A. Manchester, The role and dimensions of food advertising and the food system. In J. M. Connor and R. W. Ward, eds., *Advertising and the Food System*, NCR Project 117 Monograph, Madison, Wisc., in press.
10. M. M. Zimmerman, *The Supermarket*, Mass Distribution Publications, New York, 1937.

11. F. Presbrey, *The History and Development of Advertising*, Doubleday, Doran & Co., New York, 1929.
12. A. Gallo, J. Connor, and W. Boehm, Mass media food advertising. National Food Review 9. U.S. Department of Agriculture—ESCS, Winter 1980.
13. T. Tyebjee, Affirmative disclosure of nutrition information and consumer food preferences: A review. *J. Consumer Affairs* **13**, 206 (1979).
14. J. Gussow, Selling it! In J. Gussow, ed., *The Feeding Web: Issues in Nutritional Ecology*, Bull Publishing, Palo Alto, Calif., 1978.
15. U.S. Congress, Senate, Select Committee on Nutrition and Human Needs. *Dietary Goals for the United States*, 2nd ed., U.S. Government Printing Office, Washington, D.C., 1977.
16. L. Masover, Television food advertising: a positive or negative contribution to nutrition education? Thesis, Northwestern University, Evanston, Ill., 1977.
17. L. Kaufman, Prime-time nutrition. *J. Commun.*, Summer, 37 (1980).
18. H. Gifft, M. Washbon, and G. Harrison, *Nutrition, Behavior and Change*, Prentice-Hall, Englewood Cliffs, N.J., 1972, p. 74.
19. C. Dirksen and A. Kroeger, *Advertising Principles and Problems*, Richard D. Irwin, Homewood, Ill., 1973.
20. R. D. Buzzell, Predicting short term changes in market share as a function of advertising strategy. *J. Marketing Res.* **28**, 31 (1964).
21. W. Clement, P. Henderson, and C. Eley, The effect of different levels of promotional expenditures on sales of fluid milk. U.S. Department of Agriculture ERS 259, Washington, D.C., October 1965.
22. U.S. Department of Agriculture. Butter and cheese: sales changes associated with three levels of promotion. Agricultural Economic Report no. 322, Washington, D.C., January 1976.
23. U.S. Department of Agriculture. Promotional programs for lamb and their effects on sales. Economic Research Service Paper 522, Washington, D.C., January 1962.
24. P. Henderson and S. Brown, Effectiveness of a special promotional campaign for frozen concentrated orange juice. U.S. Department of Agricultue MRR 457, Washington, D.C., March 1961.
25. J. P Galst and M. A. White, The unhealthy persuader: the reinforcing value of television and children's purchase-influencing attempts at the supermarket. *Child Dev.* **47**, 1089 (1976).
26. S. Ward and D. Wackman, Children's purchase influence attempts and parental yielding. *J. Market Res.* **9**, 316 (1972).

27. M. Goldberg and G. Gorn, Children's reactions to television advertising: an experimental approach. *J. Consumer Res.* **1**, 69 (1974).
28. K. Clancy–Hepburn, A. Hickey, and G. Nevill, Children's behavior responses to TV food advertisements. *J. Nutr. Ed.* **6**, 93 (1974).
29. G. Falciglia and J. D. Gussow, Television commercials and eating behavior of obese and normal-weight women. *J. Nutr. Ed.* **12**, 196 (1980).
30. R. Wilder, Fads, fancies and fallacies in adult diets. *Sigma Xi Quart.* **26**, 73 (1938).
31. Virginia State Board of Pharmacy v. Virginia Citizens Consumer Council, Inc. 425 U.S. 748; 1976.
32. Clayton Act (38 Stat 730, as amended, 15 U.S.C. 12); October 15, 1914.
33. FTC Act (38 Stat 717, as amended 15 USC 41–51); September 26, 1914.
34. Wheeler–Lea amendment to the FTC Act, 1938 (Sections 12–15).
35. J. Turner, *The Chemical Feast*, Grossman Publishers, New York, 1970.
36. E. Cox, R. Fellmeth, and J. Schutz, *The Nader Report on the Federal Trade Commission*, Grove Press, New York, 1969.
37. Magnuson–Moss Warranty–Federal Trade Commission Improvements Act (15 USC 2301) (88 Stat 2183), 1975.
38. The Federal Trade Commission Food Advertising Proposed Trade Regulation Rule 16 CFR Part 437 (39 FR 39842); November 11, 1974.
39. *White House Conference on Food, Nutrition and Health. Final Report.* U.S. Government Printing Office, Washington, D.C., 1970.
40. Federal Trade Commission Food Advertising Proposed Trade Regulation Rule 16 CFR Part 437 (41 FR 8970); March 2, 1976.
41. Federal Trade Commission Food Advertising Proposed Trade Regulation Rule 16 CFR Part 437 (45 FR 23706); April 8, 1980.
42. *Statements and Decisions of the Council on Food and Nutrition*, American Medical Association, Chicago, 1957.
43. A review and perspective on advertising industry self-regulation 1971–77 NARB; May 1978.
44. J. C. Goulden, *The Best Years: 1945–1950*, Atheneum, New York, 1976.
45. National Science Foundation. *Research on the Effects of Television Advertising to Children*, U.S. Government Printing Office, Washington, D.C., 1977.

46. F. E. Barcus, *Children's Television: An Analysis of Programming and Advertising*, Praeger, New York, 1977.
47. M. Helitzer and C. Heyel, *The Youth Market*, Media Books, New York, 1970.
48. National Association of Broadcasters Children's Advertising Code, New York, 1974.
49. Federal Trade Commission v. R. F. Keppel and Bros. 291 US 304; 1934.
50. Council of Better Business Bureaus, Inc., National Advertising Division, Children's Advertising Review Unit. Children, Food Advertising and Nutrition: Draft Bibliography, December 1976.
51. National Association of Broadcasters Children's Advertising Statement of Principles, New York, April 1977.
52. Federal Trade Commission Children's Advertising Proposed Trade Regulation Rule 16 CFR Part 461 (215–60) 43 FR 17967; April 27, 1978.
53. Federal Trade Commission. Final Staff Report and Recommendation: Children's Advertising Proposed Trade Regulation Rule 16 CFR Part 461 43 FR 17967.
54. J. Vermeersch and H. Swenerton, Consumer responses to nutrition claims in food advertisements. *J. Nutr. Ed.* **11**, 22 (1979).
55. *Woman's Day Magazine*. Nutrition: a study of consumers' attitudes and behavior towards eating at home and out of home. Yankelovich, Skelly & White, New York, 1978.
56. R. L. Kohls and J. M. Uhl, *Marketing of Agricultural Products*, 5th ed., McMillan, New York, 1980: chapter 14.
57. A. Resnik and B. Stern, An analysis of information content in television advertising. *J. Marketing* **41**, 50 (1977).
58. P. Cuozzo, An inquiry into the image of food and food habits as presented by television food commercials. Thesis, University of Pennsylvania, Annenberg School of Communications, Philadelphia, 1971.
59. R. Rosenberg, An investigation of the nature, utilization, and accuracy of nutritional claims in magazine food advertising. Thesis, New York University School of Education, New York, 1955.
60. Anon., Federal expert tells food advertisers to get housewife's view. *Advertising Age* **1** (1), 1 (January 11, 1930).
61. M. Pertschuk, Remarks before the Food and Nutrition Board, NAS–NRC, Washington, D.C., December 8, 1977.
62. G. M. Hochbaum, Behavior and education. In R. Levy, B. Rifkind, B. Dennis, and N. Ernst, eds., *Nutrition Lipids and Coronary Heart Disease*, Raven Press, New York, 1979, p. 381.

63. Anon., Use nutritional info in TV ads, Choate urges food men. *Advertising Age*, March 27 (1971).
64. Anon., Nutrition education needs ad help, Senate unit hears. *Advertising Age*, December 18 (1971).
65. Anon., Nutrition education a part of food ad's role: Manoff. *Advertising Age*, September 24 (1973).
66. H. Rothman and D. Radford, Bread, advertising and scientific debate. *New Scientist*, p. 264, October 24 (1974).
67. U.S. Congress, Senate, Select Committee on Nutrition and Human Needs, National Nutrition Policy Study. Report and recommendation V prepared by a subpanel on popular nutrition education of the Panel on Nutrition and the Consumer. U.S. Government Printing Office, Washington, D.C., 1974.
68. U.S. Congress, House of Representatives, Subcommittee on Domestic Marketing, Consumer Relations, and Nutrition of the Committee on Agriculture. Hearings on National Consumer Nutrition Information Act of 1978, Ninety-fifth Congress. Parts I and II. U.S. Government Printing Office, Washington, D.C.
69. National Consumer Nutrition Information Act of 1978, H.R. 11761.
70. D. Merchant, Opportunities to enter markets using nutrition as a major product feature. *Food Processing* **39**, 28 (1978).
71. S. Cohen, Washington's view of the consumer's nutritional needs. *Food Processing* **39**, 41 (1978).
72. D. Kennedy, Food labels and advertisements are a means of educating consumers as part of a public health mission. *Food Prod. Dev.* **11**, 66 (1977).
73. K. Schlossberg, Industry should board the nutrition bandwagon. *CNI Weekly Rep.* **8** (28), 4 (1978).
74. Anon., Food industry urged to unite, communicate position to consumers. *Food Chem. News*, May 21 (1979).
75. J. S. Turner, In Alternative Advertising and Nutrition: A workshop to explore strategies for implementation. Federal Trade Commission, June 1978.
76. Proceedings of the National Conference on Nutrition Education Directions for the 80's. *J. Nutr. Ed.* **12**(2), suppl.; 1980.
77. Anon., GAO exploring funding, organization of food information panel, FTC is told. *Food Chem. News*, December 1 (1980).
78. J. Gussow, Can industry afford a healthy America? *CNI Weekly Rep.*, p. 4, June 7 (1979).
79. U.S. Department of Agriculture and U.S. Department of Health, Education and Welfare. *Nutrition and Your Health: Dietary Guidelines*

for Americans, U.S. Government Printing Office, Washington, D.C., 1980.

80. J. E. Austin, Marketing nutrition. *Cereal Foods World* **22**, 557 (1977).
81. L. Rozen, Marketers cautious about capitalizing on nutrition. *Advertising Age*, October 30 (1978).
82. D. Scammon, Information load and consumers. *J. Consumer Res.* **4**, 148 (1977).
83. J. Beltman, Issues in designing consumer information environments. *J. Consumer Res.* **2**, 169 (1975).
84. Anon., Few psa's get airing on nets, study says. *Advertising Age*, April 30 (1979).
85. W. D. Novelli, Copy testing the answer to dull health messages. *Marketing News* **11**, June 16 (1978).
86. P. Seidenman, Getting your message on the air. *Nutr. Action* **8**, 6 (1976).
87. The Advertising Council Report to the American People, 1978–1979, New York.
88. J. Farquhar, N. Maccoby, P. D. Wood, J. K. Alexander, H. Breitrose, B. W. Brown, Jr., W. L. Haskell, A. L. McAlister, A. J. Meyer, J. D. Nash, and M. P. Stern, Community education for cardiovascular health. *Lancet* **1**, 1192 (1977).
89. M. Schlinger, The role of mass communications in promoting public health. *Adv. Cons. Res.* **3**, 302 (1976).
90. T. Robertson and L. Wortzel, Consumer behavior and health care change: The role of mass media. *Adv. Cons. Res.* **5**, 525 (1978).

ADDITIONAL RECENT REFERENCE

J. Handler, The self-regulatory system—an advertiser's viewpoint. *Food Drug Cosmetic Law J.* **37**, 257–63 (1982).

INDEX